PREFACE

Although this book deals with elementary statistical methods, it is hoped that it will be widely useful to workers in the medical and allied fields. No previous study of statistics is assumed, and only a very modest knowledge of mathematics is required.

A vocabulary of symbols precedes each chapter. Each list of symbols includes all the symbols used in that chapter, not merely those employed in that chapter for the first time.

As in other books on statistics that I have written or on which I have collaborated, practically all numerical illustrations are based on actual, not hypothetical, data. Real illustrative data enhance the usefulness of a book and make it more interesting to the reader.

Thanks are due to many persons for helping in the various phases of the writing of this book. First, it is only fair to state that the able collaboration of Professor Dudley J. Cowden on previous books cannot help but be reflected, to some extent, in the present volume. Alfred J. Kana, Associate in Statistics, William A. Maloy, Instructor in Statistics, and Richard H. Ostheimer, formerly Instructor in Statistics (all of Columbia University), assisted in locating suitable illustrative material. Mr. Kana also read portions of the text and Mr. Maloy prepared some of the charts. Otto Dykstra, Jr. assisted in the preparation of charts and with the computations. Everett P. Messmer did some of the lettering of the charts. For the typing of the manuscript I am particularly indebted to Betty Ruth Austin and also to Anne M. Anderson and Eleanor A. Danker. Finally I am indebted to my wife, Rosetta R. Croxton, who helped make the lists of symbols, assisted with the preparation of the tables, and aided me with the reading of proof.

To all who have allowed me to use data from their articles and from their files, I express my appreciation. Each individual or organization is specifically mentioned at the point where the figures are used.

For permission to reproduce the tables of ordinates and areas of the normal curve, shown in Appendices I and II and taken from H. O. Rugg, *Statistical Methods Applied to Education*, I am grateful

PREFACE

to Houghton Mifflin Company. I am indebted to Professor R. A. Fisher and to Messrs. Oliver and Boyd, Ltd., of Edinburgh for permitting me to reprint in Appendices V, VI, and X portions of Tables III, IV, and V from *Statistical Tables for Biological, Agricultural, and Medical Research*. I am obligated to Professor Egon Pearson for allowing me to use, in Appendices V, VI, X, XI, and XII, tables or parts of tables originally published in Volumes XXII, XXXII, and XXXIII of *Biometrika*.

FREDERICK E. CROXTON

Leonia, New Jersey

Elementary Statistics

with
Applications in Medicine
and the
Biological Sciences

By

FREDERICK E. CROXTON, PH.D.

Professor of Statistics, Columbia University

Dover Publications, Inc.
New York

Copyright © 1953 by Frederick E. Croxton

All rights reserved under the Pan American and
International Copyright Conventions.

Published simultaneously in Canada by
McClelland & Stewart, Ltd.

This new Dover edition first published in 1959 is
an unabridged and corrected republication of the
work first published under the title, *Elementary
Statistics with Applications in Medicine.*

Library of Congress Catalog Card Number: 59-8685

Manufactured in the United States of America

Dover Publications, Inc.
180 Varick Street
New York 14, New York

CONTENTS

CHAPTER	PAGE
1. INTRODUCTION; RATES, RATIOS, AND PERCENTAGES	1
Introduction	1
Rates, Ratios, and Percentages	3
2. TABULAR AND GRAPHIC PRESENTATION OF DATA	10
Tables	10
Graphs	18
3. THE FREQUENCY DISTRIBUTION	39
Raw Data	39
The Array	40
The Frequency Distribution	41
4. MEASURES OF CENTRAL TENDENCY	59
Symbols Used in Chapter 4	57
The Arithmetic Mean	59
The Median	66
The Mode	70
Comparison of the Arithmetic Mean, the Median, and the Mode	72
Other Measures of Central Tendency	78
5. DISPERSION, SKEWNESS, AND KURTOSIS	82
Symbols Used in Chapter 5	80
Dispersion	82
Skewness	93
Kurtosis	101
6. LINEAR CORRELATION OF TWO VARIABLES	109
Symbols Used in Chapter 6	107
Introduction	109
Correlation of Ungrouped Data	112
Some Cautions	127
Correlation of Grouped Data	131
Intraclass Correlation	138
Rank Correlation	140

CONTENTS

CHAPTER	PAGE
7. NON-LINEAR AND MULTIPLE CORRELATION	148
Symbols Used in Chapter 7	144
Non-linear Correlation	148
Multiple Correlation	159
8. THE NORMAL CURVE, THE BINOMIAL, AND THE POISSON DISTRIBUTION	180
Symbols Used in Chapter 8	179
The Normal Curve	180
The Binomial	196
The Poisson Distribution	201
9. RELIABILITY AND SIGNIFICANCE OF ARITHMETIC MEANS	209
Symbols Used in Chapter 9	207
Behavior of Arithmetic Means of Random Samples	210
Significance of Difference Between $\bar{X}$ and $\bar{X}_\varphi$ When Population Values Are Known	219
Significance of Difference Between $\bar{X}$ and $\bar{X}_\varphi$ When σ Is Unknown	226
Confidence Limits of $\bar{X}_\varphi$	231
Significance of Difference Between Two Sample Means	235
Conclusion	242
10. RELIABILITY AND SIGNIFICANCE OF PROPORTIONS	246
Symbols Used in Chapter 10	245
Behavior of Proportions from Random Samples	247
The Reliability of p When π Is Known	252
Confidence Limits of π	257
The Significance of the Difference Between p_1 and p_2	263
11. THE χ^2 TEST	267
Symbols Used in Chapter 11	266
The 1 × 2 Table	267
The 2 × 2 Table	271
The 1 × 3 Table	279
2 × 3 and Larger Tables	280
Test of "Goodness of Fit"	282
12. SIGNIFICANCE TESTS FOR VARIANCES; ANALYSIS OF VARIANCE; TESTS FOR CORRELATION COEFFICIENTS AND FOR MEASURES OF SKEWNESS AND KURTOSIS	288
Symbols Used in Chapter 12	284
Sample Variances	288

CONTENTS

CHAPTER	PAGE
Analysis of Variance	295
Interrelationships Between the Normal Distribution, t, χ^2, and F	310
Correlation Coefficients	312
Skewness and Kurtosis	318

APPENDICES 321

I. Ordinates of the Normal Curve 321
II. Areas Under the Normal Curve 322
III. Areas in One Tail of the Normal Curve at Selected Values of $\frac{x}{s}$ or $\frac{x}{\sigma}$ from the Arithmetic Mean 323
IV. Areas in Two Tails of the Normal Curve at Selected Values of $\frac{x}{s}$ or $\frac{x}{\sigma}$ from the Arithmetic Mean 324
V. Values of t 326
VI. Values of χ^2 328
VII. Values of $\frac{\hat{\sigma}^2}{\sigma^2}$ for Use in Determining Sampling Limits of $\hat{\sigma}^2$ 330
VIII. Values of $\frac{\sigma^2}{\hat{\sigma}^2}$ for Use in Determining Confidence Limits of σ^2 332
IX. Values of F at Selected Upper and Lower Points . . . 334
X. Values of F at Selected Upper Points 336
XI. Upper Limits of β_1 341
XII. Upper and Lower Limits of β_2 342
XIII. Squares, Square Roots, and Reciprocals 343
XIV. Logarithms of Numbers 353

INDEX 369

Chapter 1
INTRODUCTION; RATES, RATIOS, AND PERCENTAGES

Introduction

The term *statistics*, as used in this book, refers to the methods which have been developed for working with numerical data. Sometimes, in fact too often, *statistics* is used as a synonym for *data*, but it will not be so employed in this volume.

Nearly everyone involved in any aspect of medicine needs to have some knowledge of statistics. The practitioner and the medical student will better understand the conclusions of articles in the journals if they have some grasp of the statistical methods which are used. The research worker, seeking to present his results in a clear and effective manner, should know what statistical techniques are available to him and should use the appropriate procedure which will enable him to demonstrate the validity (or lack of validity!) of his findings. This is not to argue that everyone practicing medicine or doing medical research should also be a competent statistician. He should, however, be familiar with the rudiments of statistics. Beyond that he may wish to use the services of a professional statistician.

Recently a physician mentioned that he had attended a lecture on a medical topic and that the speaker had stated that his findings had been verified by means of a chi-square test. The doctor had no idea what the chi-square test might be and requested the writer to elucidate. Readers of this book will obtain a basic idea of some of the more important aspects of the chi-square test.

During World War II a pharmaceutical concern asked the writer to serve as statistical consultant in connection with research work under way on an antibiotic. Their approach concluded with the amazing statement: "We have come to the end of our rope, chemically, or we would not be looking for a statistician." The reason for mentioning this occurrence is that the organization should have had a statistician on its staff, or, alternatively, should have had the services of a consulting statistician from the beginning. The importance of this lack was apparent when it was found that the experiments, seeking to ascertain the effectiveness of the antibiotic, had been so carelessly designed and performed that useful statistical analysis was impossible. The consulting assignment was declined.

In another instance, a group of physicians completed the laboratory portion of an extensive research undertaking involving scores of laboratory animals but, arriving at the point of analyzing their data statistically, found themselves completely helpless. Although none of them had a knowledge of statistics, their basic data were, luckily, sound and it was possible for a statistician to proceed with the statistical tests which were necessary in order to demonstrate that the findings were of value. The results of this study appeared in a leading medical journal.

The pharmaceutical company asked for the help of a statistician too late. Fortunately, statistical help was possible for the group of physicians. Sometimes, statistical analysis is not even attempted, although it is sorely needed. A published article undertook to describe a new device for measuring a certain characteristic of blood. After discussing the apparatus, the author compared the numerical results which he had obtained with those (for the same blood specimens) obtained by two other frequently used methods. That was the end of the article; there was no statistical analysis to demonstrate that his device did indeed give, as alleged, results essentially the same as those given by the customary procedures. A knowledge of the statistical methods described in this volume would have been more than adequate to enable him to analyze his data.

Illustrations of published studies which did not succeed in demonstrating the validity of their findings because of failure to use statistical methods are numerous. An article dealing with the use of antihistamines for treating head colds did not make the statistical tests which were necessary if the efficacy of the drug were to be determined. A discussion of the merits of early postoperative activity did not make the appropriate statistical tests to compare the results of early and late activity and even presented the data in such compressed form that the reader was not in a position to make the tests for himself. A moderately technical house organ of an insurance company compared similarly employed diabetics and non-diabetics in regard to absenteeism and accidents but did not test the observed differences statistically.

The reader should not get the impression that all statistical work deals with tests of significance (the subject matter of Chapters 9–12). In many other situations simpler procedures are called for. The Veterans' Administration needed to estimate the amount of X-ray film of various sizes required for each hospital. After study of the data, it was found that the different sizes constituted relatively constant proportions at the hospitals, and all that was necessary was to keep a record of the number of patients and make use of the proper ratios for each size of film. Ratios will be discussed in the following section of this chapter. In later chapters illustrative material will involve the use of averages, measures of dispersion, curve fitting, correlation, and other procedures, as well as tests of significance.

Rates, Ratios, and Percentages

Absolute vs. relative comparisons. Before proceeding to discuss rates, ratios, and percentages it may be well to point out the difference between absolute and relative comparisons, since either may be used in statistical work and since rates, ratios, and percentages are all relative figures. Consider two cities: city A, which had a population of 100,000 at a given census and 200,000 at the time the following census was taken, and city B, which had 1,000,000 inhabitants at the first census and 1,300,000 at the second census. If we compare the absolute increases of the two cities, we find that city A showed an increase of 100,000 persons while city B increased 300,000. On a relative basis, city A increased 100 per cent, while city B increased 30 per cent. City B showed the greater *absolute* increase; city A showed the greater *relative* increase. There is nothing contradictory about these two statements. They merely represent different ideas.

Rates vs. ratios. Occasionally a distinction is made between the terms *rate* and *ratio*. A rate is sometimes considered as the amount or quantity of one variable considered in relation to one unit of a different variable. Thus, 30 miles per hour is a *rate* of speed. A ratio may be thought of as the relation existing between two similar variables. For example, if a community had 2,794 births and 1,411 deaths during a year, the birth-death ratio (2,794 ÷ 1,411) would be 1.98. Here the variables were both persons. This distinction between rate and ratio is not strictly honored in general usage and we shall make no forced attempt to do so in this book.

Ratios and percentages. We shall consider a ratio as a means of expressing the relationship that one magnitude bears to another. Thus, we may say 800 is to 400 as 2 is to 1, or using : to mean "is to" and :: to mean "as," we may write, 800:400::2:1. This is a ratio to the base one. We could also say 800:400::10:5, using a ratio to the base 5; or 800:400::20:10, using a ratio to the base 10; or 800:400::200:100, using a ratio to the base 100. A ratio to the base 100 states the first of the two magnitudes per hundred or *per cent* (per centum) of the second magnitude. Thus, we might say "800 is 200 per cent of 400." Note that a percentage is merely a ratio which has employed 100 as the base.

Although 800 is 200 per cent of 400, it is also correct to say that 800 is 100 per cent *greater than* 400. The reader must always note with care which of these two types of statements is being made.

Computation of ratios and percentages. Ratios involve extremely simple arithmetic, yet many mistakes result from the computation and use of them. The rule for computing a ratio is: *always divide by the base.* For those who, not infrequently, say: "But, I don't know which number is the base," the answer is: *The base is the number to which the other number is being compared.* Suppose that in a given year there were 300 cases of measles in a community and the following year 420 cases, and that the percentage of increase from the first year to the second is desired. The *amount* of increase is 420 − 300 = 120 cases, and 300 is the base. Therefore, the *relative* increase is

$$\frac{120}{300} = 0.40, \text{ or } 40 \text{ per cent.}$$

An alternative method of computation eliminates the initial subtraction to obtain the amount of increase, substituting the subtraction of 100 per cent at the end. Thus, for our figures,

$$\frac{420}{300} = 1.40, \text{ or } 140 \text{ per cent}$$

and the percentage of increase is 140 per cent − 100 per cent = 40 per cent.

When a decrease is involved, either method may still be used. If, in a city, 350 cases of lobar pneumonia in one year are to be com-

Chap. 1]   RATES, RATIOS, AND PERCENTAGES   5

pared with 300 cases the following year, the relative change would be

$$\frac{300-350}{350} = \frac{-50}{350} = -0.1429, \text{ or } -14.3 \text{ per cent.}$$

Alternatively, we may compute

$$\frac{300}{350} = 0.8571, \text{ or } 85.71 \text{ per cent.}$$

This is the percentage that 300 is of 350, and the per cent of decrease is obtained by subtracting 100 per cent, as before, giving

$$85.71 - 100.00 = -14.3 \text{ per cent.}$$

Note that, while a percentage of increase may be indefinitely large, a percentage of decrease cannot exceed 100 per cent unless negative values are possible. For example, if 400 is increased to 1,600, the increase is 300 per cent; if 400 is increased to 4,000, the increase is 900 per cent. Now, if 400 is decreased to 0, the decrease is 100 per cent; a decrease of 120 per cent would mean that our original figure of 400 had declined to -80. Such a situation is possible when dealing with profit and loss data but not in many other situations. The failure of research workers, or of newsmen, to be fully aware of this has occasionally resulted in the publication of meaningless or misleading statements. In one instance, a new invention for the prevention of frostbite to high-altitude flyers was said to have cut cases of frostbite 1,500 per cent! The figures on which this was based were 60 per 100,000 before the use of the new device, and 4 per 100,000 after its employment. The figure of 1,500 per cent resulted from comparing 60 instead of 56 (the decrease) with the wrong base, 4. The correct percentage of decrease is 93 per cent. In another instance, the use of a new (but unspecified) treatment for malaria was said to have reduced the annual number of cases in a certain location 9,250 per cent from one year to the next. During the first year there had been 555 cases; during the second year, 6 cases. The correct percentage of reduction was 98.9. The incorrect figure was obtained by using the wrong base and relating it to 555 instead of to 549.

Rounding. When we computed the relative decrease involved in the decline of 350 to 300, we obtained 14.29 per cent, which we rounded to 14.3 per cent. The principles involved in rounding, as used in this book, are relatively simple. They are:

1. If the digit to be dropped is more than 5, the preceding digit is increased one. Thus, if we desire to show but one decimal,

> 16.78 becomes 16.8,
> 24.36 becomes 24.4, and
> 6.49 becomes 6.5.

Note that 12.3500000001 would be rounded to 12.4 if we wished to show but one decimal. In this case, we would not be likely to carry the division out as far as indicated, but would merely note that there was a remainder after the 5 in the second decimal place had been obtained.

2. If the digit to be dropped is less than 5, the preceding digit is unchanged. Thus, if we are to show one decimal,

> 43.61 becomes 43.6,
> 11.44 becomes 11.4, and
> 14.30 becomes 14.3.

3. If the digit to be dropped is *exactly* 5, it is customary to use a scheme which will result in half of the preceding digits being raised and half remaining unchanged. One way to accomplish this is to raise whenever the digit preceding the 5 is odd but make no change when the digit preceding the 5 is even.[1] Under this scheme

> 12.15 becomes 12.2,
> 7.35 becomes 7.4, and
> 37.95 becomes 38.0, but
> 4.85 becomes 4.8, and
> 22.25 becomes 22.2.

Misplaced decimals. When computing and using percentages, it is important that the decimal points be properly placed. A misplaced decimal point always involves a serious misstatement; the *least* mistake that can occur is for the decimal point to be *one* place out of position. This means that the figure is ten times as large as it should be if the decimal point is one place too far to the right; or one-tenth as large as it should be if the decimal point is one place too far to the left.

---

[1] It will be noted that this results in all final digits being even, when the dropped digit is exactly 5. There are other possible procedures, but none is thoroughly satisfactory.

An author of an article in a leading magazine[2] was making the point that the tests used by medical-legal experts are valuable but are not reliable if the technician who made the test was careless. In this connection he stated that court testimony by an expert to the effect that a man was drunk because his blood contained 2.5 per cent alcohol should not be considered conclusive. An alert state police trooper pointed out that if a man had 2.5 per cent alcohol in his blood, he not only would be dead but would hardly need to be embalmed.[3] The figure which the author intended to use was undoubtedly 0.25 per cent.

Misplaced decimal points are most likely to occur when very large or very small percentages of change are involved. To give an illustration of only the first of these: a news magazine, commenting on the decrease in the number of Chinese and the increase in the number of Japanese in the United States from 1880 to 1940, stated that the Japanese "increased from 148 to 126,947 or 845 per cent." Actually, the 1940 figure is 857.75 *times* the 1880 figure and the relative increase was 85,675 per cent.

Base should not be small. In general, percentages should not be computed unless the base is 100 or more. Percentages based upon small numbers are apt to be misleading. Consider the case of a college student who had planned to work in a lumber camp but who decided against it when he learned that in the camp "two per cent of the men were married to fifty per cent of the women." Actually, there were fifty men and two women cooks in the camp. One of the men was married to one of the women. The use of percentages with these figures could serve only to supply a joke of dubious merit.

Some medical ratios. Medical data are not infrequently relative figures. Cell volume, for example, is expressed in cubic centimeters per hundred cubic centimeters of blood and is, in fact, a percentage. Data of cell volume appear in various tables in Chapters 3, 4, and 5. In Table 8.1, red blood cell counts are shown. These are stated in terms of millions of cells per cubic millimeter of blood. Since this ratio is referred to rather frequently in Chapter 8, we have employed M^2/mm^3 to mean "millions ($M^2 = 1,000^2$) per cubic millimeter."

---

[2] See "How Murderers Beat the Law," by Pete Martin, *The Saturday Evening Post*, December 10, 1949.

[3] *Ibid.*, January 21, 1950, in a letter to the editor from Trooper M. Huffman of the Indiana State Police.

Table 6.1 includes data of intravenous injections of glucose, in terms of grams per kilogram of body weight per hour.

The ratios just mentioned are relatively simple in concept; there are others which are more complex. For example, a hemoglobin coefficient may be computed by stating the grams of hemoglobin which 100 cubic centimeters of blood would contain if the red cell count were 5 M^2/mm^3. This is obtained from the expression

$$\frac{\text{red cell count}}{5 \ M^2/mm^3} = \frac{\text{hemoglobin in grams per 100 c.c.}}{\text{hemoglobin coefficient}}$$

Vital rates. Birth rates, death rates, morbidity rates, marriage rates, and divorce rates are occasionally of interest in medicine. To give an extended description of these and of allied figures such as fertility rates, stillbirth ratios, and so forth, is beyond the scope of this book.[4] However, we shall give brief and superficial attention to death rates.

Death rates. The *crude death rate* for an area is obtained by dividing the number of deaths occurring in that area during a year by the population of the area at the middle of the year. The resulting figure is expressed as a ratio per 1,000. As an example, the number of deaths from all causes during 1951 in the five boroughs of New York City was 79,109 and the July 1, 1951 population was estimated to be 7,976,000. The crude death rate for New York City was, therefore,

$$\frac{79,109}{7,976,000} \ 1,000 = 9.9.$$

When death rates are computed for a period of less than a year, they are usually converted to an annual basis.

The crude death rate is sometimes referred to as a "recorded death rate" or "death rate by place," emphasizing that the figure for number of deaths (1) did not include the deaths of residents of the area who died elsewhere and (2) did include deaths occurring in the area of persons residing elsewhere. To rectify this situation, there may be computed a *resident death rate* which employs deaths

---

[4] For discussions, see F. E. Linder and R. D. Grove, *Vital Statistics Rates in the United States, 1900–1940*, Federal Security Agency, Public Health Service, National Office of Vital Statistics, 1947, and *Vital Statistics of the United States, 1949, Parts I and II*, Federal Security Agency, Public Health Service, National Office of Vital Statistics, 1951.

according to place of residence of the decedents. The computation of death rates according to place of residence instead of place of occurrence of the deaths does not affect rates for the entire United States and results in but little change in the rates for the individual states. The difference is important, however, for cities. Crude death rates for cities may be quite misleading. In 1935, when crude death rates for 1934 were announced, the borough of Queens, New York, was shown to have a crude death rate of 6.5. This was the lowest rate for any community during 1934 and there was newspaper comment to the effect that Queens was the healthiest place in the United States. Actually, the rate for Queens was low because Queens had proportionally fewer hospitals than the other nearby boroughs. Manhattan, with more hospitals, had a crude death rate of 16.3.

If a death rate, based at first on a preliminary population estimate, is recomputed in relation to a revised population estimate, the new death rate is referred to as a *revised death rate*. A preliminary population estimate is usually a post-censal estimate, as, for example, an estimate for July 1, 1953. A revised population estimate is ordinarily an inter-censal estimate; the July 1, 1953 estimates would become an inter-censal estimate after the 1960 census figures became available.

When death rates are computed for designated portions of the population or for particular causes of death, they are known as *specific death rates*. Thus, we may have "age-specific death rates," "sex-specific death rates," "race-specific death rates," and "cause-specific death rates." Explanations of these and of methods of adjusting death rates to "standard populations" will be found in the references given in footnote 4.

Chapter 2
TABULAR AND GRAPHIC PRESENTATION OF DATA

It is very important that the numerical findings of any study be presented clearly and concisely. Usually the data should be given by means of tables or charts, or both. It is not ordinarily desirable to embody more than just a few figures in a paragraph of text, since such an arrangement confuses most readers and fails to tell the story as effectively[1] as does a table or a chart.

This chapter will briefly discuss statistical tables and charts, mentioning a few of the more important considerations for each method of presentation. Detailed treatments may be found in other volumes.[2]

Tables

A statistical table presents the numerical findings of a study in a compact form, with the data arranged in contiguous columns and rows. Such a device is not only clear and concise, but by its very nature it facilitates comparisons. Of course, a table will not be clear and easy to understand unless it is properly designed. Ambiguous wording in a table can easily destroy its usefulness. Such situations do occur; the writer recently found it necessary to get into personal touch with an investigator to ascertain what was meant by one of the headings in a table.

Every table has at least four parts and may have as many as seven. The four necessary parts are (1) a title, which customarily appears above the table, (2) a stub, which is the column at the extreme left, including the heading of that column, (3) a box head, which includes all of the column headings and subheadings except

---

[1] For a comparison of text and tabular presentation, see F. E. Croxton and D. J. Cowden, *Applied General Statistics*, Prentice-Hall, Inc., New York, 1939, pp. 49–51.

[2] For example, *ibid.*, Chapters III, IV, V, and VI.

the heading of the first column, and (4) the body, which is all the rest of the table proper—the part which contains the figures. These may readily be identified by referring to Table 2.1 or any other table in this volume. In addition to the four essential parts, a table may have a prefatory note, one or more footnotes, and a source note. A prefatory note is placed just below the title (see Table 7.2) and refers to all or a substantial part of the table. Foot-

TABLE 2.1

EXPECTATION OF LIFE IN YEARS, BY COLOR AND SEX, FOR TOTAL PREMIUM-PAYING BUSINESS OF THE INDUSTRIAL DEPARTMENT OF THE METROPOLITAN LIFE INSURANCE COMPANY, 1949

Age in years	White		Colored	
	Males	Females	Males	Females
5	62.76	68.10	60.20	62.66
10	57.95	63.25	55.45	57.83
15	53.13	58.36	50.68	52.98
20	48.40	53.50	46.17	48.36
25	43.73	48.69	41.74	43.89
30	39.06	43.90	37.27	39.43
35	34.42	39.17	32.91	35.00
40	29.94	34.53	28.74	30.78
45	25.71	29.99	24.80	26.80
50	21.77	25.63	21.14	23.03
55	18.15	21.47	17.76	19.44
60	14.90	17.56	14.68	16.13
65	11.97	13.97	12.03	13.19
70	9.31	10.79	9.74	10.61

Source: Metropolitan Life Insurance Company, *Statistical Bulletin*, August 1950, p. 5.

notes appear just below the bottom line of a table (see Table 2.3) and provide explanations concerning individual figures or, occasionally, an entire column or row. If the data of a table were taken from another publication or were supplied by someone else, a source note, as in Table 2.1, should be included. The source note usually follows the footnote or footnotes if any are present.

Reference tables vs. text tables. A table which presents a large amount of data and which serves as a repository of information is termed a general table or a reference table. Such tables contain detailed data, are designed for ease of reference, and frequently appear in one or more appendixes at the end of a report. Text tables are relatively small tables which are included in the discussion and which are designed to present a few closely related findings as succinctly and as effectively as possible.

TABLE 2.2

EXPECTATION OF LIFE IN YEARS, BY SEX AND COLOR, FOR TOTAL PREMIUM-PAYING BUSINESS OF THE INDUSTRIAL DEPARTMENT OF THE METROPOLITAN LIFE INSURANCE COMPANY, 1949

Age in years	Males		Females	
	White	Colored	White	Colored
5	62.76	60.20	68.10	62.66
10	57.95	55.45	63.25	57.83
15	53.13	50.68	58.36	52.98
20	48.40	46.17	53.50	48.36
25	43.73	41.74	48.69	43.89
30	39.06	37.27	43.90	39.43
35	34.42	32.91	39.17	35.00
40	29.94	28.74	34.53	30.78
45	25.71	24.80	29.99	26.80
50	21.77	21.14	25.63	23.03
55	18.15	17.76	21.47	19.44
60	14.90	14.68	17.56	16.13
65	11.97	12.03	13.97	13.19
70	9.31	9.74	10.79	10.61

Source: Metropolitan Life Insurance Company, *Statistical Bulletin*, August 1950, p. 5.

Reference tables may be fairly complicated, with numerous headings and subheadings, but text tables should be as simple as practicable. Whenever possible, the detailed reference tables (if there are any) should be included so that all useful information may be available to those who want it. When full data are not given, readers who need the details find it necessary to write to the author for the desired data. Sometimes the figures are forthcoming, but sometimes the worksheets containing them have been lost or discarded or are not available because they have been put in storage. The inclusion of an appendix of reference tables in a report avoids such difficulties.

Designing a reference table. A reference table does not undertake to facilitate particular comparisons nor to emphasize one part of the data rather than any other part. Its purpose is to make it easy for a reader to find any information he desires which may be in that table. For this reason items in the stub or box head may often be arranged alphabetically, but are rarely listed according to their magnitude. Other arrangements (such as chronological, customary classes, numerical, and so forth) may be used in a general table if they make the table serve its purpose effectively.

Designing a text table. The purpose of a text table is to facilitate comparisons of data and to emphasize one or more items in the table. Considering first the matter of comparing figures, we may note that individual figures can be compared more readily if they are arranged above and below each other in a column than if they are arranged side by side in a row. For this reason Table 2.3

TABLE 2.3

NUMBER OF DEATHS IN THE UNITED STATES, EXCLUSIVE OF DEATHS AMONG THE ARMED FORCES OVERSEAS, FROM THE TEN LEADING CAUSES, 1948

Cause of death	Number of deaths
Diseases of the heart	471,469
Cancer and other malignant tumors	197,042
Intracranial lesions of vascular origin	131,036
Motor vehicle and other accidents	98,001
Nephritis	77,377
Pneumonia (all forms) and influenza	56,493
Tuberculosis (all forms)	43,833
Premature birth	39,085
Diabetes mellitus	38,638
Arteriosclerosis and high blood pressure*	27,565
Ten leading causes	1,180,539
All causes	1,444,337

* For complete title, refer to International List of Causes of Death.
Data from National Office of Vital Statistics, *United States Summary of Vital Statistics, 1948*, June 1, 1950, pp. 910–911.

consists of a single column of figures rather than a single row. If this table were to be redrawn with but one entry "Number of deaths" in the stub and with the figures arranged in a single row, comparisons would be less easy to make and the table would have an extremely awkward shape. When two or more sets of figures are to be compared, they are usually placed in contiguous columns rather than in contiguous rows. However, both methods are used, and in either case the important consideration is that series of figures which are to be compared should be so placed that the desired comparison is made easy. This point is illustrated by Table 2.1, which shows the life expectancy of industrial policy-holders of the Metropolitan Life Insurance Company by color and sex. Table 2.2 shows the same information, but here the columns are rearranged with "Male" and "Female" as the two major column headings. Table 2.1 facilitates comparison of males and females of the same color; Table 2.2 facilitates comparison of White and Colored of the same sex.

The arrangement of the entries in the stub and box head of a text table should be such that the items which are to be emphasized are in the most prominent positions. Since Occidentals read from left to right and from top to bottom, the entries first noted by the reader are those at the left in the box head and at the top in the stub. It follows, then, that a category which is to be emphasized will be placed at the left in the box head or at the top in the stub, and that other categories to be compared with it will follow. It is not necessary that the largest of a series of items be placed in the most prominent position, although the arrangement of items in order of magnitude, shown in Table 2.3, is often used. A total is sometimes placed at the right in the box head or at the bottom in the stub. However, if a total is to be emphasized, it would be given the more prominent location in box head or stub.

Chronological data, such as those shown in Table 2.7, may be arranged in the usual sequence from earliest to most recent date, as in that table. However, if it is desired to emphasize the more recent years, the listing of the years would be in reverse order: 1948, 1947, · · · , 1938, 1937. The two alternatives are, of course, also available when dates appear in the box head.

Sometimes boldface type is used for emphasis. For example, it may be desired to list the items in order of magnitude but to call particular attention to one row or column of figures. These, with their row or column heading, may be shown in boldface type.

Considerations common to reference and text tables. Without undertaking to go into the details of table construction, it is nevertheless in order to point out a few of the more important matters that must be taken into account if one is to make workmanlike tables.

Title. Each table should have a title, which is usually preceded by an identifying number if two or more tables are presented. The title is almost invariably placed above the table and should be a brief, clearly worded statement telling what the table shows. When a title consists of several lines, it may be arranged in "inverted pyramid" form, as in Table 2.1. Reference to the title of this table and others in this volume will show that the longest line of a title never exceeds the width of the table itself.

Headings. Just as it is important that a title of a table be clearly worded, so it is important that each column heading and row heading be unambiguous. If there is danger that a heading, because of its brevity, might be misunderstood, a fuller explanation should be given in a footnote.[3]

Units. Sometimes the units of measurement used for the data in a table are self-identifying. This is the case, for example, when monetary figures are being shown, since the dollar mark is customarily placed before the first figure in each column and before the total of each column. For most other units, a statement is necessary. If the units used are the same throughout the table, mention of the units may be made in the title, as in Table 3.1, or in a prefatory note, as in Table 7.2. When the units used in the various columns (or rows) of a table are different, the heading of each column (or row) should state the unit.

TABLE 2.4

EXPECTATION OF LIFE IN YEARS, BY COLOR AND SEX, FOR TOTAL PREMIUM-PAYING BUSINESS OF THE INDUSTRIAL DEPARTMENT OF THE METROPOLITAN LIFE INSURANCE COMPANY, 1949

Age in years	White		Colored	
	Males	*Females*	*Males*	*Females*
5	62.76	68.10	60.20	62.66
10	57.95	63.25	55.45	57.83
15	53.13	58.36	50.68	52.98
20	48.40	53.50	46.17	48.36
25	43.73	48.69	41.74	43.89
30	39.06	43.90	37.27	39.43
35	34.42	39.17	32.91	35.00
40	29.94	34.53	28.74	30.78
45	25.71	29.99	24.80	26.80
50	21.77	25.63	21.14	23.03
55	18.15	21.47	17.76	19.44
60	14.90	17.56	14.68	16.13
65	11.97	13.97	12.03	13.19
70	9.31	10.79	9.74	10.61

Source: Metropolitan Life Insurance Company, *Statistical Bulletin*, August 1950, p. 5.

---

[3] A footnote may also explain more fully a specific numerical entry in a table. In such a case it is important not to key the footnote to the numerical entry by means of a number, but to employ a symbol (*, †, #, ‡, or the like), as in Table 8.8, or a letter.

Source. When the data in a table were obtained from a publication or when they were supplied by an individual or an organization, a source note should give a full statement, as in Tables 2.4, 3.2 and 7.2. In Table 3.2 additional explanatory material follows the source note.

TABLE 2.5

EXPECTATION OF LIFE IN YEARS, BY COLOR AND SEX, FOR TOTAL PREMIUM-PAYING BUSINESS OF THE INDUSTRIAL DEPARTMENT OF THE METROPOLITAN LIFE INSURANCE COMPANY
1949

Age in years	White		Colored	
	Males	Females	Males	Females
5	62.76	68.10	60.20	62.66
10	57.95	63.25	55.45	57.83
15	53.13	58.36	50.68	52.98
20	48.40	53.50	46.17	48.36
25	43.73	48.69	41.74	43.89
30	39.06	43.90	37.27	39.43
35	34.42	39.17	32.91	35.00
40	29.94	34.53	28.74	30.78
45	25.71	29.99	24.80	26.80
50	21.77	25.63	21.14	23.03
55	18.15	21.47	17.76	19.44
60	14.90	17.56	14.68	16.13
65	11.97	13.97	12.03	13.19
70	9.31	10.79	9.74	10.61

Source: Metropolitan Life Insurance Company, <u>Statistical Bulletin</u>, August 1950, p. 5.

Ruling. Printed tables are ordinarily shown with horizontal and vertical rules, as given in the various tables of this volume. It is customary in the United States not to close the sides of a table by means of vertical rules. In England and in Europe, on the other hand, the sides of a table are ordinarily closed. Printed

Chap. 2] TABULAR AND GRAPHIC PRESENTATION 17

tables may be set up without rules, and Table 2.4 shows how Table 2.1 might appear with no horizontal or vertical rules.

Typewritten tables may be ruled by hand using pen and ink or with horizontal rules made on the typewriter by use of the underscore or long dash and with vertical rules made by means of colons.

TABLE 2.6

EXPECTATION OF LIFE IN YEARS, BY COLOR AND SEX,
FOR TOTAL PREMIUM-PAYING BUSINESS OF
THE INDUSTRIAL DEPARTMENT OF
THE METROPOLITAN LIFE
INSURANCE COMPANY
1949

Age in years	White		Colored	
	Males	Females	Males	Females
5	62.76	68.10	60.20	62.66
10	57.95	63.25	55.45	57.83
15	53.13	58.36	50.68	52.98
20	48.40	53.50	46.17	48.36
25	43.73	48.69	41.74	43.89
30	39.06	43.90	37.27	39.43
35	34.42	39.17	32.91	35.00
40	29.94	34.53	28.74	30.78
45	25.71	29.99	24.80	26.80
50	21.77	25.63	21.14	23.03
55	18.15	21.47	17.76	19.44
60	14.90	17.56	14.68	16.13
65	11.97	13.97	12.03	13.19
70	9.31	10.79	9.74	10.61

Source: Metropolitan Life Insurance Company, *Statistical Bulletin*, August 1950, p. 5.

Alternatively, typewritten tables may be left unruled or may be partially ruled. Table 2.5 is a typewritten table ruled with underscores and colons; Table 2.6 shows the same data but employs partial ruling.

Only one size and style of type is available when an ordinary typewriter is used. Printed tables, which may be set up using type of various sizes and styles, can be constructed with a greater degree of flexibility than can typewritten tables. Sometimes a typewritten table is made with two typewriters, one having pica and the other elite type. Even wider choice in regard to type size and style for typewritten tables may be had by using a typewriter which is capable of variable spacing with different kinds and sizes of type.

Graphs

Statistical graphs or charts are not intended to show the detailed information that is presented by a table. Rather, a graph undertakes to show a general situation *at a glance*. For this reason a chart should be made as simple and as clear as possible so that the reader may grasp its meaning without having to study it. The data from which the chart is made should not be shown on the chart itself. If it is desired to show details, a separate table should be included.

Statistical charts are of various kinds, the most important of which are: line diagrams or curves, bar charts, pie diagrams, pictographs, and statistical maps. There are also charts which are not statistical, for example, organization and procedure charts,[4] which will not be discussed in this book. Any graph, of whatever sort, should be carefully and neatly made. Such a chart is attractive and not likely to be overlooked. A sloppy, carelessly drawn chart does not inspire the reader's confidence in the facts shown, and the chart itself may often be dismissed as of no importance. If the author was not willing to take the time to do a workmanlike job of drawing a graph, the reader may, unconsciously, consider that the point made by the graph could hardly be very important. To illustrate this point, Chart 2.1 was drawn with care while Chart 2.2 shows the same information presented by a carelessly constructed chart.

Line diagrams using arithmetic scales. Most of the line diagrams or curves which one encounters are drawn with reference to arithmetic scales, an arithmetic scale being one on which a given distance (say, one inch) anywhere on that scale will represent the same numerical value. For example, on the vertical scale of Chart 2.1, seven-eighths of an inch represents 3 mg. per ml.

Like a table, each chart must have a title and, if the data upon which the chart is based have come from another source, a source

---

[4] See W. C. Brinton, *Graphic Presentation*, Brinton Associates, New York, 1939, Ch. 6. This book also discusses other kinds of non-statistical (as well as statistical) graphs.

note should be included. The title of a chart undertakes to state clearly and succinctly the nature of the information shown by the chart. Printed titles are often placed below the charts, as in this book; occasionally they are put above the chart. If a hand-lettered title is used (as on a large wall chart), the title may be above,

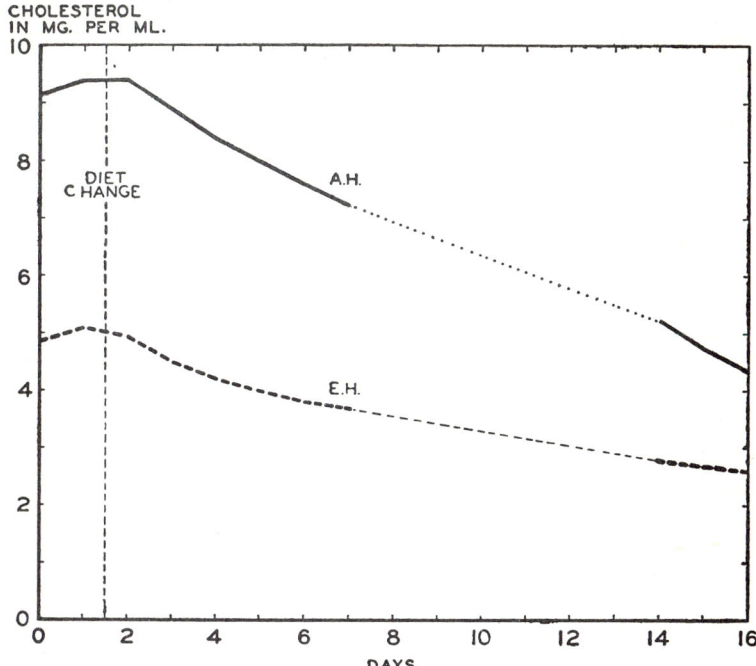

Chart 2.1. Concentration of Total Cholesterol in the Blood Serum of Two Men, A. H. and E. H., with Familial Hypercholesteremia Before and After Changing to a Fat-free Vegetarian Diet Totally Devoid of Cholesterol. The light broken portions of the curves indicate nonexistence of data between certain values. Before the diet change the two men had a moderately low cholesterol intake. Based on data from "The Relation in Man between Cholesterol Levels in the Diet and in the Blood," by Ancel Keys, *Science*, July 12, 1950, pp. 79–81.

below, or even on the grid of the chart itself. Source notes are usually placed below the chart even if the title is at the top. When the title is below the chart, the source note follows the title and is in smaller or less prominent type than the title, as in Chart 2.1.

The scales of a chart should be clearly labeled and these labels should include a statement of the units involved, as in Chart 2.1.

Occasionally a graph is seen having some lettering vertical rather than horizontal (for example, the label of the vertical scale of Chart 2.2). This usage should be avoided; all lettering on charts should be horizontal if possible.

Footnotes and prefatory notes are not often used in connection with graphic representations. If explanation is needed, it may

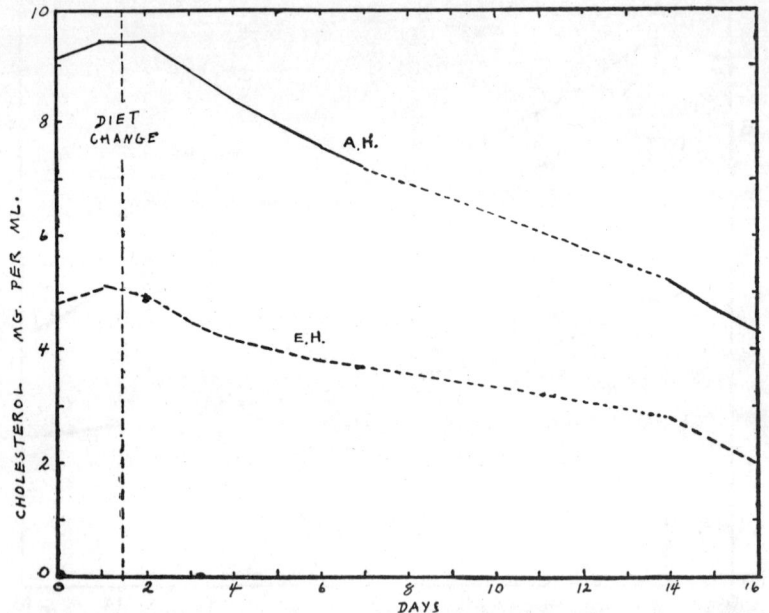

Chart 2.2. *A Carelessly Drawn Chart.* Concentration of Total Cholesterol in the Blood Serum of Two Men, A. H. and E. H., with Familial Hypercholesteremia Before and After Changing to a Fat-free Vegetarian Diet Totally Devoid of Cholesterol. The light broken portions of the curves indicate nonexistence of data between certain values. Before the diet change the two men had a moderately low cholesterol intake. Based on data from "The Relation in Man between Cholesterol Levels in the Diet and in the Blood," by Ancel Keys, *Science*, July 12, 1950, pp. 79–81.

follow the title (and precede the source note), as in Charts 2.1 and 3.6.

Observation of Chart 2.1 and of other line diagrams in this book will show that several different widths of lines are used for each chart. The heaviest line is used for the curve itself in order to make it stand out. The lightest width of ruling is used for the guide lines (see Chart 2.6). Just heavier than guide lines are the border lines and just heavier than these (but lighter than the curve itself) are the horizontal or vertical zero lines. If two or more curves appear on a graph (as in Charts 2.1 and 3.10), different types of lines, such as solid, long-dash, and short-dash, should be used. It is desirable not to have more than two or three curves on a chart. However, if more than three are shown, and particularly if the curves intertwine, it will be necessary to use lines of light or intermediate width rather than heavy lines, and also to use different types of lines. Very light broken lines are used in Chart 2.1 to indicate the nonexistence of readings between certain values.

There should not be too many guide lines on a finished chart. If a large number of horizontal and vertical guides are used, they detract from the appearance of the chart and do not permit the curve itself to be as prominent as it should be. The presence of many guide lines would enable one to read values more accurately from a chart, but a chart is not intended to serve this purpose. If it is desired that accurate values be available, a table should be used instead of a chart. Sometimes guide lines are omitted altogether and "tics" are used instead, as in Charts 2.1 and 6.7.

When charts are made for publication, a closely ruled grid printed in light blue ink may be employed. The guide, border, and base lines which are desired in the finished chart, as well as the curve, are ruled in black on this blue grid. Scale values and scale labels are then added. When the chart is reproduced by an ordinary photographic or photoengraving process, all of the blue rulings disappear. Virtually all of the charts in this book were prepared in this manner. It may be of incidental interest that the charts shown herein are smaller than the original drawings. In most cases the originals were reduced to about one-half of their linear dimensions. A reasonable reduction of the size of a chart tends to improve its appearance. This may be observed in advance by looking at the original through a reducing glass. When charts are not to be reproduced, as in the case of wall charts, closely ruled pencil guide lines may be used to aid in plotting and can later be erased.

The lettering on a chart may be freehand provided that someone with the requisite skill is available to do the work. It is usually much more satisfactory, as well as less expensive, to use lettering guides, which are available from stores selling draftsmen's and architects' supplies. Lettering guides were used to prepare the

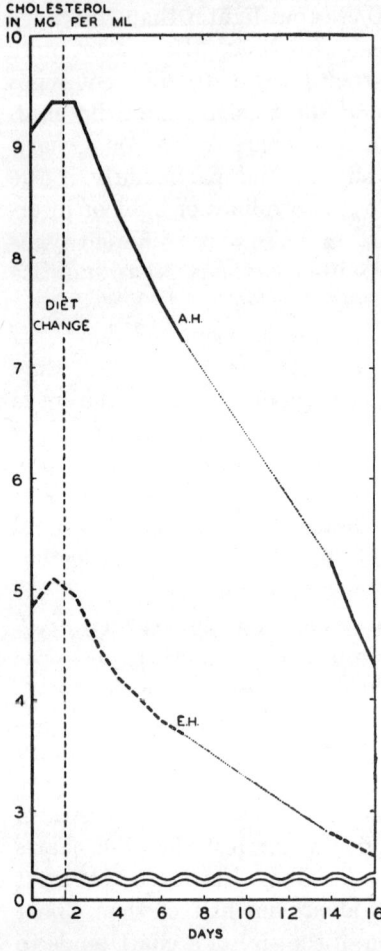

Chart 2.3. Concentration of Total Cholesterol in the Blood Serum of Two Men, A. H. and E. H., with Familial Hypercholesteremia Before and After Changing to a Fat-free Vegetarian Diet Totally Devoid of Cholesterol. The light broken portions of the curves indicate nonexistence of data between certain values. Before the diet change the two men had a moderately low cholesterol intake. Based on data from "The Relation in Man between Cholesterol Levels in the Diet and in the Blood," by Ancel Keys, *Science*, July 12, 1950, pp. 79–81.

scales and scale labels for the charts in this book, with the exception of Chart 2.2.

It is important that a line diagram (and also other types of graphs) be drawn with the horizontal and vertical dimensions bearing a reasonable proportion to each other. No exact rule can be given, since (1) there is a good deal of latitude in the term "reasonable proportion" and (2) the proportion that might be considered "reasonable" depends largely on the nature of the data being shown. Illustrations of bad proportions are given in Chart 2.3, which overexpands the vertical dimension of Chart 2.1, and in Chart 2.4, which overexpands the horizontal dimension of Chart 2.1.

It is often important that the zero on the vertical scale of a chart be shown or, if it is omitted, that its omission be clearly indicated. Consider Chart 2.5, which is a re-drawing of Chart 2.1 with the vertical scale ending just below 3 mg. per ml. A quick look at such a chart—and charts are intended to be looked at quickly—gives the visual impression that the curve for E.H. nearly reached zero at 16 days. Furthermore, the eye is not able to make a proper compari-

increases (or decreases) by a constant proportion or ratio. This cannot be ascertained from a chart of the type described in the preceding paragraphs unless the percentages of change themselves are computed and plotted. However, a line diagram using a logarithmic vertical scale, which is referred to as a "semi-logarithmic chart" or a "ratio chart," will enable the reader to recognize visually a series which is increasing or decreasing by a constant ratio, to

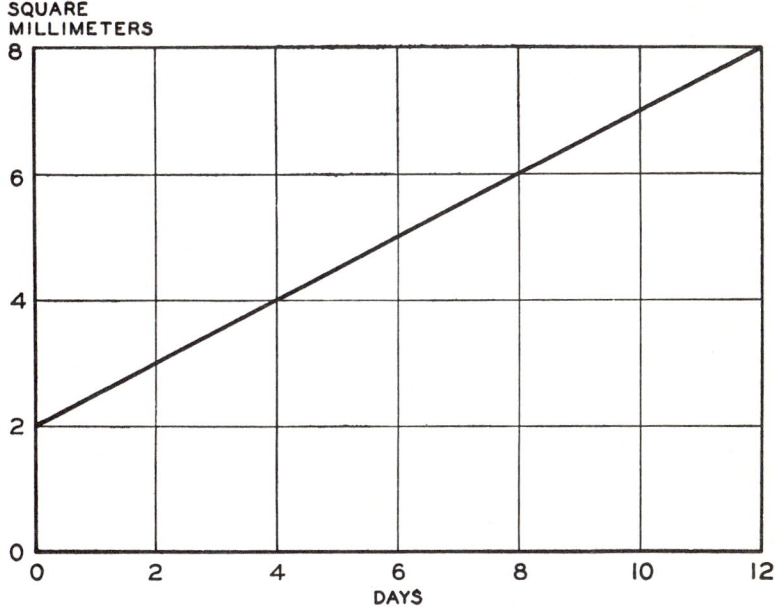

Chart 2.7. An Arithmetic Progression.

observe whether the ratio of increase or decrease is itself increasing or decreasing, and to compare the ratios of change between two or more curves or between parts of a single curve.

A line diagram using arithmetic scales makes it possible to recognize a series which is increasing or decreasing at a constant amount (an arithmetic progression), since an arithmetic progression appears as a straight line when plotted on "arithmetic paper." Chart 2.7 shows the appearance of an increasing arithmetic progression when arithmetic scales are used. An increasing arithmetic progression having a greater amount of increase would give a steeper curve; a decreasing arithmetic progression would slope downward.

A series of data having a constant ratio of increase or decrease (a geometric progression) cannot be recognized when plotted on arithmetic paper. Consider the two curves of Chart 2.8; one is a geometric progression while the other is not, but it is not possible

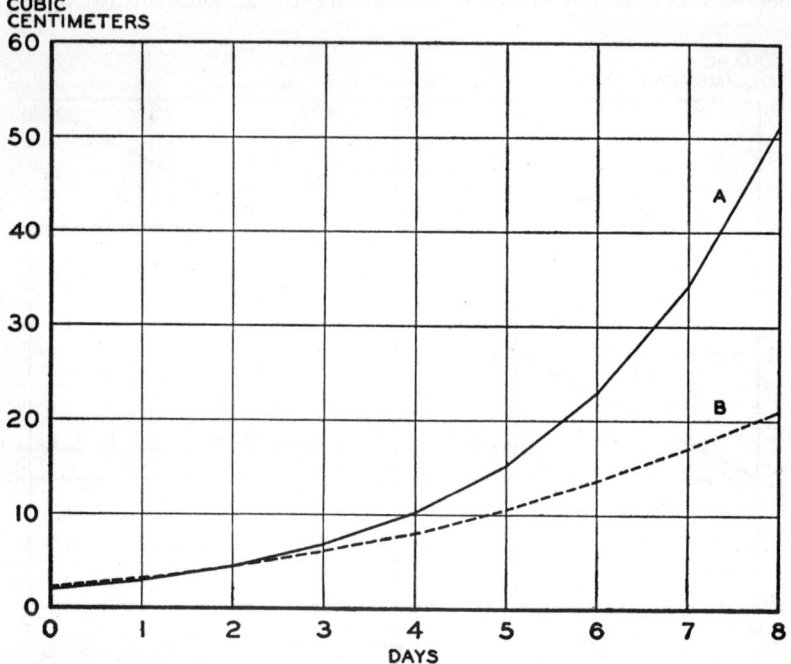

Chart 2.8. A Geometric Progression (A) and a Series Having Increasing Amounts of Increase but Decreasing Percentages of Increase (B), Shown on Arithmetic Paper.

to identify them from their appearance on this chart. If, now, the same two series are drawn on a grid having a logarithmic vertical scale and an arithmetic horizontal scale ("semi-logarithmic paper"), as in Chart 2.9, it is immediately apparent that Series A is a geometric progression while Series B is not. We are able to recognize Series A as a geometric progression because a geometric progression plotted on semi-logarithmic paper yields a straight line which slopes upward if the series is increasing and downward if it is decreasing. Chart 2.9 tells us not only that Series A is a geometric progression but also that Series B increases each period by a ratio smaller than for the preceding period.

The reason why a geometric progression yields a straight line when plotted on semi-logarithmic paper is that the logarithms of a geometric progression form an arithmetic progression. We could, of course, plot the logarithms of the values, but it is more convenient to use a vertical scale with logarithmic spacing. It is not

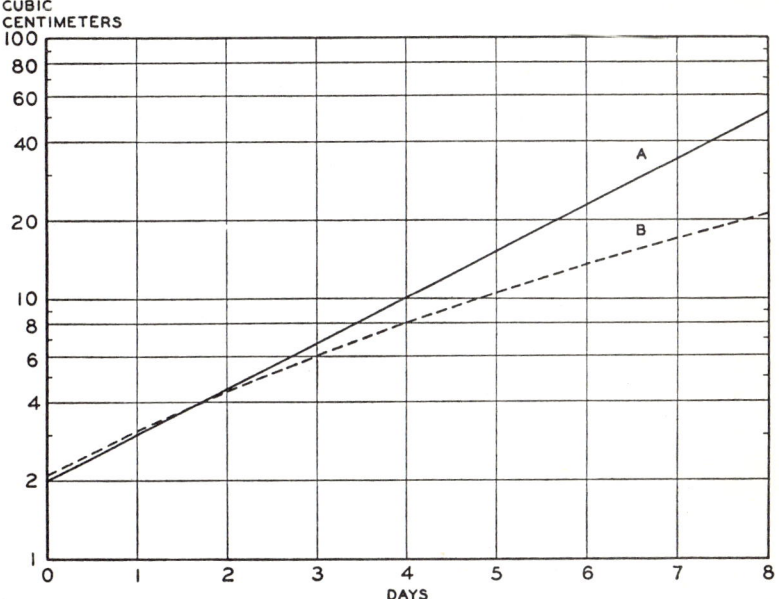

Chart 2.9. A Geometric Progression (A) and a Series Having Increasing Amounts of Increase but Decreasing Percentages of Increase (B), Shown on Semi-logarithmic Paper.

necessary to understand logarithms in order to understand the special grid of Chart 2.9. Observe that the distance from 1 to 2 is $\frac{13}{32}$ inch. Now measure $\frac{13}{32}$ inch elsewhere on the vertical scale of this chart, and it will be found that the two scale values will have the ratio 1:2. It is for this reason that the term "ratio chart" is appropriate. It is, of course, synonymous with "semi-logarithmic chart," but the former term is less imposing and is often used when such a chart is being presented to readers who might shy away from the term "semi-logarithmic."

One application of the semi-logarithmic chart may be illustrated by the data of Table 2.7, which show the number of deaths occurring

TABLE 2.7

NUMBER OF DEATHS IN THE UNITED STATES FROM CANCER AND FROM CIRRHOSIS OF THE LIVER, 1937–1948

Year	Cancer and other malignant tumors	Cirrhosis of the liver
1937	144,774	10,960
1938	149,214	10,808
1939	153,846	10,904
1940	158,335	11,286
1941	159,926	11,876
1942	163,400	12,553
1943	166,848	12,527
1944	171,171	11,485
1945	177,464	12,541
1946	182,005	13,451
1947	189,811	14,940
1948	197,042	16,512

Data from National Office of Vital Statistics, *United States Summary of Vital Statistics, 1948*, June 1, 1950, pp. 910–911.

in the United States from cancer and other malignant tumors and from cirrhosis of the liver for each year during the period 1937–1948. The data of Table 2.7 have been plotted on arithmetic paper in Chart 2.10, where it is seen that the number of deaths from cancer has shown a decided increase over the period. Deaths from cirrhosis of the liver have increased, too, but not greatly, it appears. Little can be said by way of comparing the two curves except that the curve for cancer (representing a series of large magnitude) has shown the greater absolute increase over the years. When the data are plotted on semi-logarithmic paper, as in Chart. 2.11, the two curves may be compared in regard to relative growth and it is readily seen, for example, that from 1938 to 1939 the relative increase in deaths from cancer was greater than the relative increase in deaths from cirrhosis of the liver, and that from 1944 to 1948 the relative increase in deaths from cirrhosis of the liver was greater than the relative increase in deaths from cancer. Notice that two different vertical scales were used in Chart 2.11. This is possible

CHAP. 2] TABULAR AND GRAPHIC PRESENTATION 29

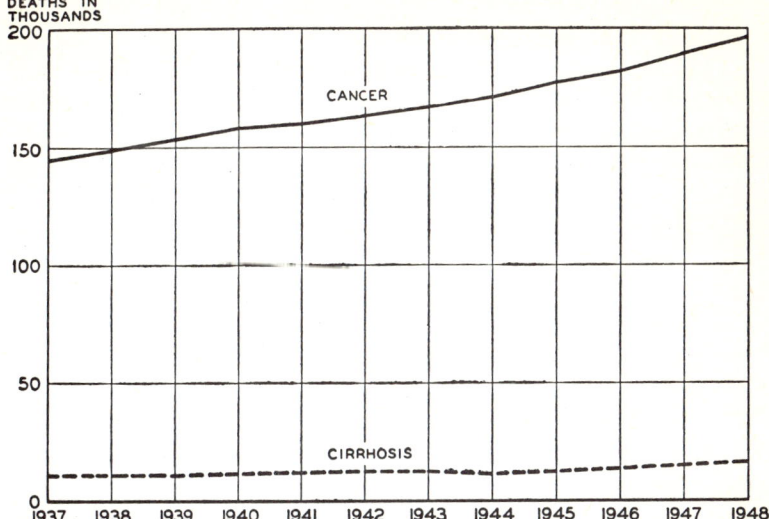

Chart 2.10. Number of Deaths in the United States from Cancer and Other Malignant Tumors and from Cirrhosis of the Liver, 1937–1948. Data from National Office of Vital Statistics, *United States Summary of Vital Statistics, 1948*, June 1, 1950, pp. 910–911.

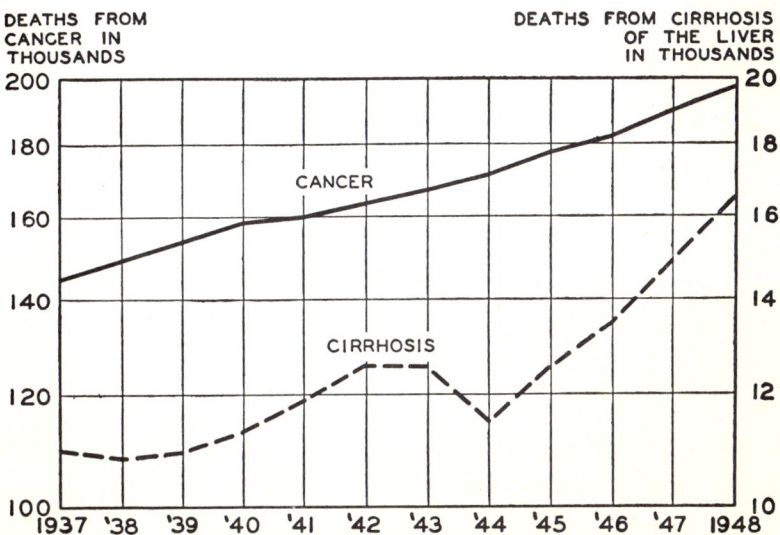

Chart 2.11. Number of Deaths in the United States from Cancer and Other Malignant Tumors and from Cirrhosis of the Liver, 1937–1948. Data from National Office of Vital Statistics, *United States Summary of Vital Statistics, 1948*, June 1, 1950, pp. 910–911.

because there is no zero on a logarithmic scale and because the slope of a curve on semi-logarithmic paper is not affected by the scale values used. To be more specific in regard to the second point: using a given logarithmic spacing on the vertical axis and a given horizontal scale, changing the values on the vertical scale can merely result in moving a curve up or down on the grid; no change occurs in the slope of any part of the curve.

Chart 2.11 illustrated the use of semi-logarithmic paper for making comparisons of the relative change of two series of different magnitude. Two or more series expressed *in different units* may also be compared on semi-logarithmic paper. This and other applications of the semi-logarithmic chart are not discussed in this volume but may be found elsewhere.[6]

The reader may have wondered if there is ever occasion to use a grid with a logarithmic horizontal scale and an arithmetic vertical scale. The answer is "Yes." Chart 7.4 has a logarithmic horizontal scale and an arithmetic vertical scale. It is not uncommon, also, to employ a grid having both scales logarithmic, although none appears in this book.[7]

Bar charts. Chronological comparisons involving a few values may be made by means of bars, as shown in Chart 2.12, which shows the expectation of life at birth among the industrial policyholders of a life insurance company at quinquennial periods since 1925. This chart contains but 6 bars. If it had been desired to show the data for each year from 1925 to 1950, a curve would have been preferable.

Note, in Chart 2.12, that the bars are arranged horizontally, the individual bars being vertical. This is the usual (but not invariable) practice when a chronological comparison is being made. For a comparison of categories, as in Chart 2.13, it is customary to arrange the bars vertically, the individual bars being horizontal. One advantage of such an arrangement is that the labels may readily be affixed to the individual bars.

In order that the reader may observe the two alternatives, Chart 2.12 has been drawn with a border, while Chart 2.13 has no border.

Chart 2.14 shows a comparison of two chronological series and, accordingly, has been made with the bars in horizontal sequence.

---

[6] A more complete discussion, as well as additional applications, will be found in F. E. Croxton and D. J. Cowden, *Applied General Statistics*, Prentice-Hall, Inc., New York, 1939, Ch. V.

[7] For an example, see *ibid.*, p. 695.

The comparison in Chart 2.15 is of two categorical series, and the bars are placed in vertical sequence. The purpose of Chart 2.15 is to point out that high (or low) values of one series are associated with low (or high) values in the other series. Note, too, that Chart 2.15 does not have the bars of one series alternating with those of the other, as was the case in Chart 2.14. This is so because the two series of Chart 2.15 are expressed in different units.

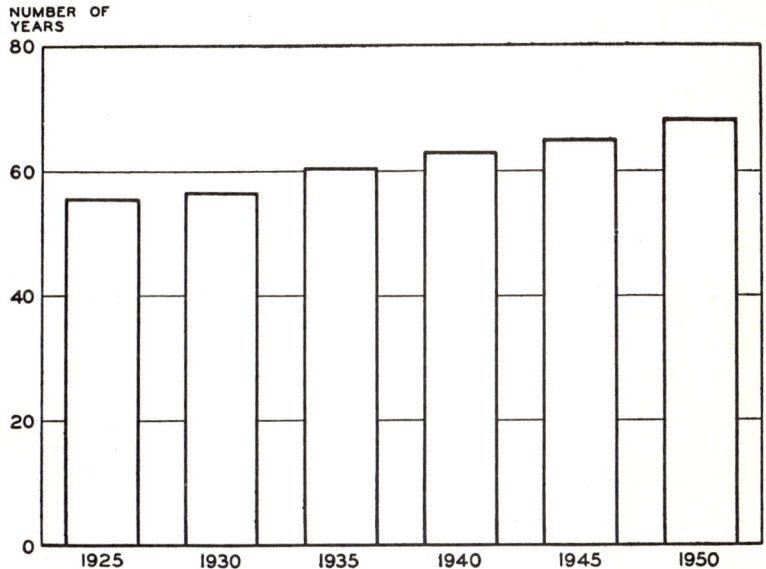

Chart 2.12. Expectation of Life at Birth of Industrial Policyholders of the Metropolitan Life Insurance Company, 1925, 1930, 1935, 1940, 1945, and 1950. Figures are for weekly premium-paying business prior to 1950, weekly and monthly business for 1950. Data from Metropolitan Life Insurance Company, *Statistical Bulletin*, August 1950, p. 4, and January 1951, p. 2.

Bars and pies for component parts. When it is desired to show the various component parts of a whole, use may be made of a bar chart, such as that of Chart 2.16, or a pie diagram, as in Chart 2.17. Either of these devices is satisfactory, but the pie diagram is often employed when the data represented are of a monetary nature, since the pie diagram may be made to resemble (not too closely!) a silver dollar. When several individual component-part diagrams are to be compared, as in Chart 2.18, it is obvious that the reader can compare bars much more readily than he can compare pies.

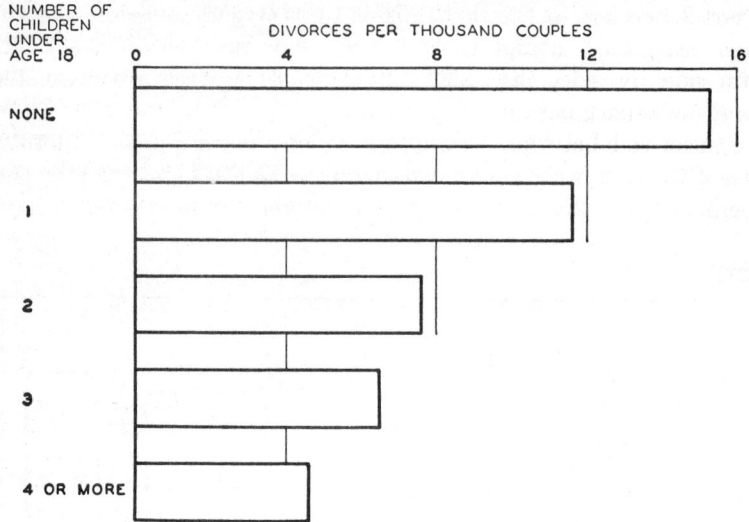

Chart 2.13. Divorces per 1,000 Married Couples in the United States, by Size of Family, 1948. Data from Metropolitan Life Insurance Company, *Statistical Bulletin*, February 1950, p. 2.

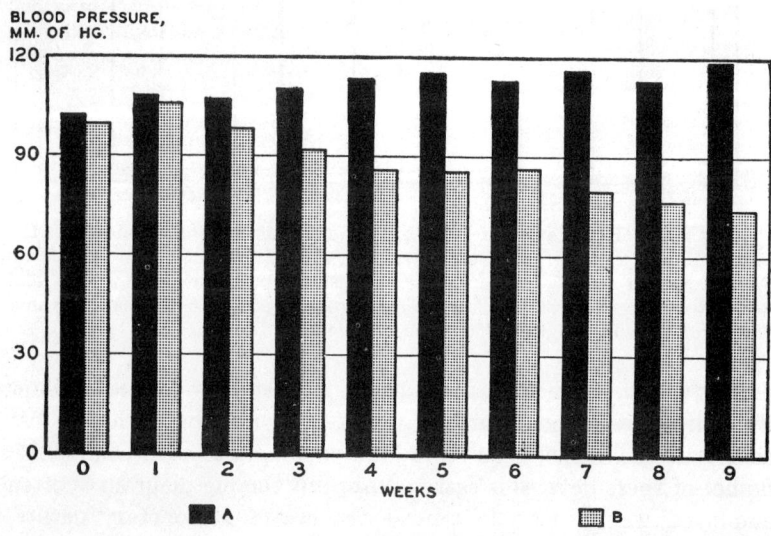

Chart 2.14. Blood Pressure of Two Groups of Rats, 0–9 weeks after Beginning Controlled Diets. Group A was permitted a 1 per cent solution of potassium chloride; group B had a potassium-free diet. Data from S. Charles Freed and Meyer Friedman, "Hypotension in the Rat Following Limitation of Potassium Intake," *Science*, Vol. 112, December 29, 1950, pp. 788–789.

Chap. 2] TABULAR AND GRAPHIC PRESENTATION 33

Chart 2.19 is similar to Chart 2.18 but involves chronological rather than categorical comparisons. Note that both charts have the bars side by side. Such an arrangement is often made of the component-part bars for a categorical comparison, since the parts are easier to label when arranged in this fashion than would be the case if the bars were above and below each other. Chart 2.20 is a component-part bar chart showing absolute values rather than

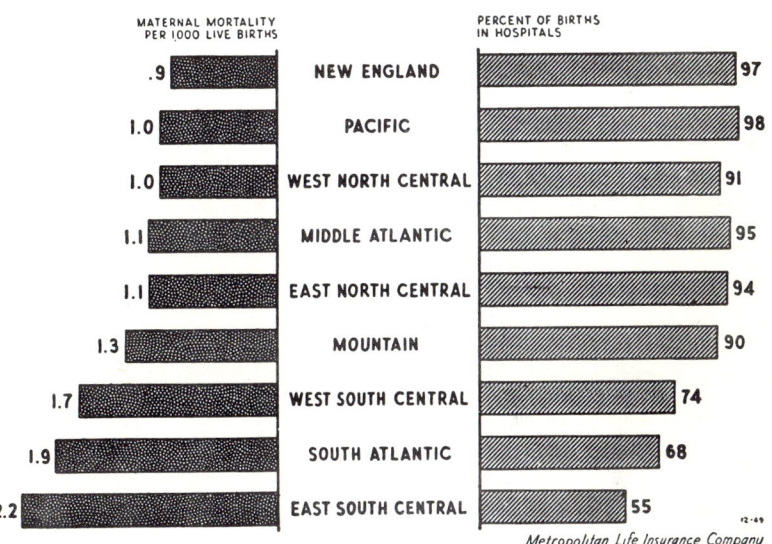

Chart 2.15.

MATERNAL MORTALITY AND HOSPITALIZATION OF BIRTHS BY REGIONS, UNITED STATES, 1947

Reproduced, by permission, from *Statistical Bulletin* of the Metropolitan Life Insurance Company, October 1949, p. 7.

percentages. An alternative method of showing component parts, which is particularly useful when a large number of years is involved, consists of using curves instead of bars. Chart 2.21 shows the number of persons in the United States in the various age categories and is similar to Chart 2.20, but covers a greater number of census periods. Curves could, of course, be used to show the proportions instead of the numbers in the five age groups, if desired.

Pictographs. Since a bar chart is not particularly effective for attracting attention, simple comparisons of a few figures are some-

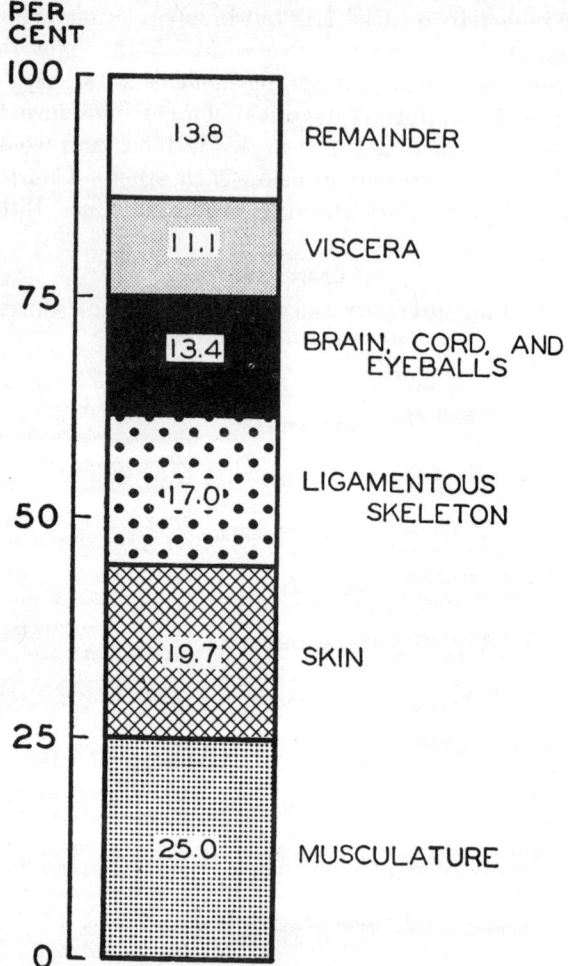

Chart 2.16. Percentages of Total Body Weight Formed by Various Parts in the Newborn Human. Data from W. J. Robbins and others, *Growth*, Yale University Press, New Haven, 1928, p. 126.

times attempted by means of large and small pictures: for example, men of various sizes to indicate the number of inhabitants in each of two or more cities. Occasionally the reader is told to compare the heights of the figures, but ordinarily he does not know whether the comparison is one of height, area, or apparent volume. It should be added that accurate comparisons of areas and of two-dimensional representations of volumes is not possible.

The pictograph or pictogram embodies the attention-getting value of a picture and the accuracy of a bar chart. Chart 2.22 shows a pictograph of the number of deaths per 100,000 policyholders of the Metropolitan Life Insurance Company from certain types of diseases of the heart during February 1952. Although the

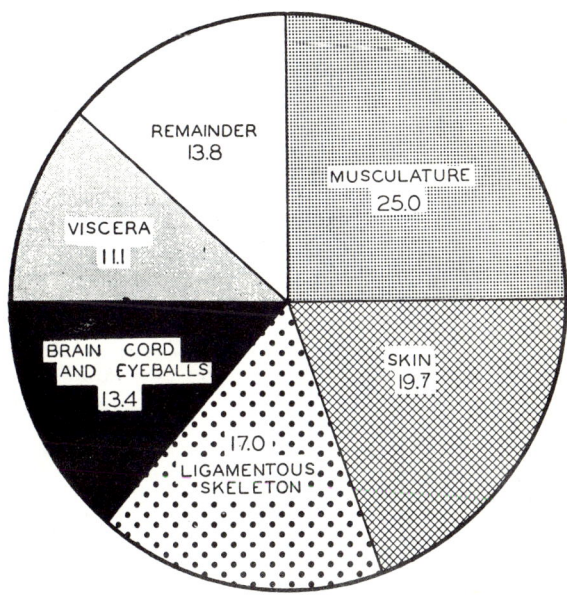

Chart 2.17. Percentages of Total Body Weight Formed by Various Parts in the Newborn Human. Data from same source as Chart 2.16.

experience referred only to February 1952, the specific death rate for that month was adjusted to an annual basis, as was pointed out in the preceding chapter to be customary. An extended discussion of pictographs is not in order here,[8] but it is worth while to note that pictographs usually have the individual pictures in rows, rarely in columns; that the picture should immediately suggest the nature of the data being shown; and that some types of data,

---

[8] For a detailed treatment, see Rudolph Modley and Dyno Lowenstein, *Pictographs and Graphs*, Harper and Brothers, New York, 1952.

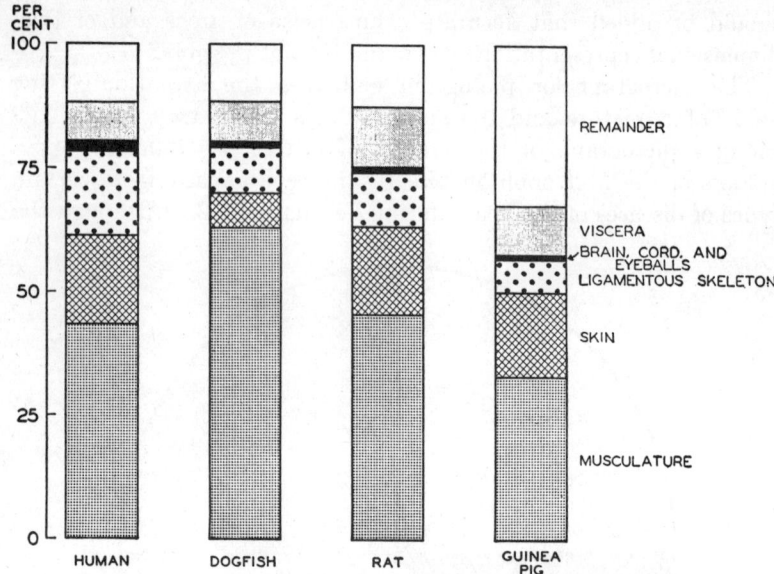

Chart 2.18. Percentages of Total Body Weight Formed by Various Parts in the Adult Human, Dogfish, Rat, and Guinea Pig. Data from same source as Chart 2.16.

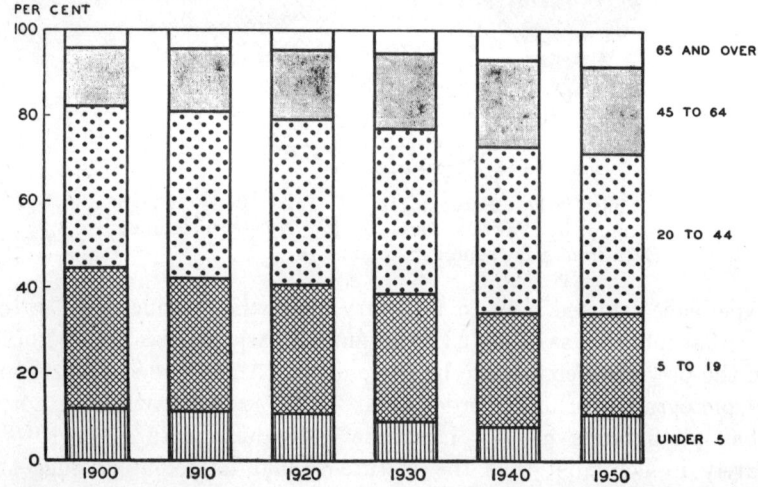

Chart 2.19. Proportion of the Population of the United States in each Specified Age Group, 1900, 1910, 1920, 1930, 1940, and 1950. Data from U. S. Bureau of the Census, *Fifteenth Census of the United States: 1930*, Population, Vol. II, p. 576, and *1950 Census of Population, Preliminary Reports*, Series PC-7, No. 1, p. 6.

CHAP. 2] TABULAR AND GRAPHIC PRESENTATION 37

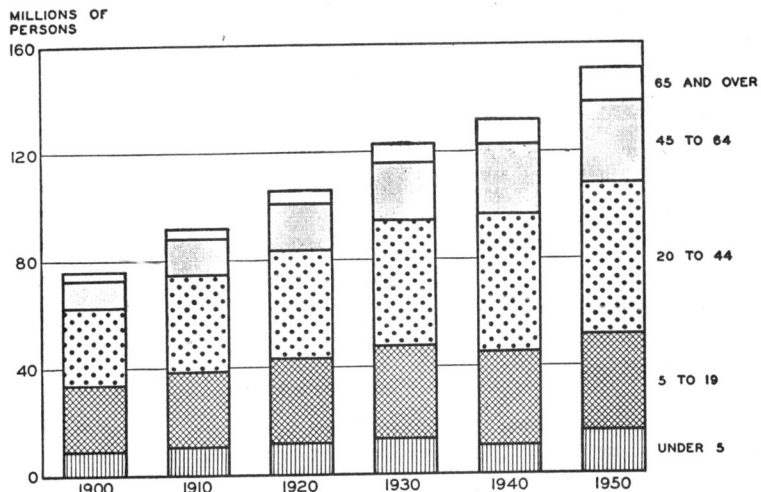

Chart 2.20. Population of the United States in Each Specified Age Group, 1900, 1910, 1920, 1930, 1940, and 1950. Data from same sources as Chart 2.19.

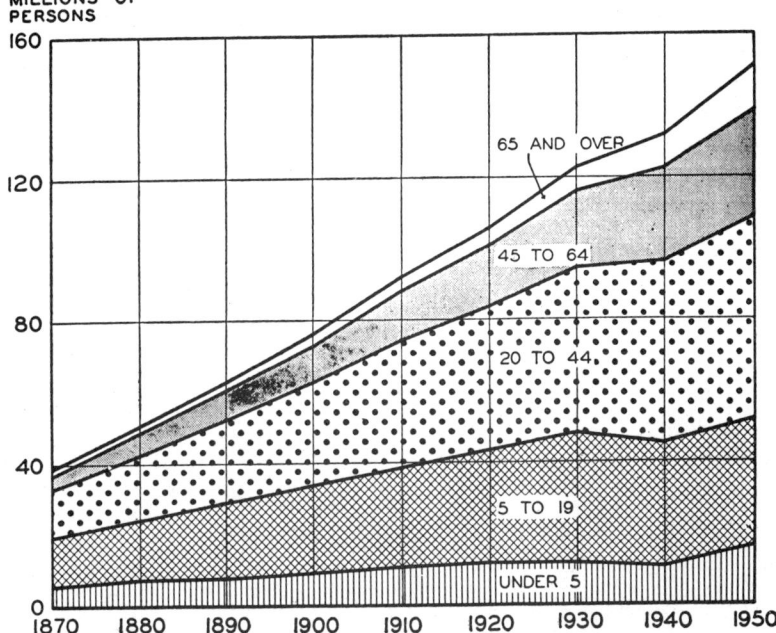

Chart 2.21. Population of the United States in Each Specified Age Group, 1870–1950, by Decades. Data from same sources as Chart 2.19.

such as blood pressure and pulse rates, cannot readily be pictured and are not suitable for portrayal by means of pictographs.

Statistical maps. Statistical maps show quantitative data by geographical location. Depending upon the purpose of the map and

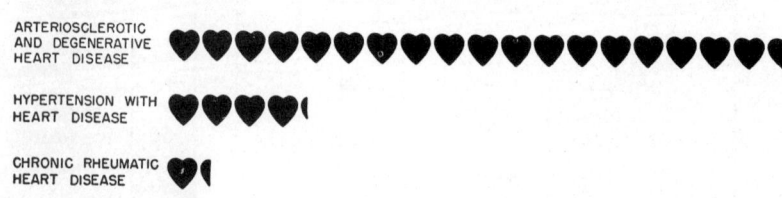

Chart 2.22. Deaths per 100,000 Policyholders of the Metropolitan Life Insurance Company from Specified Diseases of the Heart, February 1952. Data from *Statistical Bulletin*, Metropolitan Life Insurance Company, March 1952, p. 11. The rates are provisional and have been adjusted to an annual basis.

the nature of the data being presented, a map may be hatched or shaded, or the chart maker may employ dots or pins. Since few readers of this volume are likely to be interested in statistical maps, the topic will receive no further attention here.[9]

---

[9] A brief discussion, with eight maps as examples, is given in F. E. Croxton and D. J. Cowden, *Applied General Statistics*, Prentice-Hall, Inc., New York, 1939, pp. 137–145.

Chapter 3
THE FREQUENCY DISTRIBUTION

Statistical data are often presented in the form of a frequency distribution. As shown in Table 3.1, a frequency distribution

TABLE 3.1

VOLUME OF CELLS, IN CUBIC CENTIMETERS PER HUNDRED CUBIC CENTIMETERS OF BLOOD, FOR 100 NORMAL YOUNG WOMEN

Volume of cells	Number of women*
35.0–36.5	4.5
36.5–38.0	7.5
38.0–39.5	12
39.5–41.0	23.5
41.0–42.5	28
42.5–44.0	13
44.0–45.5	9.5
45.5–47.0	2
Total	100

*See page 42 for an explanation of the fractional frequencies. Source of data: see Table 3.2.

arranges the items of a series into groups or classes and indicates the number of cases occurring in each group.

Raw Data

Table 3.2 gives data of the volume of cells per 100 c.c. of blood for each of 100 normal young women. There is no apparent order in the arrangement of these 100 items, and for our purposes they may be thought of as statistically unorganized. We can obtain very little information from these 100 figures in their present form. We cannot readily note the smallest and largest values, nor can we ascertain around what value, if any, the items tend to concentrate.

40 THE FREQUENCY DISTRIBUTION [Chap. 3

This and other information may be had if we rearrange and summarize the data.

TABLE 3.2

Volume of Cells, in Cubic Centimeters per Hundred Cubic Centimeters of Blood, for 100 Normal Young Women

Subject	Volume of cells	Subject	Volume of cells	Subject	Volume of cells	Subject	Volume of cells
1	35.3	26	42.1	51	40.6	76	41.3
2	37.0	27	42.4	52	37.9	77	39.8
3	38.5	28	37.5	53	40.8	78	41.2
4	42.6	29	42.1	54	39.5	79	35.3
5	37.0	30	42.2	55	39.2	80	44.6
6	35.2	31	43.7	56	41.8	81	43.6
7	38.3	32	42.5	57	43.4	82	43.5
8	36.5	33	40.3	58	40.9	83	39.3
9	42.2	34	37.2	59	39.6	84	41.8
10	41.2	35	43.5	60	36.4	85	42.2
11	40.0	36	41.1	61	41.0	86	43.4
12	41.9	37	42.0	62	40.8	87	38.4
13	44.2	38	40.1	63	37.7	88	40.7
14	41.3	39	41.4	64	38.5	89	44.1
15	37.3	40	39.8	65	41.8	90	38.7
16	41.4	41	42.0	66	44.7	91	39.4
17	44.4	42	42.3	67	45.9	92	41.4
18	43.9	43	39.2	68	46.3	93	39.3
19	44.0	44	42.6	69	39.3	94	42.5
20	44.9	45	42.1	70	40.6	95	41.5
21	39.5	46	39.8	71	43.1	96	39.8
22	41.6	47	41.7	72	45.0	97	40.4
23	40.5	48	40.9	73	42.5	98	45.3
24	40.0	49	40.8	74	40.4	99	41.3
25	45.2	50	42.8	75	40.6	100	40.0

Data from E. E. Osgood and H. D. Haskins, "Relation Between Cell Count, Cell Volume, and Hemoglobin Content of Venous Blood of Normal Young Women," *Archives of Internal Medicine*, Vol. 39, May, 1927, pp. 643–655. The young women were 18–30 years of age. The data of volume of cells are given by Osgood and Haskins to two decimals. Many investigators contend that differences of 0.01 c.c. in volume of cells cannot be satisfactorily distinguished. Consequently, for purposes of illustration, Osgood's and Haskins' data have been rounded to one decimal and treated as if they originally had been recorded in that manner.

The Array

An array rearranges but does not summarize. It consists of a listing of the values in order of magnitude from smallest to largest or from largest to smallest, whichever is preferred. Table 3.3 is an array of the data of Table 3.2 with the figures ranging from lowest to highest. From this array it may immediately be noted that the smallest cell volume was 35.2 c.c. while the largest was 46.3 c.c. It may also be observed that there is a large number of values in the neighborhood of 40, 41, and 42 c.c. In addition, it appears that there are relatively few values below 37 and above 45 c.c. Although it gives us information which is not readily available from the raw data, an array of a large number of values is still an awkward form to work with, since all of the original items are still indi-

TABLE 3.3

Array of Volume of Cells, in Cubic Centimeters per Hundred Cubic Centimeters of Blood, for 100 Normal Young Women

35.2	39.3	40.6	41.8	43.1
35.3	39.3	40.7	41.8	43.4
35.3	39.4	40.8	41.8	43.4
36.4	39.5	40.8	41.9	43.5
36.5	39.5	40.8	42.0	43.5
37.0	39.6	40.9	42.0	43.6
37.0	39.8	40.9	42.1	43.7
37.2	39.8	41.0	42.1	43.9
37.3	39.8	41.1	42.1	44.0
37.5	39.8	41.2	42.2	44.1
37.7	40.0	41.2	42.2	44.2
37.9	40.0	41.3	42.2	44.4
38.3	40.0	41.3	42.3	44.6
38.4	40.1	41.3	42.4	44.7
38.5	40.3	41.4	42.5	44.9
38.5	40.4	41.4	42.5	45.0
38.7	40.4	41.4	42.5	45.2
39.2	40.5	41.5	42.6	45.3
39.2	40.6	41.6	42.6	45.9
39.3	40.6	41.7	42.8	46.3

vidually listed. The array is most likely to be useful for brief series of data, particularly those having too few items to warrant the construction of a frequency distribution.

The Frequency Distribution

The frequency distribution of Table 3.1 not only rearranges the data of Table 3.2 but also summarizes them by showing the number of items occurring in each of eight classes. The information is now in a more compact form than in either Table 3.2 or Table 3.3 and it will be easier to work with. The approximate minimum and maximum values of 35.0 and 47.0 c.c. may be observed; the concentration in the 41.0–42.5 c.c. class is apparent; the relatively few values at the two ends of the distribution are readily noted. It is, of course, obvious that when the data are compressed into a frequency distribution, the exact values of the individual items are no longer known.

The half-frequencies shown in four classes are due to the fact that some values occurred on the dividing line between classes. This will be clear when the entry form on page 45 is examined.

Graphic portrayal. A frequency distribution may be shown graphically by means of a column diagram, as shown in Chart 3.1.

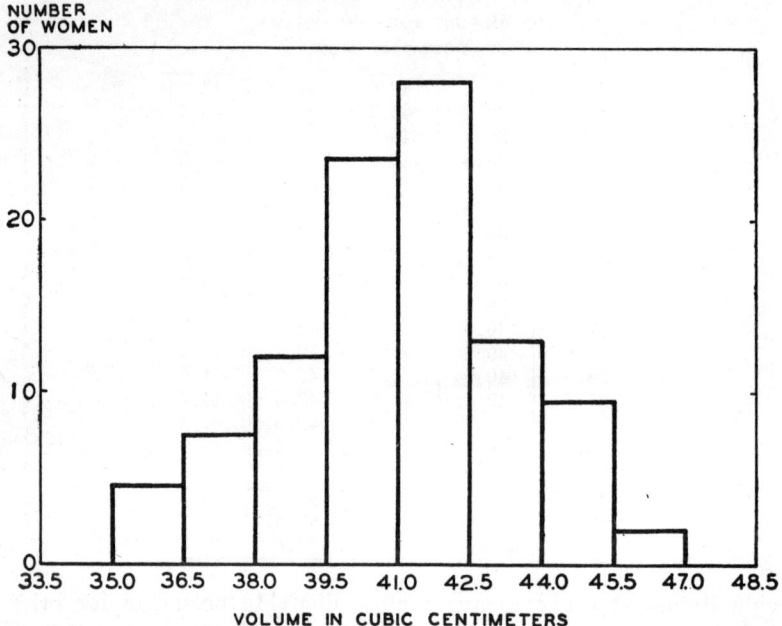

Chart 3.1. Volume of Cells, in Cubic Centimeters per Hundred Cubic Centimeters of Blood, for 100 Normal Young Women. Data of Table 3.1.

Each bar in the chart is the same width; the heights of the bars vary to indicate the number of items or frequency for each class. Alternatively, we may use a curve instead of bars to depict a frequency distribution graphically. To do this, we plot each frequency against the appropriate class mid-value, getting the curve of Chart 3.2.

The relationship existing between the column diagram of Chart 3.1 and the frequency curve of Chart 3.2 is shown in Chart 3.3, where the two types of charts are superimposed. If the curve is extended, as shown by the dotted lines, so that the curve meets the base line at 34.25 and 47.75 c.c. (which are, respectively, the mid-values of the classes 33.5–35.0 and 47.0–48.5 c.c.), the area under the curve and the area enclosed by the bars are the same. For this reason, a frequency curve is sometimes extended (using either a broken or solid line) as shown in Chart 3.3. There are, however, strong reasons for not extending a frequency curve: first, the extension conveys the impression that extreme cases had occurred in the

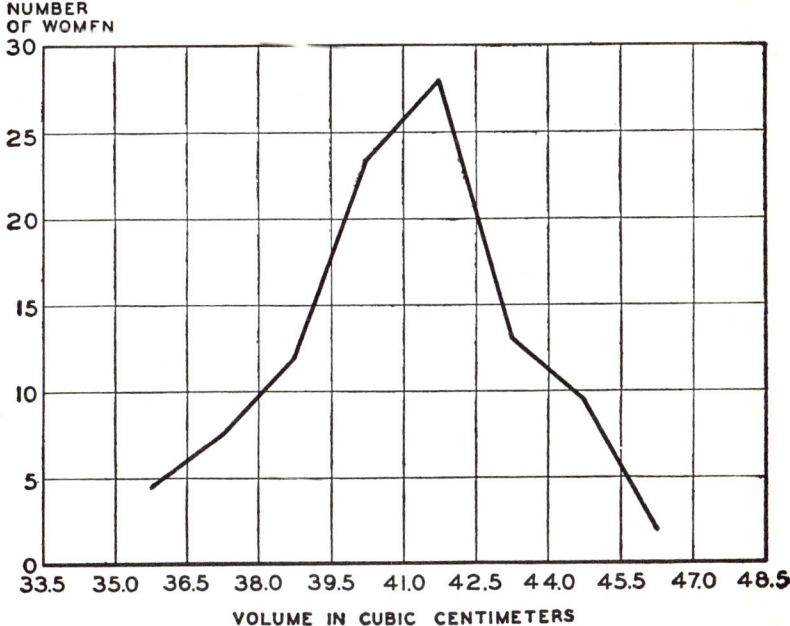

Chart 3.2. Volume of Cells, in Cubic Centimeters per Hundred Cubic Centimeters of Blood, for 100 Normal Young Women. Data of Table 3.1.

sample, when actually they had not; second, if the lower limit of the first class is zero, extending the curve at the left will make it appear that negative values have occurred, which is often impossible.

Constructing a frequency distribution. When data are already in an array, it is a simple matter to make a frequency distribution, since the items need only be counted. The array may also be useful in helping one to decide what classes to use, a topic that is discussed in the next section.

If we know at the outset what classes are desired, a frequency distribution may be made directly from raw data by the use of a tally

44 THE FREQUENCY DISTRIBUTION [Chap. 3

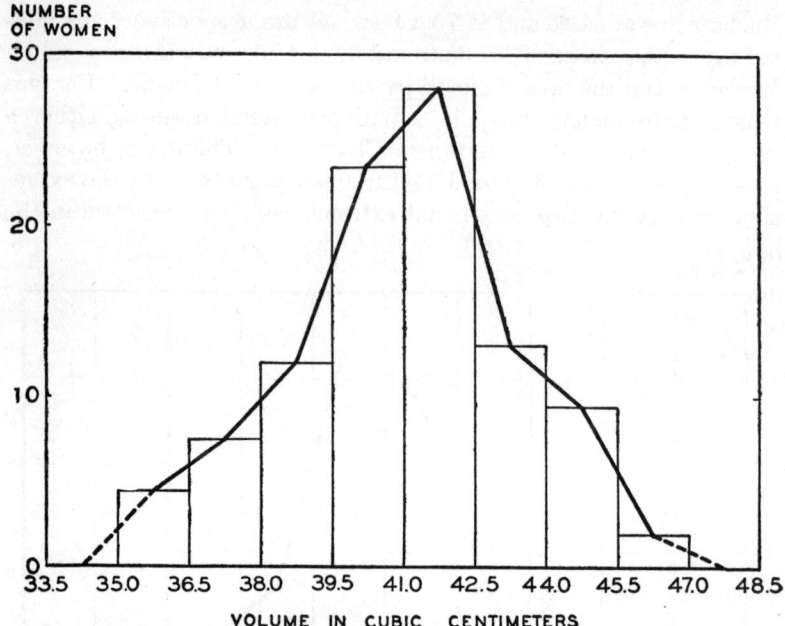

Chart 3.3. Volume of Cells, in Cubic Centimeters per Hundred Cubic Centimeters of Blood, for 100 Normal Young Women. Data of Table 3.1.

Tally Form for Volume of Cells, in Cubic Centimeters per Hundred Cubic Centimeters of Blood, for 100 Normal Young Women

Volume of cells	number of women	
35.0 – 36.5	/ ////	4.5
36.5 – 38.0	ℳ //	7.5
38.0 – 39.5	// ℳ ℳ /	12
39.5 – 41.0	/ ℳ ℳ ℳ ℳ //	23.5
41.0 – 42.5	/// ℳ ℳ ℳ ℳ ℳ /	28
42.5 – 44.0	/ ℳ ℳ /	13
44.0 – 45.5	ℳ ////	9.5
45.5 – 47.0	//	2

CHAP. 3] THE FREQUENCY DISTRIBUTION 45

form, such as that shown on page 44. When the data are recorded on cards, the frequency distribution may be obtained by hand sorting; if the information is on punch cards,[1] a frequency distribution may be constructed quickly by mechanical means.

ENTRY FORM FOR VOLUME OF CELLS, IN CUBIC CENTIMETERS PER HUNDRED CUBIC CENTIMETERS OF BLOOD, FOR 100 NORMAL YOUNG WOMEN

35.0–36.5	36.5–38.0	38.0–39.5	39.5–41.0	41.0–42.5	42.5–44.0	44.0–45.5	45.5–47.0
35.3	37.0	38.5	40.0	42.2	42.6	44.2	45.9
35.2	37.0	38.3	40.5	41.2	43.9	44.4	46.3
36.5			39.5	41.9		44.0	
36.4	37.3	39.2	40.0	41.3	43.7	44.9	
35.3	37.5	39.2	40.3	41.4	43.5	45.2	
	37.2	38.5	40.1	41.6	42.6	44.7	
	37.9	39.3	39.8	42.1	42.8	45.0	
	37.7	39.3	39.8	42.4	43.4	44.6	
		38.4	40.9	42.1	43.1	44.1	
		38.7	40.8	42.2	43.6	45.3	
		39.4	40.6	42.5			
		39.3	40.8	41.1	43.5		
			39.5	42.0	43.4		
			40.9	41.4			
			39.6	42.0			
			40.8	42.3			
			40.6	42.1			
			40.4	41.7			
			40.6	41.8			
			41.0				
			39.8	41.8			
			40.7	42.5			
			39.8	41.3			
			40.4	41.2			
			40.0	41.8			
				42.2			
				41.4			
				42.5			
				41.5			
				41.3			

If we are not certain what classes are to be used, there is a marked advantage in using the entry form shown just above, since, if it should be decided that 1-c.c. or 2-c.c. class intervals would be preferable, the change may be readily made. In addition, the entry form enables us to examine each column of figures to ascertain whether any items have been incorrectly entered.

[1] For a description, see F. E. Croxton and D. J. Cowden, *Applied General Statistics*, Prentice-Hall, Inc., New York, 1939, pp. 40–44.

The classes for a frequency distribution. When deciding upon the classes to use for a frequency distribution, consideration must be given to the number of classes to be used and to the class limits to be employed.

Number of classes. No satisfactory hard-and-fast rule can be given for the number of classes to use. It must be obvious, however, that if too many classes are used, some of the classes will have few or no frequencies and the resulting frequency distribution will be irregular. On the other hand, if there are too few classes, the data will be unduly compressed, a large proportion of the frequencies will occur in one, two, or three classes, and much information will be lost. One statistician has suggested a rule[2] for the number of classes which would result in the use of 20 classes for our data of volume of cells! This would, of course, be too many for a sample of only 100 items. It is not desirable to make a frequency distribution for fewer than about 25 or 30 items, since a smaller number of items may be studied in an array. For samples of this size, we may use 5 or 6 classes and increase the number of classes for larger samples. Frequency distributions do not often have more than 20 classes unless they are based upon very extensive data.

Another consideration may sometimes dictate the number of classes that will be used, quite aside from the number of items in a distribution. For example, a classification of amputees might show amputations of 1, 2, 3, or 4 extremities, and a frequency distribution of these data could have no more classes than these four, irrespective of the size of the sample.

Writing the classes. At this point it will be desirable to distinguish between discrete and continuous variables. The number of children in a family may be 0, 1, 2, 3, 4, 5, and so forth, and no intermediate values are possible; the values differ from each other by finite amounts, which is characteristic of a discrete variable. The values of a continuous variable may differ from each other by

---

[2] His rule is that the class interval should be not more than one-fourth of the estimated population standard deviation (see page 228). The estimated population standard deviation for our data is 2.41 c.c., and, according to this rule, our class intervals should be not more than $2.41 \div 4 = 0.6$ c.c. in width. Since the raw data ranged from 35.2 c.c. to 46.3 c.c., we would have to use 20 classes or more! See G. W. Snedecor, *Statistical Methods*, 4th edition, Collegiate Press, Ames, Iowa, 1946, p. 170.

infinitely small amounts. Volume of blood cells is a continuous variable. In Table 3.3 there is one case showing 45.2 c.c. and another having 45.3 c.c. Actually, we might have many values *between* these two, provided that we could measure cell volume accurately enough and provided that we measured enough subjects.

When working with a discrete variable, the problem of how to write the classes is sometimes quite simplified. For data of the number of children in a family, the classes might be 0, 1, 2, 3, 4, and so forth, or, if wider classes were desirable, 0 or 1, 2 or 3, 4 or 5, 6 or 7, and so forth. As another illustration, consider a frequency distribution of the wages lost by factory employees because of accidents during a year. This is also a discrete variable, since the data are in dollars and cents, and steps of less than one cent do not occur. If three dollar classes are to be used, the distribution might be:

Wages lost	Number of employees
0–$2.99	7
$3.00– 5.99	12
6.00– 8.99	15
etc.	etc.

Note that the classes are not written 0–$3.00, $3.00–$6.00, and so forth, because that would result in overlapping: a reader would not know whether $3.00 was in the first or second class. For a continuous variable, it is not always possible or desirable to avoid overlapping of class limits, since, owing to inability to measure with sufficient accuracy or because of other reasons, cases may occur which fall on class limits. Reference to the entry form shows that eight such items were present in our data of cell volume, and each of these items was divided between the two classes concerned.

The mid-value of each class (which is the average of the lower and upper limits of the class) was used to represent the class when drawing the frequency curve of Chart 3.2. We shall make use of the mid-values also when we compute various measures from frequency distributions in following chapters. It is important, therefore, that the classes of a frequency distribution be so designed that the mid-value of each class will be representative of the class. This makes it necessary to consider the manner in which data have been recorded and the presence of any concentrations in the data.

If ages have been recorded *to the last birthday* (sometimes referred to as the census method), it is clear that persons listed as 22 years of age will range from just 22 to almost 23 years old. Two-year classes should, therefore, be written:

Age in years	Number of persons
20 but less than 22	10
22 but less than 24	17
24 but less than 26	28
etc.	etc.

If ages have been recorded *to the nearest birthday* (sometimes called the insurance method), persons who are reported as 22 years of age would range from one-half year less than to one-half year more than 22. Two-year classes should be written:

Age in years	Number of persons
20–21	8
22–23	19
24–25	24
etc.	etc.

In Oriental countries and in some European countries, it is customary to report age *to the next birthday*. On this basis, persons reported as 22 years of age would range from just over 21 to 22 years old and it would be correct to write two-year classes:

Age in years	Number of persons
Over 20–22	5
Over 22–24	12
Over 24–26	21
etc.	etc.

If concentrations are present in data, it is necessary to consider them in designating the classes for a frequency distribution. For example, when age data are collected in an inquiry, such as a census, which does not require that birth certificates or other evidence be shown, there are certain concentrations which are almost certain to appear in tabulated data, the most striking of which is an excess of persons aged 30, 35, 40, 45, and so forth. There will be more persons aged 30 than aged 29 or 31, more aged 35 than 34 or 36, and so on. Consideration would be given, in writing the classes, to whether the ages were reported to the last, nearest, or next birthday, but the classes should be 5 years in width[3] and multiples of 5 should be the mid-values. Thus, if age was reported to the nearest birthday, we would have:

---

[3] Alternatively, they could be 10 or 15 years wide if the data would not be unduly compressed owing to the use of too few classes.

Age in years   Number of persons
28–32.............. 75
33–37.............. 128
38–42.............. 143
etc.   etc.

Graphic forms of frequency distributions. It has already been pointed out that a frequency distribution may be shown graphically by means of a column diagram or a curve. Sometimes, when a discrete variable is under consideration, a column diagram is used,

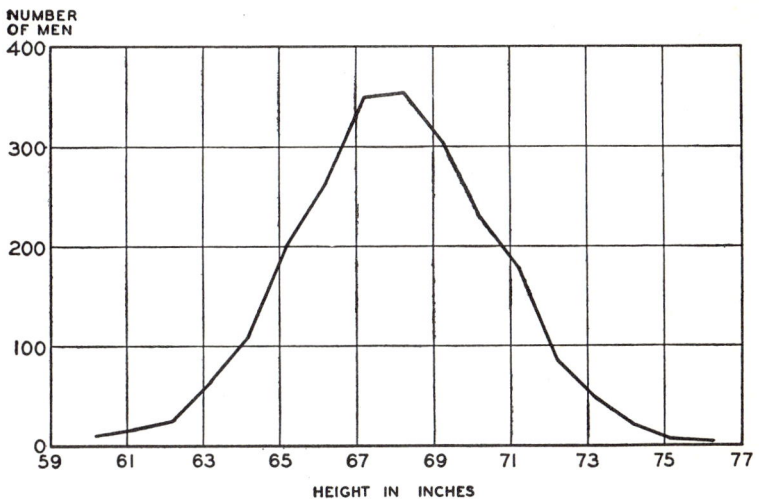

Chart 3.4. Heights of 2,266 Male Selectees, 30 but Less Than 35 Years of Age, Inducted Into the United States Army, Who Were Examined May 1943. Data from Medical Statistics Division, Office of the Surgeon General, United States Army.

with the bars slightly separated from each other to emphasize the discrete nature of the variable. This has been done in Chart 8.11, where the data shown are of the number of male live births in families which had four live births. To illustrate the more important graphic forms which frequency distributions may assume, curves are used in Charts 3.2 to 3.7.

The curve of Chart 3.2 is approximately symmetrical and is one of several curve forms that will be frequently encountered. This curve is not perfectly symmetrical, but only very roughly so. It is not likely that the reader will ever encounter a set of sample data that gives an *exactly* symmetrical curve. A second curve which is approximately symmetrical is shown in Chart 3.4, which depicts

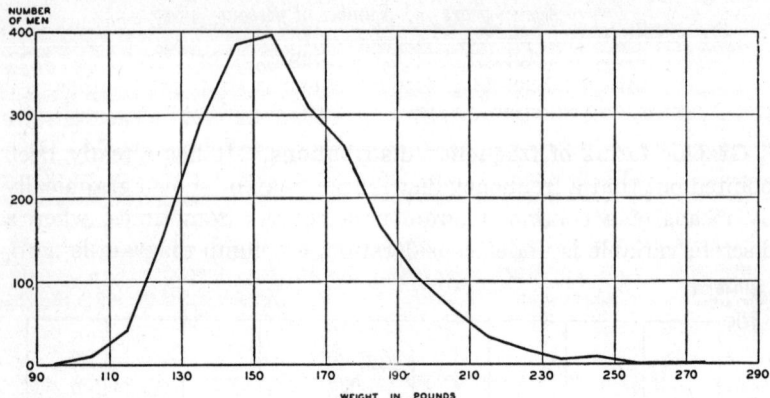

Chart 3.5. Weights of 2,266 White Selectees, 30 but Less Than 35 Years of Age, Inducted Into the United States Army, Who Were Examined May 1943. Data from Medical Statistics Division, Office of the Surgeon General, United States Army.

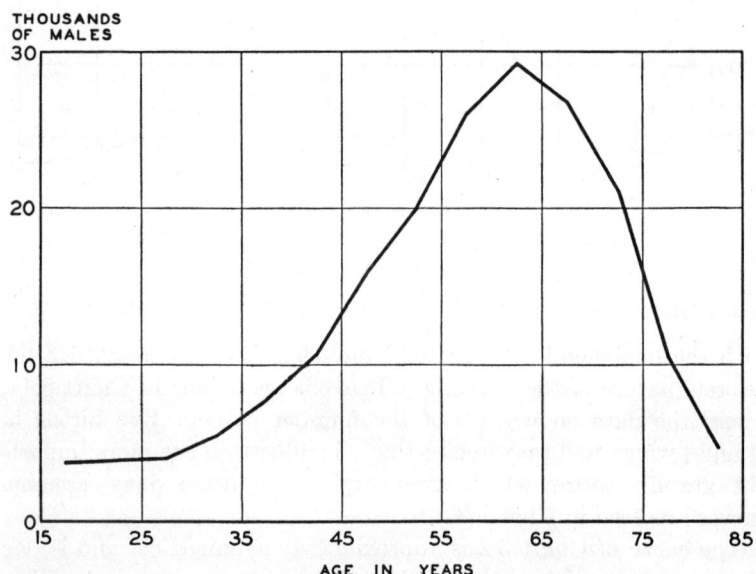

Chart 3.6. Estimated Number of Male Diabetics, 15–85 Years of Age, in the 1940 Population of the United States. Omitted from this chart are 6,600 males under 15 years of age and 1,000 males 85 or more years old. Data from Mortimer Spiegelman and Herbert H. Marks, "Age and Sex Variations in the Prevalence and Onset of Diabetes Mellitus," *American Journal of Public Health*, Vol. 36, No. 1, January 1946, pp. 26–33.

CHAP. 3] THE FREQUENCY DISTRIBUTION 51

the heights of 2,266 white selectees, 30 but less than 35 years of age, who were inducted into the United States Army and who were examined during May 1943. If we consider, not the heights, but the weights of this same group of men, we obtain the curve shown in Chart 3.5. This curve is clearly asymmetrical or skewed. It is skewed to the right.

Frequency distributions which are skewed to the left are less often encountered than those skewed to the right. In making such

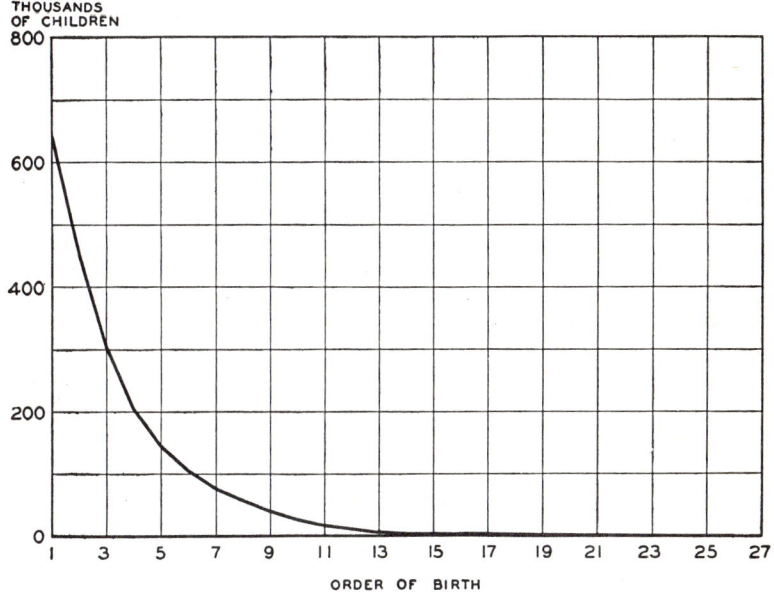

Chart 3.7. Order of Birth of 2,086,882 Children Born in the United States, 1928. Data from Barbara S. Burks, "A Statistical Method for Estimating the Distribution of Sizes of Completed Fraternities in a Population Represented by a Random Sampling of Individuals," *Journal of the American Statistical Association*, Vol. 28, No. 184, December 1933, pages 388–394.

a statement, reference is to distributions that are characteristically skewed, which is to say that they can be depended upon to show skewness in the same direction (though not necessarily to exactly the same degree) from one sample to another. A frequency distribution which is skewed to the left is shown in Chart 3.6.

In addition to curves which show concentrations in the neighborhood of the center or somewhat to one side of the center of the distribution, series are occasionally found which have a concentration at one end. A curve of such a series is shown in Chart 3.7. Since order of birth is a discrete variable, this chart might alternatively have been shown by means of separated bars, as in Chart 8.11.

Ogives. It is occasionally useful to construct cumulative frequency distributions, which when shown graphically are called *ogives*. The frequencies of a frequency distribution may be cumulated from either end of the distribution, and Table 3.4 shows the results of cumulating the frequencies of Table 3.1. Table 3.4 enables us to ascertain the number of young women who had any specified cell volume or more and any specified cell volume or less. Usually one of the cumulative distributions is of more interest than the other; if so, only that one would be given, not both. When the data of Table 3.4 are shown graphically by means of curves, we

TABLE 3.4

CUMULATIVE DISTRIBUTIONS OF VOLUME OF CELLS, IN CUBIC CENTIMETERS PER HUNDRED CUBIC CENTIMETERS OF BLOOD, FOR 100 NORMAL YOUNG WOMEN

Volume of cells	Number of women having indicated cell volume	
	Or more	Or less
35.0	100	0
36.5	95.5	4.5
38.0	88	12
39.5	76	24
41.0	52.5	47.5
42.5	24.5	75.5
44.0	11.5	88.5
45.5	2	98
47.0	0	100

obtain the two ogives of Chart 3.8. Note that, in drawing these curves, the cumulative frequencies are plotted at the class limits shown in Table 3.4, not at the mid-values of Table 3.1. In addition to providing a pictorial representation of a cumulative frequency distribution, an ogive allows us to make, by graphic approximation, an arithmetic interpolation for values not shown in the cumulative distribution. By way of illustration, it is shown in Chart 3.8 that about 68 normal young women could be assumed to have had 40 c.c. or more of cells per 100 c.c. of blood. This was accomplished by drawing a line perpendicular to the horizontal axis at 40 c.c. and extending this line until it intersected the "or more" curve.

CHAP. 3] THE FREQUENCY DISTRIBUTION 53

At the point of intersection a line was drawn perpendicular to the vertical axis until it intersected the vertical axis. At this point of intersection the frequency is seen to be 68.

Graphic comparison of frequency distributions. For purposes of comparison, two frequency curves may be drawn on the same chart,

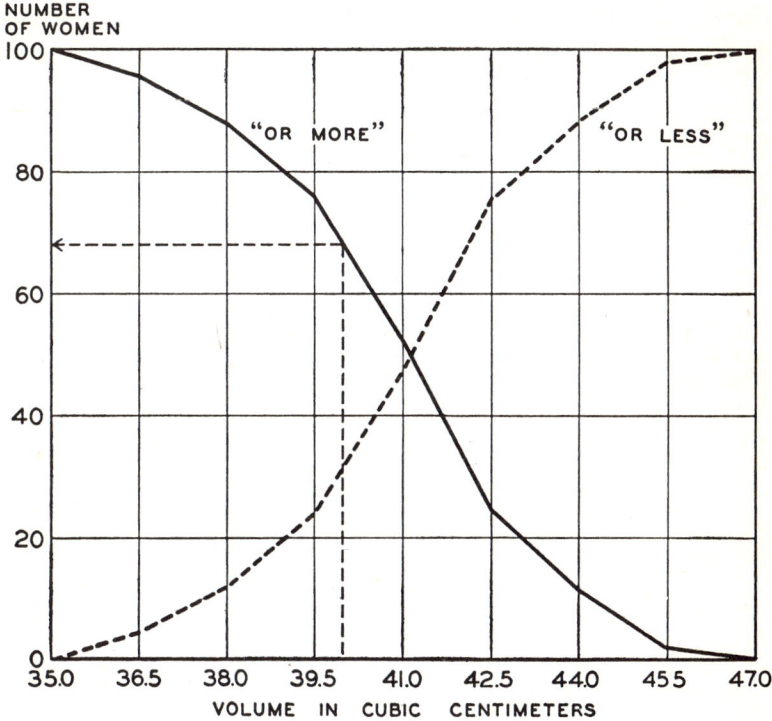

Chart 3.8. Cumulative Distributions of Volume of Cells, in Cubic Centimeters per Hundred Cubic Centimeters of Blood, for 100 Normal Young Women. Data of Table 3.4.

but difficulty arises when the two series consist of markedly different numbers of items. Chart 3.9 shows frequency distributions of the blood pressure of 2,565 male industrial workers aged 30–39 and of 734 male industrial workers aged 50–59, based on the data of Table 3.5. Comparison of these two curves is difficult because one has a much larger area than the other. If we compute percentage frequencies, which are shown in Table 3.6, and then draw

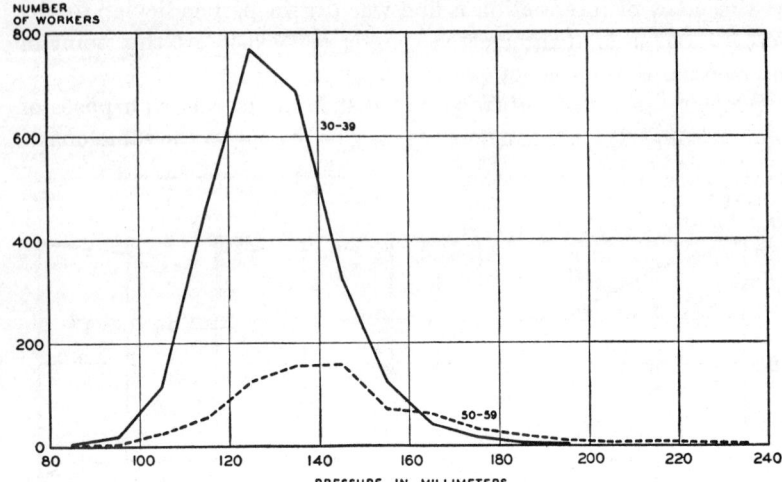

Chart 3.9. Systolic Blood Pressure, in Millimeters of Mercury, for 2,565 Male Industrial Workers 30-39 Years of Age and for 734 Male Industrial Workers 50-59 Years of Age. Data from Table 3.5.

TABLE 3.5

Distribution of Systolic Blood Pressures, in Millimeters of Mercury, of Male Industrial Workers 30-39 and 50-59 Years of Age

Blood pressure	Number of workers	
	30-39 years of age	50-59 years of age
Less than 90	3	1
90- 99	18	2
100-109	117	24
110-119	461	56
120-129	767	127
130-139	688	156
140-149	323	158
150-159	123	71
160-169	43	62
170-179	16	32
180-189	4	21
190-199	2	10
200-209		4
210-219		6
220-229		3
230-239		1
Total	2,565	734

Data from R. H. Britten and L. R. Thompson, *A Health Study of Ten Thousand Male Industrial Workers*, Public Health Bulletin No. 162, p. 155.

THE FREQUENCY DISTRIBUTION

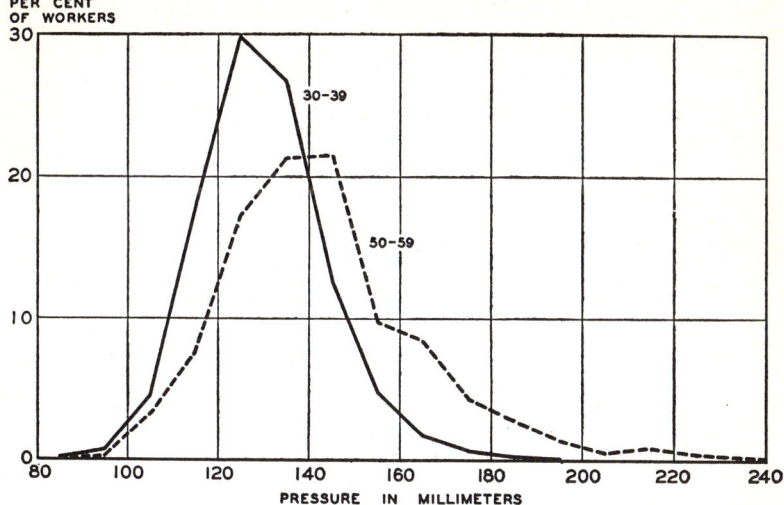

Chart 3.10. Percentage Distributions of Systolic Blood Pressure, in Millimeters of Mercury, for 2,565 Male Industrial Workers 30–39 Years of Age and 734 Male Industrial Workers 50–59 Years of Age. Data from Table 3.6.

TABLE 3.6

Percentage Distribution of Systolic Blood Pressures, in Millimeters of Mercury, of Male Industrial Workers 30–39 and 50–59 Years of Age

Blood pressure	Per cent of workers	
	30–39 years of age	50–59 years of age
Less than 90	0.1	0.1
90– 99	.7	.3
100–109	4.6	3.3
110–119	18.0	7.6
120–129	29.9	17.3
130–139	26.8	21.3
140–149	12.6	21.5
150–159	4.8	9.7
160–169	1.7	8.4
170–179	.6	4.4
180–189	.2	2.9
190–199	.1	1.4
200–209		.5
210–219		.8
220–229		.4
230–239		.1
Total	100.0	100.0

Data from R. H. Britten and L. R. Thompson, *A Health Study of Ten Thousand Male Industrial Workers*, Public Health Bulletin No. 162, p. 155.

the two curves as in Chart 3.10, the difficulty is resolved and it is easy to see the relative number in the two age groups for any specified pressure.

In the event that ogives based on different numbers of items are to be compared, the cumulative frequencies should similarly be put into percentage form before the curves are drawn.

Symbols Used in

CHAPTER 4

d: deviation of an X value from $\overline{X}_d$.

d': deviation, in terms of class intervals, of an X value from $\overline{X}_d$.

$D_1, D_2, \cdots, D_9$: the deciles.

Δ_1: upper-case Greek delta, the difference between the frequency of the modal class and the frequency of the class graphically to the left of the modal class.

Δ_2: upper-case Greek delta, the difference between the frequency of the modal class and the frequency of the class graphically to the right of the modal class.

f: a frequency.

$f_1, f_2, f_3, \cdots$: the frequencies associated with $X_1, X_2, X_3, \cdots$.

G: the geometric mean.

H: the harmonic mean.

i: the class interval.

l_1: the lower limit of a class.

l_2: the upper limit of a class.

Med: the median.

Mo: the mode.

N: the number of items in a sample. In a frequency distribution, $N = \Sigma f$. In later chapters, where two or more samples are under consideration, the number of items in the samples will be designated $N_1, N_2, N_3, \cdots$ and $N = N_1 + N_2 + N_3 + \cdots$.

$P_1, P_2, \cdots, P_{99}$: the percentiles.

Q_1, Q_2, Q_3: the quartiles. $Q_2 = $ Med.

Qu_1, Qu_2, Qu_3, Qu_4: the quintiles.

Σ: upper-case Greek sigma, meaning "take the sum of."

Σ_1: when used in conjunction with f, $\Sigma_1 f$, the sum of the frequencies in the classes graphically to the left of l_1.

Σ_2: when used in conjunction with f, $\Sigma_2 f$, the sum of the frequencies in the classes graphically to the right of l_2.

$x_1, x_2, x_3, \cdots$: deviations of $X_1, X_2, X_3, \cdots$ from $\overline{X}$.

X: a value in a series; also, the mid-value of a class in a frequency distribution.

SYMBOLS USED IN CHAPTER 4

$X_1, X_2, X_3, \cdots$: the values in a series; also, the mid-values of the classes of a frequency distribution.

$\overline{X}_d$: a designated mean used as a first approximation to facilitate the computation of $\overline{X}$ of a frequency distribution.

$\overline{X}$: the arithmetic mean. In later chapters, we shall distinguish between the arithmetic mean of a sample, $\overline{X}$, and the arithmetic mean of the population, $\overline{X}_\wp$.

$|\ |$: disregard signs; thus, $\Sigma|x|$ means "take the sum of the x values without regard to signs."

Chapter 4
MEASURES OF CENTRAL TENDENCY

A glance at the curves of Charts 3.2, 3.4, 3.5, and 3.6 will reveal that the items exhibit a "central tendency." There are various ways in which this tendency may be measured. This chapter will concern itself with the more important measures of central tendency: the arithmetic mean, the median, and the mode. Brief mention will be made of other measures of central tendency. The measures which we shall examine will be useful to describe not only distributions of the type pictured in Charts 3.2, 3.4, 3.5, and 3.6, but also distributions such as that of Chart 3.7, although one of the measures of central tendency (the mode) will not actually be centrally located for such a series.

In Chapter 5 we shall consider other aspects of frequency distributions: (1) dispersion, which refers to the extent to which the values of a series differ from each other; (2) skewness, departure from symmetry; and (3) kurtosis, the "peakedness" of a series.

The Arithmetic Mean

Ungrouped data. The arithmetic mean is so well known that it is not unusual for it to be referred to as "the average" or "the mean," and many laymen are aware of no other measure of central tendency. When various means, such as the arithmetic mean, the geometric mean, the harmonic mean, and others are under consideration, it is, of course, important to specify the mean to which one is referring in order to avoid confusion.

The arithmetic mean of a series is obtained by adding the values of the items and dividing by the number of items. Thus, if five figures of the volume of cells in the blood of normal young women are, respectively, 38.8, 39.6, 40.9, 42.0, and 44.2 c.c. per 100 c.c. of blood, the arithmetic mean would be

$$\frac{38.8 + 39.6 + 40.9 + 42.0 + 44.2}{5} = \frac{205.5}{5} = 41.1 \text{ c.c.}$$

If we use $\bar{X}$ to represent the arithmetic mean, N the number of items, and X_1, X_2, X_3, X_4, and so forth, to indicate the values of the various items, we may write, for any number of items,

$$\bar{X} = \frac{X_1 + X_2 + X_3 + X_4 + \cdots}{N}.$$

Or, using the symbol Σ, which means "take the sum of," we have

$$\bar{X} = \frac{\Sigma X}{N}.$$

In the foregoing illustration, each figure of cell volume occurred but once. If one or more of the values had occurred more than once, that would, of course, be taken into consideration. Suppose that the five values listed before had each occurred 1, 2, 3, 2, and 1 times, respectively. We should then compute

$$\bar{X} = \frac{(1 \times 38.8) + (2 \times 39.6) + (3 \times 40.9) + (2 \times 42.0) + (1 \times 44.2)}{1 + 2 + 3 + 2 + 1},$$

$$= \frac{368.9}{9} = 41.0 \text{ c.c.}$$

Using f_1, f_2, f_3, f_4, and so forth, to indicate the frequency of occurrence of each value, the symbolic expression would be

$$\bar{X} = \frac{f_1 X_1 + f_2 X_2 + f_3 X_3 + f_4 X_4 + \cdots}{f_1 + f_2 + f_3 + f_4 + \cdots} = \frac{\Sigma f X}{\Sigma f} = \frac{\Sigma f X}{N}.$$

There are two properties of the arithmetic mean that are of interest to us. The first is that the algebraic sum of the deviations of the various values from the arithmetic mean equals zero. The second is that the sum of the *squares* of the deviations of the values from the arithmetic mean is less than the sum of the squares of the deviations around any other value. More briefly, we say that the sum of the squares of the deviations around $\bar{X}$ is a minimum. If we use $x_1 = X_1 - \bar{X}$, $x_2 = X_2 - \bar{X}$, $x_3 = X_3 - \bar{X}$, $x_4 = X_4 - \bar{X}$, and so forth, we have

$$\Sigma x = 0$$

and

$$\Sigma x^2 = \text{a minimum}.$$

Because $\Sigma x = 0$, we can devise a short method for computing $\bar{X}$

MEASURES OF CENTRAL TENDENCY

from a frequency distribution. The fact that Σx^2 is a minimum will be referred to again in Chapter 5.

As an illustration[1] of the fact that $\Sigma x = 0$, consider the five figures of cell volume for which $\bar{X} = 41.1$ c.c.

X	$x = X - \bar{X}$
38.8	−2.3
39.6	−1.5
40.9	− .2
42.0	+ .9
44.2	+3.1
	0

Now, if we take the deviations (d) from some value *other than* $\bar{X}$, say from 40.9 c.c., we have

X	d
38.8	−2.1
39.6	−1.3
40.9	0
42.0	+1.1
44.2	+3.3
	1.0

Grouped data. If we were working with the 100 original readings of volume of cells in the blood of 100 normal young women shown in Tables 3.2 and 3.3, we would compute the value of the arithmetic mean by adding the 100 values and dividing by 100. This would give us

$$\bar{X} = \frac{4{,}103.1}{100} = 41.0 \text{ c.c.}$$

When the data are in the form of a frequency distribution, as in Table 3.1 or Table 4.1, it is not possible to determine the arithmetic mean in this manner, and we must take the mid-value of each class as representative of the class, multiply each mid-value by the

---

[1] To prove that $\Sigma x = 0$ for any set of values, we write

$$\Sigma x = \Sigma(X - \bar{X}),$$
$$= \Sigma X - N\bar{X}.$$

Now, $\bar{X} = \dfrac{\Sigma X}{N},$ and therefore $\Sigma X = N\bar{X}.$

Substituting,

$$\Sigma x = \Sigma X - \Sigma X = 0.$$

appropriate frequency (f), add the products, and divide by N. That is to say, we use the expression previously given

$$\bar{X} = \frac{\Sigma fX}{N}.$$

The computation of $\bar{X}$ for the cell volume data is shown in Table 4.1, where it is seen that $\bar{X} = 41.0$ c.c., the same as obtained for

TABLE 4.1

COMPUTATION OF THE ARITHMETIC MEAN OF THE FREQUENCY DISTRIBUTION OF VOLUME OF CELLS IN THE BLOOD OF 100 NORMAL YOUNG WOMEN BY USE OF THE EXPRESSION

$$\bar{X} = \frac{\Sigma fX}{N}$$

Volume of cells in cubic centimeters	Number of women f	Mid-value of class X	fX
35.0–36.5	4.5	35.75	160.875
36.5–38.0	7.5	37.25	279.375
38.0–39.5	12	38.75	465.000
39.5–41.0	23.5	40.25	945.875
41.0–42.5	28	41.75	1,169.000
42.5–44.0	13	43.25	562.250
44.0–45.5	9.5	44.75	425.125
45.5–47.0	2	46.25	92.500
Total	100	...	4,100.000

$$\bar{X} = \frac{\Sigma fX}{N} = \frac{4,100.000}{100} = 41.0 \text{ c.c.}$$

the 100 individual values. The agreement between these two figures indicates that *in general* the mid-values adequately represented the classes; if one or more of the mid-values were incorrect, there was a balancing by others which were off in the opposite direction. This may be seen more clearly in Table 4.2, where the mid-value of each class is compared with the arithmetic mean of the values in that class. Here it appears that the mid-value exceeds the mean of the class for four of the classes, while the reverse is true for the other four classes.

The agreement between the arithmetic mean for ungrouped data and the arithmetic mean for the same data when in frequency-distribution form will not always be as close as in our illustration. However, for series of the sort shown in Charts 3.2, 3.4, 3.5, and

TABLE 4.2

COMPARISON OF CLASS MID-VALUES AND CLASS MEANS FOR THE FREQUENCY DISTRIBUTION OF VOLUME OF CELLS IN THE BLOOD OF 100 NORMAL YOUNG WOMEN

Volume of cells in cubic centimeters	Mid-value of class	Computation of arithmetic mean for each class		
		Total of values in each class	Number of women	Arithmetic mean
35.0–36.5	35.75	160.45	4.5	35.66
36.5–38.0	37.25	279.85	7.5	37.31
38.0–39.5	38.75	167.60	12	38.97
39.5–41.0	40.25	947.20	23.5	40.31
41.0–42.5	41.75	1,169.55	28	41.77
42.5–44.0	43.25	561.85	13	43.22
44.0–45.5	44.75	424.40	9.5	44.67
45.5–47.0	46.25	92.20	2	46.10
Total	...	4,103.10	100	41.03

3.6, we can expect a negligible error in the arithmetic mean because of grouping. This is important, since one does not often have available the raw data from which a frequency distribution has been made.

The fact that $\Sigma x = 0$ enables us to compute $\bar{X}$ for a frequency distribution by a method which is shorter than that used in Table 4.1. We shall designate a convenient value (the mid-value of any class) as an approximation of $\bar{X}$, calling it $\bar{X}_d$, "the designated mean," ascertain how much $\bar{X}_d$ is incorrect, and thus obtain $\bar{X}$. Before proceeding to compute $\bar{X}$ by this method for the data of cell volume, let us refer to page 61, where the deviations of the five cell-volume figures were taken from 40.9 c.c. The five d values were -2.1, -1.3, 0, $+1.1$, and $+3.3$ c.c. Their total, Σd, is $+1.0$ c.c. On the average, then, these five d values were too large by

$$\frac{\Sigma d}{N} = \frac{+1.0}{5} = +0.2 \text{ cc.}$$

If $\dfrac{\Sigma d}{N}$ is added algebraically to $\bar{X}_d = 40.9$ c.c., we have $40.9 + 0.2 = 41.1$ c.c., which is $\bar{X}$ for the five items. What we have done may be stated symbolically

$$\bar{X} = \bar{X}_d + \frac{\Sigma d}{N}.$$

We shall use this procedure to compute $\bar{X}$ for the frequency distribution of volume of cells, but first we shall introduce the symbol f because frequencies are present. The expression now is

$$\bar{X} = \bar{X}_d + \frac{\Sigma fd}{N},$$

and the value of $\bar{X}$ is computed in Table 4.3. It is, of course, 41.0 c.c., the same as obtained in Table 4.1.

TABLE 4.3

COMPUTATION OF THE ARITHMETIC MEAN OF THE FREQUENCY DISTRIBUTION OF VOLUME OF CELLS IN THE BLOOD OF 100 NORMAL YOUNG WOMEN BY USE OF THE EXPRESSION

$$\bar{X} = \bar{X}_d + \frac{\Sigma fd}{N}$$

Volume of cells in cubic centimeters	Number of women f	d	fd	
35.0–36.5	4.5	−4.5	−20.25	
36.5–38.0	7.5	−3.0	−22.50	
38.0–39.5	12	−1.5	−18.00	− 60.75
39.5–41.0	23.5	0		
41.0–42.5	28	+1.5	+42.00	
42.5–44.0	13	+3.0	+39.00	
44.0–45.5	9.5	+4.5	+42.75	
45.5–47.0	2	+6.0	+12.00	+135.75
Total	100	...	...	+ 75.00

$$\bar{X} = \bar{X}_d + \frac{\Sigma fd}{N} = 40.25 + \frac{75.00}{100},$$
$$= 40.25 + 0.75,$$
$$= 41.0 \text{ c.c.}$$

The d values in Table 4.3 are −4.5, −3.0, −1.5, 0, +1.5, +3.0, +4.5, and +6.0 c.c. We can further simplify our work by expressing these values in terms of class intervals, and this has been done in Table 4.4. Actually, what we have done is to divide each of the d values in Table 4.3 by 1.5 c.c., the class interval. Our formula now becomes

$$\bar{X} = \bar{X}_d + \frac{\Sigma fd'}{N} i,$$

where d' indicates that the deviations from $\bar{X}_d$ are in terms of classes, and i is the class interval. The computation of $\bar{X} = 41.0$ c.c. is performed in Table 4.4, and it is clear that this is a quicker method of obtaining $\bar{X}$ than either that of Table 4.1 or that of Table 4.3.

TABLE 4.4

Computation of the Arithmetic Mean of the Frequency Distribution of Volume of Cells in the Blood of 100 Normal Young Women by Use of the Expression

$$\bar{X} = \bar{X}_d + \frac{\Sigma fd'}{N} i$$

Volume of cells in cubic centimeters	Number of women f	d'	fd'	
35.0–36.5	4.5	−3	−13.5	
36.5–38.0	7.5	−2	−15.0	
38.0–39.5	12	−1	−12.0	−40.5
39.5–41.0	23.5	0		
41.0–42.5	28	+1	+28.0	
42.5–44.0	13	+2	+26.0	
44.0–45.5	9.5	+3	+28.5	
45.5–47.0	2	+4	+ 8.0	+90.5
Total	100	...	...	+50.0

$$\bar{X} = \bar{X}_d + \frac{\Sigma fd'}{N} i = 40.25 + \frac{50}{100} 1.5,$$
$$= 40.25 + 0.75,$$
$$= 41.0 \text{ c.c.}$$

The procedure shown in Table 4.4 for obtaining $\bar{X}$ is useful only when the class intervals are uniform throughout a distribution, and this is usually, although by no means always, true. When the class intervals vary, use may be made of either

$$\bar{X} = \frac{\Sigma fX}{N}$$

or

$$\bar{X} = \bar{X}_d + \frac{\Sigma fd}{N}.$$

Averaging percentages or averages. Two groups of laboratory animals received injections of a drug. In one group of 200 animals 50, or 25 per cent, died; in the other group of 150 animals 45, or 30 per cent, died. If we were to average the two percentages, ignoring the sizes of the two groups, we should obtain

$$\frac{0.25 + 0.30}{2} = \frac{0.55}{2} = 0.275, \text{ or } 27.5 \text{ per cent.}$$

If the two groups are of more or less the same importance, this procedure would be valid. On the other hand, if the two groups are not of the same importance, we should use appropriate weights, which might be the numbers in our two samples or might be proportional to the numbers of the two types of animals believed to exist in the entire population. If we used the numbers in the two groups as weights, the combined percentage would be

$$\frac{(0.25 \times 200) + (0.30 \times 150)}{200 + 150} = \frac{50 + 45}{350} = \frac{95}{350}$$
$$= 0.271, \text{ or } 27.1 \text{ per cent,}$$

or, using the numbers dying instead of weighting the percentages,

$$\frac{50 + 45}{350} = \frac{95}{350} = 0.271, \text{ or } 27.1 \text{ per cent.}$$

The problem of averaging two or more averages is essentially the same as that of averaging percentages. If the groups being combined are of varying importance, weights should be used; if the groups do not differ in importance, or if a difference in importance exists but is not relevant[2] to our problem, the averages may be combined with equal weights.

Neither percentages nor averages of different groups should be combined, unless the groups are of such a nature that combining them is meaningful. To take a somewhat far-fetched illustration, it would be meaningless to combine the average weights of a group of native-white males 30 years of age and of a group of native-white male babies at birth.

The Median

Ungrouped data. The median is usually defined as that *value* which divides a distribution so that an equal number of items occurs

---

[2] Testing the significance of the difference between the averages of two samples is discussed in Chapter 9. The significance of the difference between two percentages is considered in Chapter 10.

on either side of it. Thus, for the five figures of cell volume used previously: 38.8, 39.6, 40.9, 42.0, and 44.2 c.c., the median is 40.9 c.c. Two items have values less than 40.9 c.c. and two exceed 40.9 c.c. If, now, we have six figures instead of 5, say six systolic blood pressure readings, 122, 124, 125, 127, 129, and 131 m.m. of mercury, the median could be any value greater than 125 but less than 127 m.m. In such a situation, the median is usually stated as the average of the two middle values, in this case 126 m.m.

If we undertake to ascertain the median for a series of values such as 124, 125, 126, 127, 127, 127, 129, and 130 m.m., we are unable to find a value which will divide the series so that 4 items are less than it and 4 items are greater. The value 127 m.m. would be designated the median, but three values are less than 127 m.m. while only two values are greater. The difficulty is that the definition given at the outset is not exact enough to cover a situation such as this, so we rephrase the definition to read: *the median is that value which divides a series so that one-half or more of the items are equal to or less than it and one-half or more of the items are equal to or greater than it.*

It is perhaps obvious that the median cannot be determined for ungrouped data which are not arrayed. For example, the median cannot be ascertained from the cell-volume data of Table 3.2. When these same data are arrayed in Table 3.3, it is readily seen that the median is 41.2 c.c. Actually, it is not necessary to array all of the items in such a series; it is merely necessary to array a few items at the middle and then to know how many are smaller and how many are larger.

Grouped data. To determine the median for the cell-volume data given in frequency-distribution form in Table 4.1, we ascertain $\frac{N}{2}$ and, working from either end of the distribution, interpolate to determine the value at this point. Proceeding from smaller to larger values, as is usually done, the expression is

$$\text{Med} = l_1 + \frac{\frac{N}{2} - \Sigma_1 f}{f_{\text{med}}} i,$$

where l_1 is the lower limit of the class in which the median falls, $\Sigma_1 f$ is the sum of the frequencies in the classes below l_1, and f_{med} is the frequency of the class in which the median falls. For the data of cell volume,

$$\text{Med} = 41.0 + \frac{\frac{100}{2} - 47.5}{28} 1.5,$$

$$= 41.0 + \frac{2.5}{28} 1.5 = 41.1 \text{ c.c.}$$

Note that this value agrees very closely with that just obtained from the array.

When proceeding in reverse fashion, from larger to smaller values, the expression for the median is

$$\text{Med} = l_2 - \frac{\frac{N}{2} - \Sigma_2 f}{f_{\text{med}}} i,$$

where l_2 is the upper limit of the class in which the median falls and $\Sigma_2 f$ is the sum of the frequencies in the classes above l_2. For our data,

$$\text{Med} = 42.5 - \frac{\frac{100}{2} - 24.5}{28} 1.5 = 41.1 \text{ c.c.}$$

The median may be located graphically from an ogive by drawing a perpendicular to the vertical axis at $\frac{N}{2}$ and extending this line until it intersects the ogive. From this point of intersection a perpendicular is drawn to the horizontal axis until it intersects, giving the median. This procedure is illustrated in Chart 4.1, which gives 41.1 c.c. (the same value as that obtained arithmetically) as the median for the data of volume of cells. Either ogive may be used, and reference to Chart 3.8 will reveal that, when both ogives are drawn on one chart, they intersect at $\frac{N}{2}$ on the vertical axis and at the median on the horizontal axis.

Related measures. Although they are not measures of central tendency, there are certain other measures which are akin to the median in that they, too, are "position measures." It is for that reason that the quartiles, quintiles, deciles, and percentiles are briefly mentioned at this point.

There are three quartiles, Q_1, Q_2, and Q_3, which divide a distribution into four equal parts. Q_1 is the quartile of lowest value, Q_2 is the median, and Q_3 is the quartile of highest value. There are four quintiles (Qu_1, Qu_2, Qu_3, and Qu_4), which divide a distribution into five equal parts, nine deciles (D_1, D_2, $\cdots$, D_9), which divide a distribution into 10 equal parts, and ninety-nine percentiles (P_1,

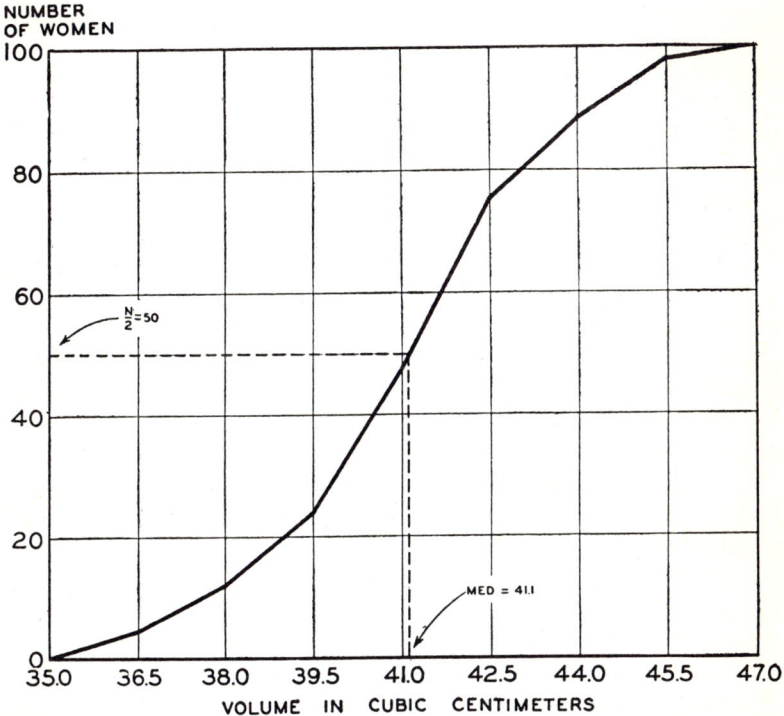

Chart 4.1. Graphic Determination of the Value of the Median for the Data of Table 4.4. The cumulative frequencies are from Table 3.4.

P_2, $\cdots$, P_{99}), which divide a distribution into one hundred equal parts. Other similar measures could be set up to divide a distribution into any desired number of parts, but position measures, other than those listed, are rarely used.

The procedure for determining the values of the quartiles, quintiles, deciles, and percentiles is similar to that for computing the median. Starting from the lower-valued end of a series, we would make interpolations for the quartiles Q_1, Q_2, and Q_3 at $\frac{N}{4}$, $\frac{2N}{4} = \frac{N}{2}$, and $\frac{3N}{4}$; for the quintiles Qu_1, Qu_2, Qu_3, and Qu_4 we would interpolate at $\frac{N}{5}$, $\frac{2N}{5}$, $\frac{3N}{5}$, and $\frac{4N}{5}$; for the deciles D_1, D_2, $\cdots$, and D_9 we would interpolate at $\frac{N}{10}$, $\frac{2N}{10} = \frac{N}{5}$, $\cdots$, and $\frac{9N}{10}$; for the percentiles P_1, P_2, $\cdots$, and P_{99} we would interpolate at $\frac{N}{100}$, $\frac{2N}{100} = \frac{N}{50}$, $\cdots$, and $\frac{99N}{100}$.

It should be fairly obvious that not all of the percentiles would be computed for even a very extensive distribution. However, use is frequently made of P_5, P_{10}, P_{15}, $\cdots$, P_{90}, and P_{95}, as well as of P_1, P_2, P_{98}, P_{99}, and some others, although not all of these would be likely to be determined for a single series.

A clear distinction should be made between the *value of a position measure* and the *portion of a distribution in which an item falls*. For example, Qu_1, Qu_2, Qu_3, and Qu_4 each has a specific value for a given set of data and they divide the series into five equal portions. The term "quintile" is sometimes misused, as when it is stated that a student's grade is "in the highest quintile." What is meant is that the grade is *in the portion of the distribution above* Qu_4. It would be much better if the five portions of a distribution which are separated by the quintiles were referred to as "lowest fifth," "next-to-lowest fifth," "middle fifth," "next-to-highest fifth," and "highest fifth." Similar misuses of quartiles, deciles, and percentiles occur; when a *portion* of a distribution is meant, it is desirable to say, respectively, "fourths," "tenths," and "hundredths." It is also not confusing to say "above the fourth quintile," "below the third decile," "between the second and ninety-eighth percentile," and so forth.

The Mode

Ungrouped data. *The mode of a series is the value around which the items tend to concentrate.* To use a very simple illustration: the values 123, 124, 125, 125, 126, and 127 mm. have as their mode

125 mm. For a series of values such as 122, 124, 126, 128, 130, and 132 mm., it is clear that there is no mode. For the more extensive array of Table 3.3, the mode is not immediately apparent. It will be necessary to group the data in order to ascertain the value around which the items tend to concentrate.

Grouped data. The data of volume of cells are in frequency-distribution form in Table 4.4, and from this table it may be seen that the modal group is 41.0–42.5 c.c. Where, between these limits, do the items tend to concentrate? One way of answering this question consists of fitting an appropriate curve to the series and determining the value on the horizontal scale which is directly below the peak of the fitted curve.[3] We shall use a simpler procedure, illustrated in Chart 4.2, which considers Δ_1, the difference between the frequency of the class to the left of the modal class (graphically) and the frequency of the modal class, as a force pulling upward from l_1, the lower limit of the modal class, and Δ_2, the difference between the frequency of the class to the right of the modal class and the frequency of the modal class, as a force pulling downward from l_2, the upper limit of the modal class. As explained below Chart 4.2, the formula for the mode (Mo) is

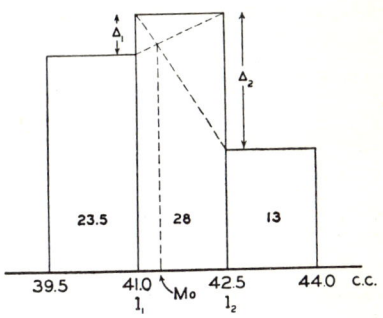

Chart 4.2. Determination of the Value of the Mode for the Data of Table 4.3. The value of the mode is located between l_1 and l_2 so that $\Delta_1:\Delta_2::\mathrm{Mo}-l_1:l_2-\mathrm{Mo}$. From this we write

$\Delta_2(\mathrm{Mo}-l_1) = \Delta_1(l_2-\mathrm{Mo})$,
$\Delta_1\mathrm{Mo} + \Delta_2\mathrm{Mo} = \Delta_2 l_1 + \Delta_1 l_2$.

Since $l_2 = l_1 + i$, we have

$\mathrm{Mo}(\Delta_1+\Delta_2) = \Delta_2 l_1 + \Delta_1 l_1 + \Delta_1 i$,

$$\mathrm{Mo} = \frac{l_1(\Delta_1+\Delta_2)}{\Delta_1+\Delta_2} + \frac{\Delta_1 i}{\Delta_1+\Delta_2},$$

$$= l_1 + \frac{\Delta_1}{\Delta_1+\Delta_2} i.$$

$$\mathrm{Mo} = l_1 + \frac{\Delta_1}{\Delta_1+\Delta_2} i.$$

---

[3] Three types of fitted curves are discussed in Chapter 8. Others are treated in F. E. Croxton and D. J. Cowden, *Applied General Statistics*, Prentice-Hall, Inc., New York, 1939, pp. 293–303.

For the data of Table 4.4, this gives

$$\text{Mo} = 41.0 + \frac{4.5}{4.5 + 15} \, 1.5,$$
$$= 41.0 + 0.3 = 41.3 \text{ c.c.}$$

The mode may also be obtained by using l_2 (the upper limit of the modal class) instead of l_1. Thus,

$$\text{Mo} = l_2 - \frac{\Delta_2}{\Delta_1 + \Delta_2} \, i,$$
$$= 42.5 - \frac{15}{4.5 + 15} \, 1.5,$$
$$= 42.5 - 1.2 = 41.3 \text{ c.c.}$$

Infrequently a distribution having two modes will occur. The curve of such a series would show two points of concentration, although they would not necessarily be of equal prominence. Usually, a bi-modal frequency distribution is the result of failure to separate two different groups, such as males and females, children and adults, or sick and healthy individuals. Bi-modality could also be present fortuitously.

Comparison of the Arithmetic Mean, the Median, and the Mode

Since the arithmetic mean, the median, and the mode are the most commonly used measures of central tendency, it is worth while pausing to compare their characteristics before we briefly consider some of the minor means. As previously mentioned, the arithmetic mean is the measure with which most people are already at least vaguely familiar. It is the most frequently used measure of central tendency and, as will be seen later, it is often used when it should not have been used, when the median or mode should have been employed instead.

The basic ideas. The three measures of central tendency embody completely different ideas. The arithmetic mean is the sum of the values divided by the number of items. The median is the value which divides a series so that one-half or more of the items are equal to or less than it and one-half or more of the items are equal to or greater than it. The mode is the value around which the items tend to concentrate. There is no "best measure of central tendency"; no one of these is the measure which should always be used under all conditions. The measure to use depends on the idea which one wishes to convey and on the nature of the data.

No matter what data we may be dealing with, an arithmetic mean may be computed. However, it may be meaningless. For the four figures 3, 5, 100, and 112 pounds, $\bar{X} = 55$ pounds, yet the figures are so divergent that $\bar{X}$ has no useful meaning. For these

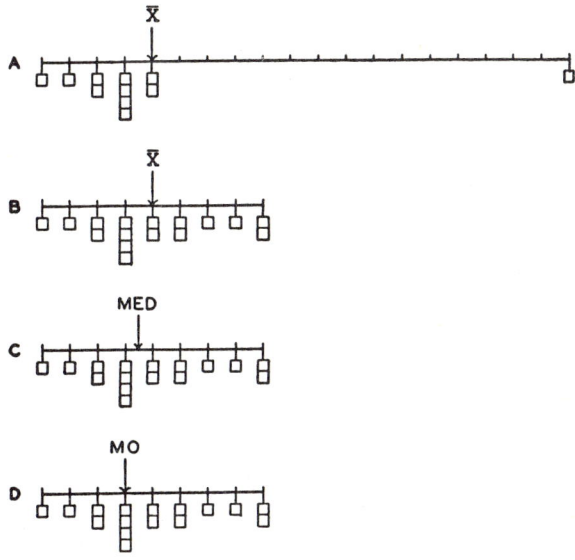

Chart 4.3. Diagrammatic Representation of the Arithmetic Mean, the Median, and the Mode. Arrangements A and B are different, but have the same $\bar{X}$ value. Sections B, C, and D involve the same arrangement but show, respectively, the location of the arithmetic mean, the median, and the mode. From F. E. Croxton and D. J. Cowden, *Practical Business Statistics*, 2nd ed., page 167, Prentice-Hall, Inc., New York, 1948.

same figures, a median of 52.5 pounds (or any figure greater than 5 but less than 100 pounds) could be computed, but it, too, would be useless. Of course, there is no mode, since each value occurred but once. A less bizarre illustration, such as 4, 5, 6, and 7 cm., would have a useful arithmetic mean or median, but no mode.

In the case of frequency distributions such as that of Chart 3.7 or the reverse of such a series, the mode is not a measure of *central* tendency, since it occurs at the end of the distribution.

The concept of the arithmetic mean is akin to the "center of mass" (often called "center of gravity") idea of physics, except that the arithmetic mean is concerned with variables in one dimension rather than three. Sections A and B of Chart 4.3 show two different sets of values having the same arithmetic mean. Note that the one value to the right of the arithmetic mean in Section A balances all of the eight values to the left of the arithmetic mean. The same eight values to the left of the arithmetic mean are repeated in Section B but are now balanced by six items to the right of the arithmetic mean. Sections B, C, and D of Chart 4.3 all show the same arrangement of values but indicate, respectively, the locations of the arithmetic mean, the median, and the mode. The median is seen to divide the series in equal parts; the mode is at the point of concentration.

Chart 4.4 shows the location of the three measures of central tendency in a frequency distribution which is skewed to the right. The arithmetic mean is still at the point where the values to the right of $\bar{X}$ balance the values to the left of $\bar{X}$, but this is not so easy to see as in Chart 4.3. An ordinate erected at the median divides the curve so that equal areas are on either side of that ordinate. The mode is below the peak of the curve.

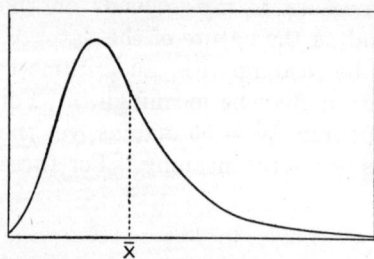

A. The values to the right of $\bar{X}$ balance the values to the left of $\bar{X}$.

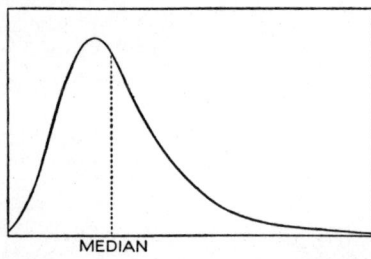

B. One half of the area under the curve is on each side of the ordinate erected at the median.

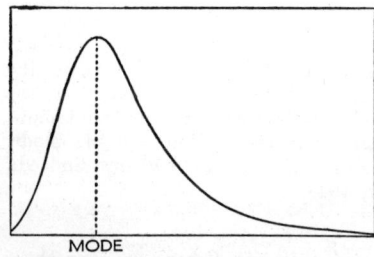

C. The mode is below the peak of the curve.

Chart 4.4. The Arithmetic Mean, the Median, and the Mode of a Frequency Distribution Skewed to the Right.

Effect of extreme values and of skewness. The presence of an extreme value (that is, a very large value or a very small value) in a series of data will have a pronounced effect upon $\overline{X}$, but will affect the median less, and the mode least of all, often having no effect on the mode. This is illustrated in Chart 4.5, Section A of which shows a series of 16 values having $\overline{X} = 4$ c.c., Med = 3.5 c.c., and Mo = 3 c.c. Section B shows the same 16 values plus an additional value much larger than any of the others. Now we have $\overline{X} = 5$ c.c., Med = 4 c.c., and Mo = 3 c.c. The arithmetic mean, because it is influenced by the magnitude of the added value, was increased from 4 to 5 c.c. If the added value in Section B were larger than 21 c.c., the arithmetic mean would be larger than 5 c.c.

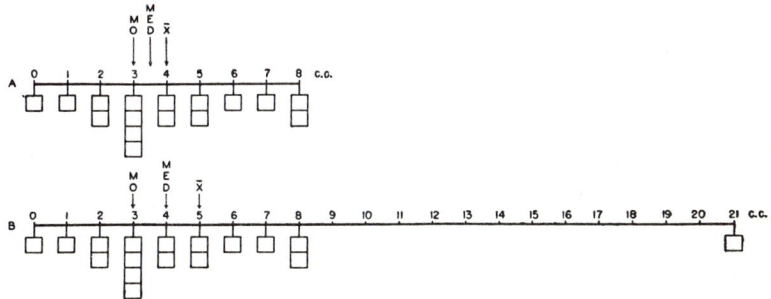

Chart 4.5. Diagram Illustrating the Effect Upon the Arithmetic Mean, the Median, and the Mode of the Addition of an Extremely Large Value.

The median, which is influenced by only the position of the added value, was slightly increased from 3.5 to 4 c.c. The added value could have been any other value, greater than 4, and the value of the median in Section B would still be 4 c.c. The value of the mode was unaffected by the presence of the extremely large value.

The presence of skewness in a frequency distribution brings about a somewhat similar situation. If a distribution is exactly symmetrical, the values of the arithmetic mean, the median, and the mode coincide. When skewness occurs, the arithmetic mean and the median are displaced from the mode toward the direction in which the curve is skewed. This displacement is greater for the arithmetic mean than for the median and is illustrated, for a series skewed to the right, in Chart 4.4. The data of volume of cells are slightly skewed to the left, and we previously computed $\overline{X} = 41.0$ c.c., Med = 41.1 c.c., and Mo = 41.3 c.c.

Because of the foregoing there are occasions when the arithmetic mean may convey a misleading impression. For example, a study was made of the incomes of a group of college graduates, and it was found that $\overline{X}$ = $13,958. This was the only figure that was released to the newspapers. The distribution of incomes was skewed to the right, and the arithmetic mean was also influenced by the presence in the distribution of several extremely large incomes. The median was $7,500, and the mode approximately $5,000. In situations such as this, it is desirable not to give the arithmetic mean alone, but to state also the value of the median and, possibly, the mode as well. Sometimes only the median is given.

Mathematical properties and algebraic treatment. It has already been mentioned that the sum of the deviations of a series of values from their arithmetic mean equals zero, $\Sigma x = 0$, and that the sum of the squared deviations of a series of values is a minimum when taken around their arithmetic mean: Σx^2 is a minimum. The first of these was useful in setting up a short method for the computation of $\overline{X}$ for a frequency distribution, the second will enable us to use short methods for computing the standard deviation (a measure of dispersion) of ungrouped data or of a frequency distribution in the following chapter. If the deviations of a series of values from their arithmetic mean are added without regard to sign, $\Sigma|x|$, the sum will not be a minimum. The sum of a series of deviations is a minimum when taken from the median of the values. As a result, the average deviation (another measure of dispersion) is sometimes computed in relation to the median instead of the arithmetic mean.

Since $\overline{X} = \dfrac{\Sigma X}{N}$, we may also write $\Sigma X = N\overline{X}$ and $N = \dfrac{\Sigma X}{\overline{X}}$. In other words, when any two of three terms (N, ΣX, and $\overline{X}$) are known, the third may be computed. No similar treatment is possible for the median or the mode.

It was previously noted that arithmetic means of two or more series may be averaged to produce one arithmetic mean for the combined series. This cannot be done with medians or modes.

Necessity for rearranging or classifying raw data. The arithmetic mean may be computed from raw data without any rearrangement. In the case of the volume of cell data, ΣX = 4,103.1 c.c. and $\overline{X}$ = 41.0 c.c., whether computed from Table 3.2 or from Table 3.3. The arithmetic mean may also be computed from a frequency distribution with little loss of accuracy. The median cannot be computed unless the raw data have been (at least partly) arrayed or put into frequency-distribution form. To ascertain the value of the mode, it is often necessary to construct a frequency distribution. This was true in the case of the data of volume of cells. Sometimes it is possible to determine the mode from an array (or partial array), but not from raw data.

Effect of extremes of unknown value. Grouped data (and, rarely, ungrouped data) may be encountered having items at either or both ends of a series but without a specific statement of the values of the items. For example, the frequency distribution of volume of cells shown in Table 4.4 might have an additional class "47.0 or more" in which there were two items. Unless we have some way of determining an appropriate mid-value for such a class, we cannot satisfactorily compute the value of the arithmetic mean. One solution is for the maker of such a frequency distribution to give, in a footnote below the table, either the arithmetic mean or the total value of the items in the "open-end" class. The presence of open-end classes does not cause any difficulty in the determination of the values of the median or the mode. If the mode occurred at one end of a series, as in Chart 3.7, there would not be an open-end class at that end of the series.

Open-end classes are present because the frequencies have become sparse. That situation occurs most frequently at the right (graphically) of a series skewed to the right and at the left (graphically) of a series skewed to the left. However, frequencies may become sparse at both ends of a series, resulting in the use of open-end classes at both ends of a series.

Effect of unequal class intervals. When a series is decidedly skewed, it is not unusual for a frequency distribution to be constructed with varying class intervals, the intervals being wider in the extended tail of the distribution. While the arithmetic mean may be computed for such a series, the offsetting of the errors which occur as a result of using the mid-values of the classes is not so closely realized as for a distribution which is more nearly symmetrical. The median may be determined without difficulty for a distribution having class intervals which vary. The mode may also be readily obtained provided the modal class and those on either side of it are the same width. This is usually the case.

Other Measures of Central Tendency

There are many other measures of central tendency, but only three more—the geometric mean, the harmonic mean, and the quadratic mean—will be briefly mentioned here.

The geometric mean is the Nth root of the product of the values. That is,

$$G = \sqrt[N]{X_1 \cdot X_2 \cdot X_3 \cdot X_4 \cdot \text{etc.}}$$

The logarithm of the geometric mean is the arithmetic mean of the logarithms of the values, or, in symbols,

$$\log G = \frac{\log X_1 + \log X_2 + \log X_3 + \log X_4 + \cdots}{N}.$$

For purposes of computation, we use

$$G = \text{antilog}\, \frac{\log X_1 + \log X_2 + \log X_3 + \log X_4 + \cdots}{N},$$

or, if the frequencies are present,

$$G = \text{antilog}\, \frac{f_1 \log X_1 + f_2 \log X_2 + f_3 \log X_3 + f_4 \log X_4 + \cdots}{N}.$$

The geometric mean of a series of values which are not all the same is smaller than the arithmetic mean. For example, the arithmetic mean of 5, 10, and 20 is $11\frac{2}{3}$, but

$$G = \sqrt[3]{5 \cdot 10 \cdot 20} = \sqrt[3]{1{,}000} = 10.$$

The geometric mean embodies a basic concept different from that of the arithmetic mean. In the case of the arithmetic mean, series which have the same number of items and the same total have the same arithmetic mean. On the other hand, series having the same number of items and the same product have the same geometric mean. To take a very simple illustration: the two values 4 and 12 total 16 and have an arithmetic mean of 8; the two values 6 and 10 have the same total and the same arithmetic mean. Consider, now, the two values 2 and 18, which have 36 as their product and 6 as their geometric mean. Also, 3 and 12 have the same product and the same geometric mean.

There are other characteristics of the geometric mean which might be discussed, but, since most of the applications of the geometric mean are in non-medical fields, a further treatment is not warranted here.[4]

The harmonic mean is the reciprocal of the arithmetic mean of the reciprocals of a series of values, that is,

$$H = \frac{1}{\left(\dfrac{1}{X_1} + \dfrac{1}{X_2} + \dfrac{1}{X_3} + \dfrac{1}{X_4} + \cdots\right) \div N}$$

or,

$$H = \frac{N}{\dfrac{1}{X_1} + \dfrac{1}{X_2} + \dfrac{1}{X_3} + \dfrac{1}{X_4} + \cdots}.$$

For a detailed discussion of this measure, the reader is referred to pages 226–232 of the publication mentioned in footnote 4.

The quadratic mean is the square root of the arithmetic mean of the squares of the values. Symbolically it is

$$\sqrt{\frac{X_1^2 + X_2^2 + X_3^2 + X_4^2 + \cdots}{N}}.$$

Very little use is made of this measure, but the quadratic mean of the *deviations* of values from their arithmetic mean

$$\sqrt{\frac{x_1^2 + x_2^2 + x_3^2 + x_4^2 + \cdots}{N}}$$

will be used in the following chapter as a measure of dispersion and is called the *standard deviation*.

---

[4] For a more detailed discussion, together with a consideration of the applications of the geometric mean, see F. E. Croxton and D. J. Cowden, *Applied General Statistics*, Prentice-Hall, Inc., New York, 1939, pp. 176–180.

Symbols Used in
CHAPTER 5

A.D.: the average (or mean) deviation.

β_1: lower-case Greek beta, a measure of skewness using the third powers of the x values.

β_2: lower-case Greek beta, a measure of kurtosis using the fourth powers of the x values.

d': deviation, in terms of class intervals, of an X value from $\bar{X}_d$.

f: a frequency.

i: the class interval.

Med: the median.

Mo: the mode.

$\mu_1, \mu_2, \mu_3, \mu_4$: lower-case Greek mu, respectively, the first, second, third, and fourth moments about $\bar{X}$, with Sheppard's corrections. $\mu_1 = \pi_1 = 0$ and $\mu_3 = \pi_3$.

N: the number of items in a sample.

$\nu_1, \nu_2, \nu_3, \nu_4$: lower-case Greek nu, respectively, the first, second, third, and fourth moments about $\bar{X}_d$.

$P_1, P_2, \cdots, P_{99}$: the percentiles.

$\pi_1, \pi_2, \pi_3, \pi_4$: lower-case Greek pi, respectively, the first, second, third, and fourth moments about $\bar{X}$. $\pi_1 = 0$.

Q: the semi-interquartile range.

Q_1, Q_2, Q_3: the quartiles. $Q_2 =$ Med.

s: the standard deviation of a sample.

s^2: the variance of a sample.

s_{cor}: the standard deviation of a sample, with Sheppard's correction.

Sk: the Pearsonian measure of skewness.

Sk_Q: a measure of skewness based on the quartiles.

$\hat{\sigma}$: lower-case Greek sigma, "sigma caret" or "sigma hat," estimate of the standard deviation of a population.

σ: lower-case Greek sigma, the standard deviation of a population.

Σ: upper-case Greek sigma, meaning "take the sum of."

V: the coefficient of variation.

x: deviation of X from $\bar{X}$.

X: a value in a series; also, the mid-value of a class in a frequency

SYMBOLS USED IN CHAPTER 5

distribution.

$\bar{X}$: the arithmetic mean. In later chapters we shall distinguish between the arithmetic mean of a sample, $\bar{X}$, and the arithmetic mean of the population, $\bar{X}_\mathcal{P}$.

$\bar{X}_d$: a designated mean.

$|\ \ |$: disregard signs; thus, $\Sigma|x|$ means "take the sum of the x values without regard to signs."

Chapter 5

DISPERSION, SKEWNESS, AND KURTOSIS

Dispersion

During January and May of 1943, slightly more than 88,000 white selectees were examined at induction centers for the United States Army. Some of these selectees were inducted into the Army, while some were rejected. The arithmetic mean of the weights of the men who were accepted was 151.0 pounds, while that of the men who were rejected was 150.2 pounds. Although there was not much difference between the two arithmetic means, the men who were rejected showed a larger proportion of very light and very heavy men than did the men who were accepted. In other words, the dispersion was greater for the rejected group than for the accepted group. A comparison limited only to the two arithmetic means would carry no hint of the fact that the two series differed in regard to dispersion.

The range. The simplest and sometimes the least satisfactory measure of dispersion is *the range*, which is the difference between the largest and smallest values of a series. For the frequency distribution of volume of cells (Table 5.3), the range is $47.0 - 35.0 = 12.0$ mm. When ungrouped but arrayed data are available, the range may be obtained more accurately. Referring to Table 3.3, the range for the ungrouped data of volume of cells is seen to be $46.3 - 35.2 = 11.1$ mm. When stating the value of a range, it is a good idea to give also the two values from which the range is obtained. This gives the reader additional useful information, since the range of 11.1 mm., just mentioned, could represent the difference between 35.2 and 46.3 mm., between 38.0 and 49.1 mm., or between many other possible pairs of values.

The simplicity of the range is at the same time its weakness. Being determined from the smallest and largest values in a series, the range fails to give any consideration to the arrangement of the

CHAP. 5] DISPERSION, SKEWNESS, AND KURTOSIS 83

values between the two extremes[1] and is obviously influenced by an extraordinarily large or an extraordinarily small value (or both), if such a value is present.

Measures of dispersion based on quartiles and percentiles. Any of the position measures mentioned in Chapter 4 might be used for obtaining a measure of dispersion. One such measure, employing the first and third quartiles, is known as Q, *the semi-interquartile range*, and

$$Q = \frac{Q_3 - Q_1}{2}.$$

For the data of volume of cells, shown in Table 5.3, we compute

$$Q_1 = 39.6 \text{ c.c.},$$
$$Q_3 = 42.5 \text{ c.c., and}$$
$$Q = \frac{42.5 - 39.6}{2} = 1.45 \text{ c.c.}$$

For a series that is symmetrical, it is clear that 50 per cent of the items occur between Med $\pm Q$, since Med $- Q = Q_1$ and Med $+ Q = Q_3$. When a series is not symmetrical, Med $- Q \neq Q_1$ and Med $+ Q \neq Q_3$, but Med $\pm Q$ will, nevertheless, include very nearly 50 per cent of the items, unless the series is markedly skewed or broken. For the data of Table 5.3,

$$\text{Med} \pm Q = 41.1 \pm 1.45 = 39.65 \text{ and } 42.55 \text{ cc.}$$

Between these two values we would expect to find $\frac{1.35}{1.5}$ of the 23.5 frequencies in the class 39.5–41.0 c.c., all of the 28 frequencies in the following class, and $\frac{0.05}{1.5}$ of the frequencies in the class 42.5 – 44.0 c.c. The total is 50.1 frequencies, or 50.1 per cent, since $N = 100$.

The semi-interquartile range is simple of concept and easy to compute, but it has a serious limitation: it is unaffected by the distribution of the values below Q_1, between Q_1 and Q_3, or above Q_3.

---

[1] This objection is of no weight when $N = 2$ and is of minor importance for very small samples drawn from a normal population.

To be more specific, the 25 values above Q_3 in Table 5.3 could be arranged in any fashion as long as they were all 42.5 c.c. or greater.

The 10–90 percentile range gives the limits between which the central 80 per cent of the values in a distribution occur. For the data of volume of cells,

$$P_{10} = 37.5 \text{ c.c.}$$

and

$$P_{90} = 44.2 \text{ c.c.}$$

A measure similar to Q could be computed from these two values, but it is more usual merely to state the values of P_{10} and P_{90}.

The average deviation. *The average deviation* or *the mean deviation* differs from the measures of dispersion previously mentioned in that it takes into consideration the values of all of the items in a distribution. It is computed from the expression

$$\text{A.D.} = \frac{\Sigma |x|}{N}$$

where | | means "without regard to sign." (It was pointed out in Chapter 4 that, if the deviations are added algebraically, the sum is zero; that is, $\Sigma x = 0$.) For a frequency distribution that is normal,[2] 57.5 per cent of the items are included within the limits of $\bar{X} \pm \text{A.D.}$

Since the average deviation is much less useful than the standard deviation, which also considers the values of all of the items in a distribution, we shall give no further attention to it but merely note that, since the sum of the deviations without regard to sign is a minimum around the median rather than around $\bar{X}$, the average deviation is sometimes computed around the median.

The standard deviation. All of the values of a series enter into the computation of the standard deviation. The deviation of each value from $\bar{X}$ is obtained and is then squared, so that all signs are positive. The squared deviations are then summed and divided by N, and the square root taken, giving the standard deviation, s. Symbolically,[3]

$$s = \sqrt{\frac{\Sigma x^2}{N}}.$$

---

[2] Chapter 8 discusses the normal curve.

[3] The square of the standard deviation, $s^2 = \dfrac{\Sigma x^2}{N}$, is referred to as the *variance*.

Before proceeding further, it may be well to point out that s measures the dispersion *in the sample*. At a later point (Chapter 9) we shall consider σ, the population standard deviation, and $\hat{\sigma}$, an estimate of the population standard deviation based upon a sample.

The standard deviation is not only a most useful measure of dispersion, but s, or some aspect of it, will be employed in connection with methods to be described later. To be specific: s or s^2 will be

TABLE 5.1

COMPUTATION OF THE STANDARD DEVIATION FOR DATA OF SYSTOLIC BLOOD PRESSURE, BEFORE EXERCISE, FOR 12 YOUNG MEN BY USE OF THE EXPRESSION

$$s = \sqrt{\frac{\Sigma x^2}{N}}$$

Pressure in millimeters of mercury	x	x^2
116	− 7.2	51.84
130	+ 6.8	46.24
126	+ 2.8	7.84
110	−13.2	174.24
114	− 9.2	84.64
142	+18.8	353.44
140	+16.8	282.24
132	+ 8.8	77.44
120	− 3.2	10.24
112	−11.2	125.44
118	− 5.2	27.04
118	− 5.2	27.04
1,478	...	1,267.68

The 12 values shown above were taken from a longer list supplied by Dr. Clark W. Heath of Harvard University. They are used for illustrative purposes only and are not necessarily representative of any group of men.

$$\bar{X} = \frac{\Sigma X}{N} = \frac{1{,}478}{12},$$

$$= 123.2 \text{ mm.}$$

$$s = \sqrt{\frac{\Sigma x^2}{N}},$$

$$= \sqrt{\frac{1{,}267.68}{12}} = \sqrt{105.6},$$

$$= 10.3 \text{ mm.}$$

TABLE 5.2

COMPUTATION OF THE STANDARD DEVIATION FOR DATA OF SYSTOLIC BLOOD PRESSURE, BEFORE EXERCISE, FOR 12 YOUNG MEN BY USE OF THE EXPRESSION

$$s = \sqrt{\frac{\Sigma X^2}{N} - \left(\frac{\Sigma X}{N}\right)^2}$$

Pressure in millimeters of mercury X	X^2
116	13,456
130	16,900
126	15,876
110	12,100
114	12,996
142	20,164
140	19,600
132	17,424
120	14,400
112	12,544
118	13,924
118	13,924
1,478	183,308

Source of data is given in Table 5.1.

$$s = \sqrt{\frac{\Sigma X^2}{N} - \left(\frac{\Sigma X}{N}\right)^2},$$

$$= \sqrt{\frac{183{,}308}{12} - \left(\frac{1{,}478}{12}\right)^2},$$

$$= \sqrt{105.6} = 10.3 \text{ mm.}$$

used in connection with the measurement of skewness and kurtosis; s will be necessary to enable us to fit a normal curve; the sum of squared deviations will provide a basis for an explanation of the correlation coefficient; σ and $\hat{\sigma}$ ($\hat{\sigma}$ is the same as s except that $N - 1$ is used instead of N) will be used in making certain tests of statistical significance.

Ungrouped data. Table 5.1 gives data of systolic blood pressure for twelve young men and indicates how the value of s is computed from the expression

CHAP. 5] DISPERSION, SKEWNESS, AND KURTOSIS 87

$$s = \sqrt{\frac{\Sigma x^2}{N}}.$$

It will be seen that this expression requires us to determine $\bar{X}$, to ascertain x for each of the values, to square each x value, sum them, divide by N, and take the square root. It is possible to set up a procedure which will make it unnecessary for us to compute each x value. If we substitute $X - \bar{X}$ for x in the expression for s, the formula may be reduced to

$$s = \sqrt{\frac{\Sigma X^2}{N} - \left(\frac{\Sigma X}{N}\right)^2}.$$

This means that, for a set of ungrouped data, we need only the values themselves and the square of each value. Table 5.2 shows the computation of s for the twelve figures of systolic blood pressure by use of this expression.

Grouped data. To compute the value of the standard deviation for the data of volume of cells in frequency-distribution form, we may use $s = \sqrt{\dfrac{\Sigma fx^2}{N}}$, as shown in Table 5.3. This expression

TABLE 5.3

COMPUTATION OF THE STANDARD DEVIATION OF THE FREQUENCY DISTRIBUTION OF VOLUME OF CELLS IN THE BLOOD OF 100 NORMAL YOUNG WOMEN BY USE OF THE EXPRESSION

$$s = \sqrt{\frac{\Sigma fx^2}{N}}$$

Volume of cells in cubic centimeters	Number of women f	Mid-values X	x	x^2	fx^2
35.0–36.5	4.5	35.75	−5.25	27.5625	124.03125
36.5–38.0	7.5	37.25	−3.75	14.0625	105.46875
38.0–39.5	12	38.75	−2.25	5.0625	60.75000
39.5–41.0	23.5	40.25	− .75	.5625	13.21875
41.0–42.5	28	41.75	+ .75	.5625	15.75000
42.5–44.0	13	43.25	+2.25	5.0625	65.81250
44.0–45.5	9.5	44.75	+3.75	14.0625	133.59375
45.5–47.0	2	46.25	+5.25	27.5625	55.12500
Total	100	...	...	...	573.75000

$\bar{X} = 41.0$ c.c.

$$s = \sqrt{\frac{\Sigma fx^2}{N}} = \sqrt{\frac{573.75}{100}} = \sqrt{5.7375} = 2.4 \text{ c.c.}$$

involves determining x for the mid-value for each class, squaring each x value and multiplying by the appropriate frequency, adding the products, dividing by N, and extracting the square root. To eliminate the unnecessary labor of obtaining the x values, and also to enable us to work with smaller figures, it is preferable to compute s by means of the expression

$$s = i \sqrt{\frac{\Sigma f(d')^2}{N} - \left(\frac{\Sigma f d'}{N}\right)^2}.$$

Because of the fact (mentioned in Chapter 4) that Σx^2 is a minimum, the correction term $\left(\dfrac{\Sigma f d'}{N}\right)^2$ used here [and also the correction term $\left(\dfrac{\Sigma X}{N}\right)^2$, used when computing s for ungrouped data] will always

TABLE 5.4

COMPUTATION OF THE STANDARD DEVIATION OF THE FREQUENCY DISTRIBUTION OF VOLUME OF CELLS IN THE BLOOD OF 100 NORMAL YOUNG WOMEN BY USE OF THE EXPRESSION

$$s = i \sqrt{\frac{\Sigma f(d')^2}{N} - \left(\frac{\Sigma f d'}{N}\right)^2}$$

Volume of cells in cubic centimeters	Number of women f	d'	fd'	$f(d')^2$
35.0–36.5	4.5	−3	−13.5	40.5
36.5–38.0	7.5	−2	−15	30
38.0–39.5	12	−1	−12	12
39.5–41.0	23.5	0		
41.0–42.5	28	+1	+28	28
42.5–44.0	13	+2	+26	52
44.0–45.5	9.5	+3	+28.5	85.5
45.5–47.0	2	+4	+ 8	32
Total	100	...	+50	280

$$s = i \sqrt{\frac{\Sigma f(d')^2}{N} - \left(\frac{\Sigma f d'}{N}\right)^2},$$

$$= 1.5 \sqrt{\frac{280}{100} - \left(\frac{50}{100}\right)^2},$$

$$= 1.5 \sqrt{2.80 - 0.25},$$

$$= 1.5 \sqrt{2.55} = 2.4 \text{ c.c.}$$

be subtracted. Table 5.4 shows the use of this shorter formula for the computation of s for the data of volume of cells. As before, $s = 2.4$ c.c.

The peculiar advantage of s as a measure of dispersion is that, if a distribution is normal,[4] a fixed proportion of the items will occur within the limits given by $\overline{X} \pm$ any desired multiple of s. To be more specific, for a normal distribution, 68.27 per cent of the items will occur within the limits given by $\overline{X} \pm s$, 95.45 per cent will fall

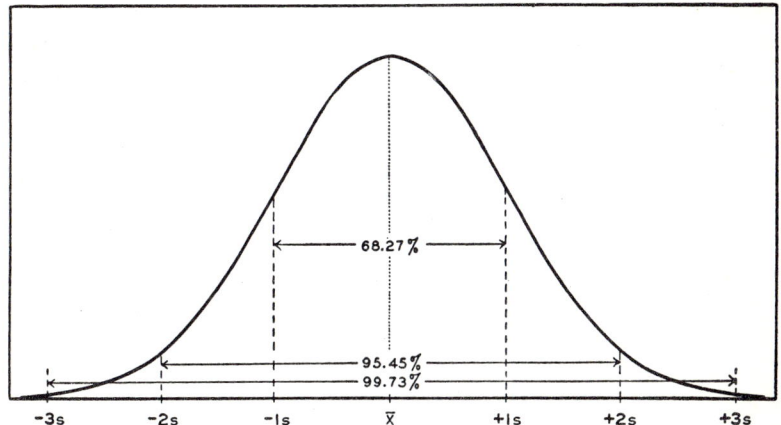

Chart 5.1. Proportions of Items in a Normal Curve Included Between $\overline{X} \pm 1s$, $\overline{X} \pm 2s$, and $\overline{X} \pm 3s$.

between $\overline{X} \pm 2s$, and 99.73 per cent will be found betwixt $\overline{X} \pm 3s$, as shown in Chart 5.1. It is also of interest that the ordinates erected at $\overline{X} \pm s$ in this chart intersect the curve at the points of inflection. Limits other than the three just given will be useful to us in later chapters. Particularly we shall be interested in $\overline{X} \pm 1.96s$, which include 95 per cent (and exclude 5 per cent) of the items, and $\overline{X} \pm 2.58s$, which include 99 per cent (and exclude 1 per cent) of the items.

Even though a distribution is not normal, these proportions may be approximately realized.[5] For the data of volume of cells,

---

[4] The normal curve is discussed in Chapter 8.

[5] No matter how a series is distributed, $\overline{X} \pm 2s$ will include 75 per cent or more of the items and $\overline{X} \pm 3s$ will include 89 per cent or more. These percentages are obtained from Tchebycheff's inequality. If a smooth distribution is unimodal, and if the mode is within s of the arithmetic mean, $\overline{X} \pm s$ will

$$\bar{X} \pm s = 41.0 \pm 2.4,$$
$$= 38.6 \text{ and } 43.4 \text{ c.c.}$$

Interpolating to estimate the number of items between 38.6 c.c. and 39.5 c.c. (the upper limit of the class within which 38.6 c.c. occurs) yields $\frac{0.9}{1.5} \times 12 = 7.2$ frequencies; including all of the frequencies in the next two classes gives 23.5 and 28 frequencies; interpolating to approximate the number of items between 42.5 (the lower limit of the class within which 43.4 c.c. falls) and 43.4 c.c. results in $\frac{0.9}{1.5} \times 13 = 7.8$ frequencies. Now adding these four figures gives $7.2 + 23.5 + 28 + 7.8 = 66.5$ frequencies, or 66.5 per cent of the 100 items. Considering that this distribution is not normal (it may be seen to be slightly skewed in Chart 3.2), this is reasonably close agreement with the figure of 68.27 per cent for a normal curve. Similar computations for the data of volume of cells show that 94.8 per cent of the items are between $\bar{X} \pm 2s$ and 100 per cent between $\bar{X} \pm 3s$.

Sheppard's correction. It was shown in Table 4.2 that, for the data of volume of cells, the mid-values of the classes did not agree with the arithmetic means of the values in the classes. In the accompanying discussion it was pointed out that the disagreements were not serious, as they tended to offset each other, and this was further borne out by the fact that the values of $\bar{X}$ from the 100 individual items and from the frequency distribution were in agreement. For frequency distributions dealing with continuous variables (or discrete variables, if there are no gaps in the data), the mid-values of classes which are graphically to the left of the mode tend to be too small while the mid-values of the classes which are graphically to the right of the mode tend to be too large. The result of these discrepancies is that when x values are computed, giving the deviations of the class mid-values from $\bar{X}$, they are too great in absolute size, and when squared for the computation of s, the errors do not offset each other but accumulate. The result is that the value of s for a frequency distribution is usually larger than the value of s for the same data in ungrouped form. In an attempt to allow for this tendency, W. F. Sheppard has designed a correction[6] which

---

include 56 per cent or more of the items, $\bar{X} \pm 2s$ will include 89 per cent or more, and $\bar{X} \pm 3s$ will include 95 per cent or more, as given by the Camp-Meidell inequality.

[6] A correction may also be in order when x^4 values are computed, but not for x^3 values. Toward the end of this chapter we shall use Σfx^3 and Σfx^4. For a development of the corrections, see W. F. Sheppard, "On the Calculation of the

CHAP. 5] DISPERSION, SKEWNESS, AND KURTOSIS 91

is applicable to continuous variables provided both tails of the curve of the frequency distribution have "high contact" with the horizontal axis. That is to say, the ends of the curve taper off gradually. Using s_{cor} to indicate that s has been corrected for grouping error,

$$s_{cor} = i\sqrt{\frac{\Sigma f(d')^2}{N} - \left(\frac{\Sigma fd'}{N}\right)^2 - 0.0833}.$$

In general, it is better not to employ Sheppard's correction unless we are reasonably sure that it is applicable. If the correction is used when it is not appropriate, it may overcorrect, resulting in an s_{cor} value that is *smaller* than s for the ungrouped data from which the frequency distribution was made. For the data of the frequency distribution of volume of cells, $s = 2.40$ c.c. If the standard deviation is computed from the ungrouped data of Table 3.2 or Table 3.3, it is found to be 2.39 c.c. Applying Sheppard's correction to the computations shown below Table 5.4 gives

$$\begin{aligned} s_{cor} &= 1.5\sqrt{2.80 - 0.25 - 0.0833}, \\ &= 1.5\sqrt{2.4667} = 1.5(1.571), \\ &= 2.36 \text{ c.c.} \end{aligned}$$

This is not particularly conclusive, since all three figures round to 2.4 c.c. (the second decimal not being significant),[7] but s_{cor} is nevertheless smaller than s from the ungrouped data. Reference to Chart 3.2 shows that high contact is not present, so that, if we had not wished to compare s_{cor} with s for the ungrouped data, we would not have felt justified in applying Sheppard's correction in this instance.

Comparing dispersions of two or more series. It is often necessary to compare the dispersions present in several series. Using only two series in each case, we shall illustrate the three sorts of situations which may occur.

1. The data of Table 5.5 refer to the heights of 2,266 white selectees, 30 but less than 35 years of age, who were examined in May, 1943, and inducted into the United States Army. For these men, $s = 2.61$ inches. Table 5.8 gives data of the heights of 1,575

Most Probable Values of Frequency Constants for Data Arranged According to Equidistant Divisions of a Scale," *Proceedings of the London Mathematical Society*, Vol. 29, 1898, pp. 353–380. More generally available is the development in H. L. Rietz (editor), *Handbook of Mathematical Statistics*, Houghton Mifflin Company, Boston, 1924, pp. 92–94.

[7] For a treatment of significant digits and rounding, see F. E. Croxton and D. J. Cowden, *Practical Business Statistics*, 2nd ed., Prentice-Hall, Inc., New York, 1948, pp. 503–506.

white boys, 12 but less than 13 months old, and for these boys $s = 1.43$ inches. The selectees show a larger standard deviation than do the boys, but this is to be expected, since the selectees are themselves larger than the boys. To allow for this, we compare s with $\bar{X}$, computing a measure of relative dispersion, the coefficient of variation, V, from the expression

$$V = \frac{s}{\bar{X}},$$

which is usually written as a percentage. For the selectees, $\bar{X} = 67.96$ inches, so

$$V = \frac{2.61}{67.96} = 0.038, \text{ or } 3.8 \text{ per cent.}$$

For the boys, $\bar{X} = 29.36$ inches and

$$V = \frac{1.43}{29.36} = 0.049, \text{ or } 4.9 \text{ per cent.}$$

Although the selectees show the greater absolute dispersion (s), the boys have the greater relative dispersion (V).

2. During May, 1943, there were 2,501 white selectees, 30 but less than 35 years of age, who were examined and subsequently rejected by the army. For the height of these men, $s = 2.73$ inches. This is greater than the value of s for the inductees mentioned in the preceding paragraph. If we compute the coefficient of variation for the men who were rejected ($\bar{X} = 67.71$ inches), we have

$$V = \frac{2.73}{67.71} = 0.040, \text{ or } 4.0 \text{ per cent,}$$

and the relative dispersion of their heights is also greater than the relative dispersion of the heights of the inductees.

3. The weights of the 2,266 inductees are shown in Table 5.6, and s is seen to be 24.27 pounds. If we wish to compare the dispersion of the heights and the dispersion of the weights of this group of inductees, we cannot use $s = 2.61$ inches for heights and $s = 24.27$ pounds for weights, since unlike units are involved. We can, however, compare the coefficients of variation giving:

For heights,

$$V = \frac{2.61}{67.96} = 0.038, \text{ or } 3.8 \text{ per cent};$$

For weights ($\overline{X} = 159.02$ pounds),

$$V = \frac{24.27}{159.02} = 0.153, \text{ or } 15.3 \text{ per cent}.$$

The relative dispersion of the weights of the inductees is much greater than the relative dispersion of their heights.

Summarizing what has been illustrated in the preceding paragraphs: (1) When comparing the dispersions of two or more series expressed in the same units but having different arithmetic means, we may make a comparison of absolute dispersions using standard deviations or a comparison of relative dispersions using coefficients of variation. (2) When comparing the dispersions of two or more series expressed in the same units and having the same (or approximately the same) arithmetic means, the conclusion is the same whether we compare standard deviations or coefficients of variation. (3) When comparing the dispersions of two or more series expressed in different units, it is not possible to compare standard deviations; therefore we must compare coefficients of variation.

Skewness

Skewness is the tendency of a distribution to depart from a symmetrical form. Illustrations of skewed series were given in Charts 3.5 and 3.6. At this point we are interested in measuring the amount of skewness present in a frequency distribution.

If a distribution is symmetrical, the values of Q_1 and Q_3 will be equidistant from the median; if skewness to the right is present (as in Chart 3.5), Q_3 will be farther from the median than will be Q_1; in the case of skewness to the left (Chart 3.6), Q_1 will be farther from the median than will be Q_3. Consequently it is possible to devise a measure of skewness based on the quartiles, such as

$$\text{Sk}_Q = \frac{(Q_3 - \text{Med}) - (\text{Med} - Q_1)}{Q_3 - Q_1},$$

which is a measure of relative skewness, as are all measures of skewness in common use. A relative measure is preferred because skewness is almost invariably measured in order to compare the asymmetry of a series with that of another series or to ascertain whether the skewness in the series is significantly greater than zero. A measure of absolute skewness, such as the numerator of the expression for Sk_Q, would not be useful for these purposes, since it would always be in terms of the units in which the series was expressed. All measures of relative skewness are "pure numbers." The measure of skewness based upon the quartiles is subject to the same shortcomings as the measure of dispersion, Q, mentioned earlier in this chapter. We shall not even compute the value of Sk_Q for a distribution, but merely note in passing that if no skewness is present, $Sk_Q = 0$ while its maximum value approaches ± 1 as a limit. Similar measures of skewness may be based upon quintiles, deciles, or percentiles, but the same criticism applies to them as to Sk_Q.

A measure of skewness,[8] sometimes referred to as the Pearsonian measure of skewness, because it was suggested by Karl Pearson, is

$$Sk = \frac{3(\overline{X} - \text{Med})}{s}.$$

If no skewness is present, this expression has a value of zero; its maximum value approaches ± 3 as a limit. Series of observed data are not likely to show values in excess of ± 1.

For the data of the heights of 2,266 inductees, shown in Table 5.5 and Chart 3.4, $\overline{X} = 67.96$ inches, Med $= 67.96$ inches, and $s = 2.61$ inches, so that

$$Sk = \frac{3(67.96 - 67.96)}{2.61} = 0,$$

---

[8] Ideally this measure would be $\dfrac{\overline{X} - \text{Mo}}{s}$, since the mode is affected by skewness less than either $\overline{X}$ or Med. However, since the simpler methods of locating the value of the mode are not too satisfactory, Pearson suggested an empirical formula for determining the mode. Based upon his observation that for a moderately skewed distribution of a continuous variable, the median tends to fall two-thirds of the distance, on the horizontal scale of a chart, from the mode toward $\overline{X}$, the formula is Mo $= \overline{X} - 3(\overline{X} - \text{Med})$. If this expression is substituted for the mode, we have

$$Sk = \frac{\overline{X} - \text{Mo}}{s} = \frac{\overline{X} - [\overline{X} - 3(\overline{X} - \text{Med})]}{s} = \frac{3(\overline{X} - \text{Med})}{s}.$$

TABLE 5.5

COMPUTATION OF β_1 FOR DATA OF HEIGHTS OF 2,266 WHITE SELECTEES, 30 BUT LESS THAN 35 YEARS OF AGE, INDUCTED INTO THE UNITED STATES ARMY, WHO WERE EXAMINED IN MAY, 1943

Height in inches (mid-values)	Number of men f	d'	fd'	$f(d')^2$	$f(d')^3$
60.2	10	−8	− 80	640	− 5,120
61.2	17	−7	−119	833	− 5,831
62.2	25	−6	−150	900	− 5,400
63.2	65	−5	−325	1,625	− 8,125
64.2	110	−4	−440	1,760	− 7,040
65.2	202	−3	−606	1,818	− 5,454
66.2	263	−2	−526	1,052	− 2,104
67.2	349	−1	−349	349	− 349
68.2	353	0			
69.2	305	+1	+305	305	+ 305
70.2	227	+2	+454	908	+ 1,816
71.2	178	+3	+534	1,602	+ 4,806
72.2	85	+4	+340	1,360	+ 5,440
73.2	47	+5	+235	1,175	+ 5,875
74.2	21	+6	+126	756	+ 4,536
75.2	6	+7	+ 42	294	+ 2,058
76.2	3	+8	+ 24	192	+ 1,536
Total	2,266	...	−535	15,569	−13,051

Data from Medical Statistics Division, Office of the Surgeon General, United States Army.

$$\bar{X} = 68.2 - \frac{535}{2,266} \cdot 1.0 = 68.2 - 0.24 = 67.96 \text{ inches.}$$

$$\nu_1 = \frac{\Sigma fd'}{N} = \frac{-535}{2,266} = -0.236099.$$

$$\nu_2 = \frac{\Sigma f(d')^2}{N} = \frac{15,569}{2,266} = 6.870697.$$

$$\nu_3 = \frac{\Sigma f(d')^3}{N} = \frac{-13,051}{2,266} = -5.759488.$$

$\pi_1 = 0.$

$\pi_2 = \nu_2 - \nu_1^2 = 6.870697 - (-0.236099)^2,$
$\quad = 6.870697 - 0.055743 = 6.814954.$

$s = i\sqrt{\pi_2} = 1.0\sqrt{6.814954} = 2.61$ inches.

$\pi_3 = \nu_3 - 3\nu_1\nu_2 + 2\nu_1^3,$
$\quad = -5.759488 - 3(-0.236099)(6.870697) + 2(-0.236099)^3,$
$\quad = -5.759488 + 4.866495 - 0.026322 = -0.919315.$

$$\beta_1 = \frac{\pi_3^2}{\pi_2^3} = \frac{(-0.919315)^2}{(6.814954)^3} = \frac{0.845140}{316.510984} = 0.00267.$$

Using Sheppard's correction:

$\mu_2 = \pi_2 - 0.083333 = 6.814954 - 0.083333 = 6.731621.$

$\mu_3 = \pi_3 = -0.919315.$

$$\beta_1 = \frac{\mu_3^2}{\mu_2^3} = \frac{(-0.919315)^2}{(6.731621)^3} = \frac{0.845140}{305.041527} = 0.00277.$$

96   DISPERSION, SKEWNESS, AND KURTOSIS [Chap. 5

indicating no skewness. The distribution of the weights of these same men (Table 5.6 and Chart 3.5) shows skewness to the right, or positive. For this series, $\bar{X} = 159.02$ pounds, Med = 156.19 pounds, $s = 24.27$ pounds, and

$$\text{Sk} = \frac{3(159.02 - 156.19)}{24.27} = \frac{8.49}{24.27} = +0.350.$$

In the preceding chapter the data of volume of cells (shown graphically in Chart 3.2) were found to have $\bar{X} = 41.0$ c.c. and Med = 41.1 c.c. In this chapter, s was computed to be 2.4 c.c. Consequently,

$$\text{Sk} = \frac{3(41.0 - 41.1)}{2.4} = \frac{-0.3}{2.4} = -0.125.$$

The most satisfactory measure of skewness employs the cubes of the deviations of the various values of a series from $\bar{X}$. Before proceeding to describe this measure, which is called β_1, it is desirable to illustrate the fact that Σx^3 (or $\Sigma f x^3$) is zero when a series of values is symmetrical around $\bar{X}$ but not zero when a series of values is not symmetrical around $\bar{X}$.

For the following series of five values, which are symmetrical around $\bar{X} = 7$, it is seen that $\Sigma x = 0$ and $\Sigma x^3 = 0$.

X	x	x^3
3	-4	-64
4	-3	-27
7	0	
10	$+3$	$+27$
11	$+4$	$+64$
	0	0

Another set of five values which also have $\bar{X} = 7$, but which are not symmetrical around $\bar{X}$, show $\Sigma x = 0$ but $\Sigma x^3 \neq 0$.

X	x	x^3
3	-4	-64
4	-3	-27
7	0	
9	$+2$	$+8$
12	$+5$	$+125$
	0	$+42$

Since skewness is ordinarily computed for data which are in the form of a frequency distribution rather than for ungrouped data, we shall employ the symbol f in our expressions from this point on.

The first moment about the arithmetic mean of a frequency distribution is

$$\pi_1 = \frac{\Sigma fx}{N},$$

and we already know that this always equals zero.

The second moment about the arithmetic mean of a frequency distribution is

$$\pi_2 = \frac{\Sigma fx^2}{N},$$

and this will be recognized as s^2.

The third moment about the arithmetic mean of a frequency distribution is

$$\pi_3 = \frac{\Sigma fx^3}{N}.$$

From π_3 and π_2 we obtain the measure of skewness, β_1, by use of the expression

$$\beta_1 = \frac{\pi_3^2}{\pi_2^3}.$$

Just as we previously made use of short methods for computing $\bar{X}$ and s, so we shall want a short method for computing π_3. We are already familiar with $\frac{\Sigma fd'}{N}$, which we shall now call ν_1 (the first moment about $\bar{X}_d$), and $\frac{\Sigma f(d')^2}{N} = \nu_2$ (the second moment about $\bar{X}_d$). To these we shall add $\nu_3 = \frac{\Sigma f(d')^3}{N}$ (the third moment about $\bar{X}_d$). We may now write

$$\pi_2 = \frac{\Sigma f(d')^2}{N} - \left(\frac{\Sigma fd'}{N}\right)^2,$$
$$= \nu_2 - \nu_1^2,$$

which is the same as the portion under the radical in the expression for computing s for a frequency distribution. In somewhat similar fashion,[9] we may obtain π_3.

---

[9] For a development of this short method, see F. E. Croxton and D. J. Cowden, *Applied General Statistics*, Prentice-Hall, Inc., New York, 1939, pp. 832–833.

$$\pi_3 = \frac{\Sigma f(d')^3}{N} - 3\frac{\Sigma fd'}{N}\frac{\Sigma f(d')^2}{N} + 2\left(\frac{\Sigma fd'}{N}\right)^3,$$
$$= \nu_3 - 3\nu_1\nu_2 + 2\nu_1^3.$$

Note that π_2 is in terms of class intervals squared while π_3 is in terms of class intervals cubed. When β_1 is computed, both the numerator and the denominator will be in terms of class intervals raised to the sixth power, thus cancelling and making it unnecessary to consider i when computing β_1.

For the data of heights of inductees, which are shown in Table 5.5 and Chart 3.4, and which are very nearly symmetrical, it is found that $\pi_2 = 6.814954$ and $\pi_3 = 0.919315$, giving

$$\beta_1 = \frac{\pi_3^2}{\pi_2^3} = \frac{(-0.919315)^2}{(6.814954)^3},$$
$$= \frac{0.845140}{316.510984} = 0.00267.$$

Note that β_1 has no sign and therefore does not indicate the direction of skewness. The direction of skewness is shown by the sign of π_3, a positive sign indicating skewness to the right and a negative sign skewness to the left.

The data of the weights of the same inductees, which are given in Table 5.6 and shown graphically in Chart 3.5, and which are decidedly skewed to the right, have $\pi_2 = 5.892653$ and $\pi_3 = 9.310297$, with

$$\beta_1 = \frac{(9.310297)^2}{(5.892653)^3} = \frac{86.681630}{204.612706},$$
$$= 0.424.$$

The data of volume of cells, which are slightly skewed to the left, are in Table 5.7 and Chart 3.2. From the table, π_2 is found to be 2.55, while $\pi_3 = -0.72$.

$$\beta_1 = \frac{(-0.72)^2}{(2.55)^3} = \frac{0.5184}{16.5814},$$
$$= 0.0313.$$

A question which we are not in a position to answer at this point is whether a given value of β_1 is *significantly* greater than zero. This will be briefly considered in Chapter 12.

TABLE 5.6

COMPUTATION OF β_1 FOR DATA OF WEIGHTS OF 2,266 WHITE SELECTEES, 30 BUT LESS THAN 35 YEARS OF AGE, INDUCTED INTO THE UNITED STATES ARMY, WHO WERE EXAMINED IN MAY, 1943

Weight in pounds (mid-values)	Number of men f	d'	fd'	$f(d')^2$	$f(d')^3$
95	1	− 6	− 6	36	− 216
105	10	− 5	− 50	250	− 1,250
115	44	− 4	−176	704	− 2,816
125	158	− 3	−474	1,422	− 4,266
135	290	− 2	−580	1,160	− 2,320
145	385	− 1	−385	385	− 385
155	396	0			
165	310	+ 1	+310	310	+ 310
175	263	+ 2	+526	1,052	+ 2,104
185	166	+ 3	+498	1,494	+ 4,482
195	107	+ 4	+428	1,712	+ 6,848
205	66	+ 5	+330	1,650	+ 8,250
215	34	+ 6	+204	1,224	+ 7,344
225	18	+ 7	+126	882	+ 6,174
235	6	+ 8	+ 48	384	+ 3,072
245	10	+ 9	+ 90	810	+ 7,290
255	1	+10	+ 10	100	+ 1,000
265		+11			
275	1	+12	+ 12	144	+ 1,728
Total	2,266	...	+911	13,719	+37,349

Data from Medical Statistics Division, Office of the Surgeon General, United States Army.

$$\bar{X} = 155 + \frac{911}{2,266} \cdot 10 = 155 + 4.02 = 159.02 \text{ pounds.}$$

$$\nu_1 = \frac{\Sigma fd'}{N} = \frac{+911}{2,266} = +0.402030.$$

$$\nu_2 = \frac{\Sigma f(d')^2}{N} = \frac{13,719}{2,266} = 6.054281.$$

$$\nu_3 = \frac{\Sigma f(d')^3}{N} = \frac{+37,349}{2,266} = +16.482348$$

$\pi_1 = 0.$

$\pi_2 = \nu_2 - \nu_1^2 = 6.054281 - (0.402030)^2,$
$\quad = 6.054281 - 0.161628 = 5.892653.$

$s = i \sqrt{\pi_2},$
$\quad = 10 \sqrt{5.892653},$
$\quad = 24.27 \text{ pounds.}$

$\pi_3 = \nu_3 - 3\nu_1\nu_2 + 2\nu_1^3,$
$\quad = 16.482348 - 3(0.402030)(6.054281) + 2(0.402030)^3,$
$\quad = 16.482348 - 7.302009 + 0.129958,$
$\quad = 9.310297.$

$$\beta_1 = \frac{\pi_3^2}{\pi_2^3} = \frac{(9.310297)^2}{(5.892653)^3} = \frac{86.681630}{204.612706} = 0.424.$$

TABLE 5.7

COMPUTATION OF β_1 FOR THE FREQUENCY DISTRIBUTION OF VOLUME OF CELLS IN THE BLOOD OF 100 NORMAL YOUNG WOMEN

Volume of cells in cubic centimeters	Number of women f	d'	fd'	$f(d')^2$	$f(d')^3$
35.0–36.5	4.5	−3	−13.5	40.5	−121.5
36.5–38.0	7.5	−2	−15	30	− 60
38.0–39.5	12	−1	−12	12	− 12
39.5–41.0	23.5	0			
41.0–42.5	28	+1	+28	28	+ 28
42.5–44.0	13	+2	+26	52	+104
44.0–45.5	9.5	+3	+28.5	85.5	+256.5
45.5–47.0	2	+4	+ 8	32	+128
Total	100	...	+50	280	+323

$$\bar{X} = 40.25 + \frac{50}{100} 1.5 = 40.25 + 0.75 = 41.0 \text{ c.c.}$$

$$\nu_1 = \frac{\Sigma fd'}{N} = \frac{+50}{100} = +0.5.$$

$$\nu_2 = \frac{\Sigma f(d')^2}{N} = \frac{280}{100} = 2.80.$$

$$\nu_3 = \frac{\Sigma f(d')^3}{N} = \frac{+323}{100} = 3.23.$$

$\pi_1 = 0.$

$\pi_2 = \nu_2 - \nu_1^2 = 2.80 - (0.5)^2 = 2.80 - 0.25 = 2.55.$

$\pi_3 = \nu_3 - 3\nu_1\nu_2 + 2\nu_1^3 = 3.23 - 3(0.5)(2.80) + 2(0.5)^3,$
$= 3.23 - 4.20 + 0.250 = -0.72.$

$$\beta_1 = \frac{\pi_3^2}{\pi_2^3} = \frac{(-0.72)^2}{(2.55)^3} = \frac{0.5184}{16.5814} = 0.0313.$$

It was pointed out in the discussion of the standard deviation that Sheppard's correction is sometimes appropriate. No correction is necessary for the first or third moment about the mean, and, using μ to indicate a moment with Sheppard's correction, we may write

$$\mu_1 = \pi_1 = 0,$$
$$\mu_2 = \pi_2 - 0.083333, \text{ and}$$
$$\mu_3 = \pi_3.$$

The correction applied to π_2 is $\frac{1}{12}$ of a squared class interval.

There is doubt as to the applicability of Sheppard's correction to the data of weights of inductees and to the data of volume of cells, since high contact is not present at both ends of the series (see Charts 3.2 and 3.5). However, it seems reasonable to apply the correction to the data of heights of inductees, shown in Table 5.5 and Chart 3.4. For these data,

$$\mu_2 = \pi_2 - 0.083333,$$
$$= 6.814954 - 0.083333 = 6.731621.$$
$$\mu_3 = \pi_3 = -0.919315.$$
$$\beta_1 = \frac{\mu_3^2}{\mu_2^3} = \frac{(-0.919315)^2}{(6.731621)^3},$$
$$= \frac{0.845140}{305.041527} = 0.00277.$$

This value of β_1 is only slightly different from that obtained for the same data without the use of Sheppard's correction.

Kurtosis

A curve of a frequency distribution may conceivably be perfectly symmetrical yet differ from a normal curve by being leptokurtic

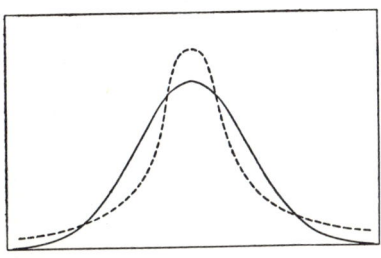

Chart 5.2. A Leptokurtic Curve and a Normal Curve. The solid line is the normal curve.

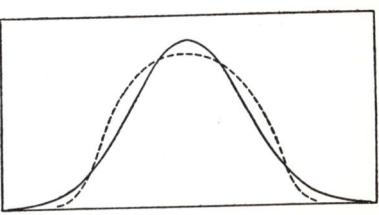

Chart 5.3. A Platykurtic Curve and a Normal Curve. The solid line is the normal curve.

or platykurtic. Chart 5.2 shows a normal (mesokurtic) curve and a leptokurtic curve. The leptokurtic curve has a narrower modal portion and higher tails than does the normal curve. Chart 5.3 shows a normal curve and a platykurtic curve. The platykurtic curve has a broader modal portion than the normal curve and may have lower tails or may not taper off gradually but may be "bob-tailed."

Kurtosis is reflected in the fourth powers of the deviations of the values of a frequency distribution from their arithmetic mean, Σfx^4. Dividing by N gives the fourth moment about the arithmetic mean

$$\pi_4 = \frac{\Sigma fx^4}{N}.$$

To compute the value of π_4, we first obtain

$$\nu_4 = \frac{\Sigma f(d')^4}{N},$$

the fourth moment around $\overline{X}_d$, and then employ the expression

$$\pi_4 = \frac{\Sigma f(d')^4}{N} - 4 \frac{\Sigma fd'}{N} \frac{\Sigma f(d')^3}{N} + 6 \left(\frac{\Sigma fd'}{N}\right)^2 \frac{\Sigma f(d')^2}{N} - 3 \left(\frac{\Sigma fd'}{N}\right)^4,$$
$$= \nu_4 - 4\nu_1\nu_3 + 6\nu_1^2\nu_2 - 3\nu_1^4.$$

Having obtained π_4, we may now determine β_2, the measure of kurtosis, from

$$\beta_2 = \frac{\pi_4}{\pi_2^2}.$$

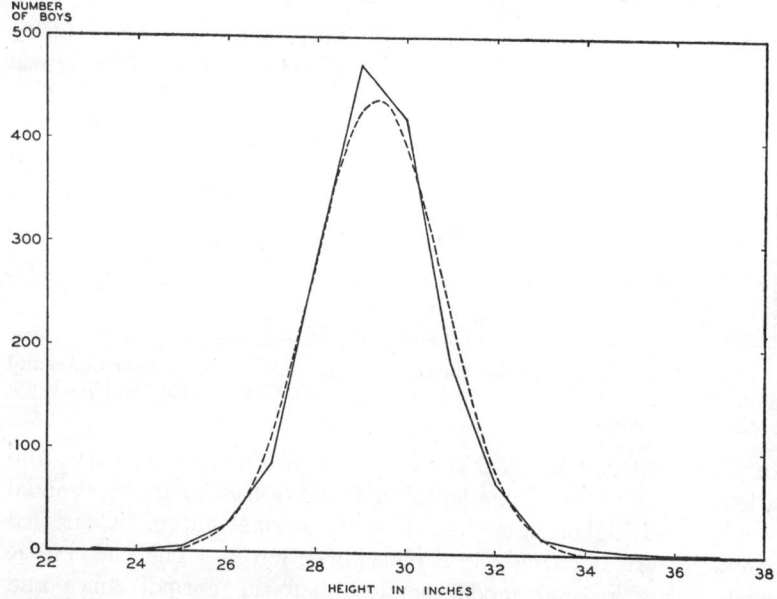

Chart 5.4. Frequency Distribution of Heights of 1,575 White Boys, 12 but Under 13 Months Old, Compared with a Normal Curve Having the Same N, $\overline{X}$, and s. The broken line is the normal curve. Based on data of Table 5.8.

CHAP. 5] DISPERSION, SKEWNESS, AND KURTOSIS   103

As in the case of β_1, all computations are in terms of class intervals.

For the same reason that it is sometimes necessary to correct π_2 for grouping error, π_4 should sometimes be corrected. Sheppard's correction is applicable here under the same conditions that were mentioned before, and

$$\mu_4 = \pi_4 - \frac{1}{2}\pi_2 + \frac{7}{240}.$$

When Sheppard's corrections have been used,

$$\beta_2 = \frac{\mu_4}{\mu_2^2}.$$

For a distribution that is normal, $\beta_2 = 3.0$. A leptokurtic distribution will have $\beta_2 > 3.0$, while a platykurtic distribution will show $\beta_2 < 3.0$.

The frequency distribution of the heights of 1,575 white boys 12 but less than 13 months old, in Table 5.8, is leptokurtic. This may be seen in Chart 5.4, where the curve of this frequency distribution

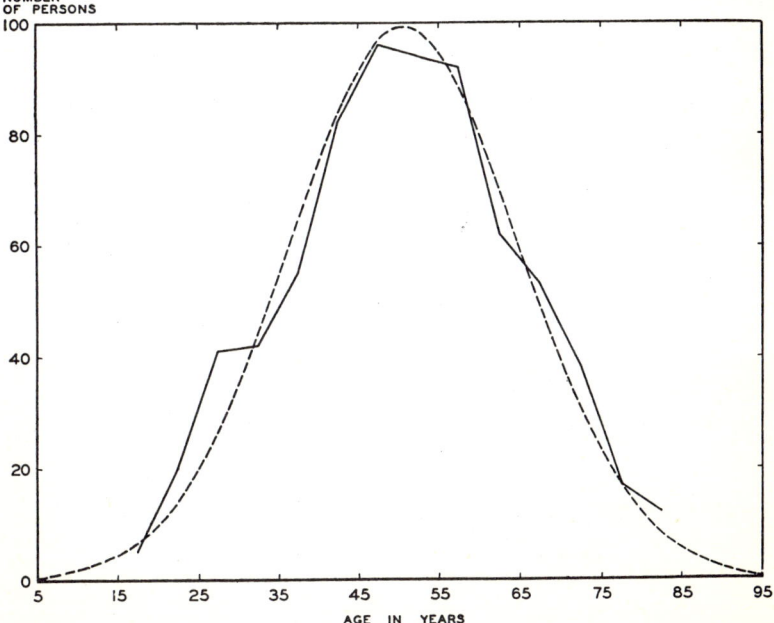

Chart 5.5. An Illustrative Platykurtic Distribution Compared with a Normal Curve Having the Same N, $\bar{X}$, and s. The broken line is the normal curve. Based on data of Table 5.9.

is shown in comparison with a normal curve having the same $\bar{X}$, the same s (or π_2), and the same area. The computations performed in Table 5.8 give

$$\pi_4 = 19.289828,$$
$$\pi_2 = 2.047365, \text{ and}$$
$$\beta_2 = 4.60,$$

indicating that the distribution is clearly leptokurtic. For thees data. of the heights of white boys, the assumptions underlying

TABLE 5.8

COMPUTATION OF β_2 FOR DATA OF HEIGHTS OF 1,575 WHITE BOYS, 12 BUT UNDER 13 MONTHS OLD

Height in inches (mid-values)	Number of boys f	d'	fd'	$f(d')^2$	$f(d')^3$	$f(d')^4$
23	1	−6	− 6	36	− 216	1,296
24	1	−5	− 5	25	− 125	625
25	5	−4	− 20	80	− 320	1,280
26	26	−3	− 78	234	− 702	2,106
27	86	−2	−172	344	− 688	1,376
28	281	−1	−281	281	− 281	281
29	473	0				
30	420	+1	+420	420	+ 420	420
31	186	+2	+372	744	+1,488	2,976
32	68	+3	+204	612	+1,836	5,508
33	16	+4	+ 64	256	+1,024	4,096
34	7	+5	+ 35	175	+ 875	4,375
35	3	+6	+ 18	108	+ 648	3,888
36	1	+7	+ 7	49	+ 343	2,401
37	1	+8	+ 8	64	+ 512	4,096
Total	1,575	...	+566	3,428	+4,814	34,724

Data from Robert Morse Woodbury, *Statures and Weights of Children under Six Years of Age*, U.S. Children's Bureau, p. 87.

$$\bar{X} = 29 + \frac{566}{1,575} 1.0 = 29 + 0.36 = 29.36 \text{ inches.}$$

$$\nu_1 = \frac{\Sigma fd'}{N} = \frac{+566}{1,575} = +0.359365.$$

$$\nu_2 = \frac{\Sigma f(d')^2}{N} = \frac{3,428}{1,575} = 2.176508.$$

$$\nu_3 = \frac{\Sigma f(d')^3}{N} = \frac{+4,814}{1,575} = +3.056508.$$

$$\nu_4 = \frac{\Sigma f(d')^4}{N} = \frac{34,724}{1,575} = 22.046984.$$

(*Computation continued on page 105.*)

CHAP. 5] DISPERSION, SKEWNESS, AND KURTOSIS   105

$\pi_1 = 0.$

$\pi_2 = \nu_2 - \nu_1^2 = 2.176508 - (0.359365)^2,$
$= 2.176508 - 0.129143 = 2.047365.$

$s = i\sqrt{\pi_2},$
$= 1.0\sqrt{2.047365},$
$= 1.43 \text{ inches}.$

$\pi_3 = \nu_3 - 3\nu_1\nu_2 + 2\nu_1^3,$
$= 3.056508 - 3(0.359365)(2.176508) + 2(0.359365)^3,$
$= 3.056508 - 2.346483 + 0.092818 = 0.802843.$

$\pi_4 = \nu_4 - 4\nu_1\nu_3 + 6\nu_1^2\nu_2 - 3\nu_1^4,$
$= 22.046984 - 4(0.359365)(3.056508)$
$\qquad + 6(0.359365)^2(2.176508) - 3(0.359365)^4,$
$= 22.046984 - 4.393608 + 1.686486 - 0.050034,$
$= 19.289828.$

$$\beta_2 = \frac{\pi_4}{\pi_2^2} = \frac{19.289828}{(2.047365)^2} = \frac{19.289828}{4.191703} = 4.60.$$

Using Sheppard's corrections:

$\mu_2 = \pi_2 - 0.083333 = 2.047365 - 0.083333 = 1.964032.$

$\mu_4 = \pi_4 - \frac{1}{2}\pi_2 + \frac{7}{240},$
$= 19.289828 - 0.5(2.047365) + 0.029167,$
$= 18.295313.$

$$\beta_2 = \frac{\mu_4}{\mu_2^2} = \frac{18.295313}{(1.964032)^2} = \frac{18.295313}{3.857422} = 4.74.$$

Sheppard's correction seem to be met, and we have

$$\mu_4 = 18.295313,$$
$$\mu_2 = 1.964032, \text{ and}$$
$$\beta_2 = 4.74,$$

a value little different from that obtained without the use of the corrections. At this point we are not in a position to ascertain whether β_2 is significantly larger than 3.0, but we shall do so in Chapter 12.

As a final illustration for this chapter, Table 5.9 presents an illustrative frequency distribution which is platykurtic and Chart 5.5 shows a curve of this frequency distribution together with a normal curve having the same $\overline{X}$, the same s, and the same area. From the computations shown in the table, it is seen that $\beta_2 = 2.48$ for the illustrative frequency distribution.

TABLE 5.9

Computation of β_2 for Illustrative Frequency Distribution

Age in years	Number of persons f	d'	fd'	$f(d')^2$	$f(d')^3$	$f(d')^4$
15 but less than 20	5	−7	− 35	245	−1,715	12,005
20 but less than 25	20	−6	−120	720	−4,320	25,920
25 but less than 30	41	−5	−205	1,025	−5,125	25,625
30 but less than 35	42	−4	−168	672	−2,688	10,752
35 but less than 40	55	−3	−165	495	−1,485	4,455
40 but less than 45	82	−2	−164	328	− 656	1,312
45 but less than 50	96	−1	− 96	96	− 96	96
50 but less than 55	94	0				
55 but less than 60	92	+1	+ 92	92	+ 92	92
60 but less than 65	62	+2	+124	248	+ 496	992
65 but less than 70	53	+3	+159	477	+1,431	4,293
70 but less than 75	38	+4	+152	608	+2,432	9,728
75 but less than 80	17	+5	+ 85	425	+2,125	10,625
80 but less than 85	12	+6	+ 72	432	+2,592	15,552
Total	709	...	−269	5,863	−6,917	121,447

$$\bar{X} = 52.5 - \frac{269}{709} 5 = 52.5 - 1.9 = 50.6 \text{ years}.$$

$$\nu_1 = \frac{\Sigma fd'}{N} = \frac{-269}{709} = -0.379408.$$

$$\nu_2 = \frac{\Sigma f(d')^2}{N} = \frac{5{,}863}{709} = 8.269394.$$

$$\nu_3 = \frac{\Sigma f(d')^3}{N} = \frac{-6{,}917}{709} = -9.755994.$$

$$\nu_4 = \frac{\Sigma f(d')^4}{N} = \frac{121{,}447}{709} = 171.293371.$$

$\pi_1 = 0.$

$\pi_2 = \nu_2 - \nu_1^2 = 8.269394 - 0.143950 = 8.125444.$

$\pi_3 = \nu_3 - 3\nu_1\nu_2 + 2\nu_1^3,$
   $= -9.755994 - 3(-0.379408)(8.269394) + 2(-0.379408)^3,$
   $= -0.452804,$

$\pi_4 = \nu_4 - 4\nu_1\nu_3 + 6\nu_1^2\nu_2 - 3\nu_1^4,$
   $= 171.293371 - 4(-0.379408)(-9.755994)$
   $\qquad + 6(-0.379408)^2 (8.269394) - 3(-0.379408)^4,$
   $= 163.567471.$

$$\beta_2 = \frac{\pi_4}{\pi_2^2} = \frac{163.567471}{(8.125444)^2},$$

$$= \frac{163.567471}{66.022840} = 2.48.$$

Symbols Used in

CHAPTER 6

a: the value of Y_c when $X = 0$ in the equation $Y_c = a + bX$.
a': the value of X_c when $Y = 0$ in the equation $X_c = a' + b'Y$.
b: the slope of the estimating equation $Y_c = a + bX$.
b': the slope of the estimating equation $X_c = a' + b'Y$.
d'_X: deviation of a cell, in terms of classes, from $\overline{X}_d$.
d'_Y: deviation of a cell, in terms of classes, from $\overline{Y}_d$.
D: difference between the ranks of paired values.
f: a frequency; in grouped correlation, a frequency in a cell.
f_X: a frequency of the X series; in grouped correlation, a column frequency.
f_Y: a frequency of the Y series; in grouped correlation, a row frequency.
i_X: class interval of the X series.
i_Y: class interval of the Y series.
k: coefficient of alienation.
k^2: coefficient of non-determination.
N: the number of items in a sample. In two-variable correlation, N is the number of pairs of items.
r: coefficient of correlation.
r^2: coefficient of determination.
r': intraclass correlation coefficient.
r_{rank}: coefficient of rank correlation.
s^2: in intraclass correlation, the standard deviation squared of all of the $2N$ values.
s_X: standard deviation of the X series.
s_Y: standard deviation of the Y series.
$s_{Y.X}$: standard error of estimate for the estimating equation $Y_c = a + bX$.
$\hat{\sigma}_Y$: lower-case Greek sigma, "sigma caret" or "sigma hat," estimated population standard deviation for the Y variable.
Σ: upper-case Greek sigma, meaning "take the sum of."

SYMBOLS USED IN CHAPTER 6

$x: X - \bar{X}$.

X: the X series, also an observed value in the X series. Thus, we refer to correlating X and Y, but ΣX means "sum the values in the X series."

X axis: the horizontal axis.

X_c: a computed X value.

$\bar{X}$: the arithmetic mean of the X series.

$\bar{X}_d$: designated mean of the X series.

$\overline{XY}$: in intraclass correlation, the arithmetic mean of all of the $2N$ values.

$y: Y - \bar{Y}$. Σy^2 is the total variation in the Y series.

$y_c: Y_c - \bar{Y}$. Σy_c^2 is the explained variation in the Y series.

$y_s: Y - Y_c$. Σy_s^2 is the unexplained variation in the Y series.

Y: the Y series, also an observed value in the Y series. Thus, we refer to correlating X and Y, but ΣY means "sum the values in the Y series."

Y axis: the vertical axis.

Y_c: a computed Y value.

$\bar{Y}$: the arithmetic mean of the Y series.

$\bar{Y}_d$: designated mean of the Y series.

Chapter 6

LINEAR CORRELATION OF TWO VARIABLES

Introduction

The most elementary aspect of correlation has to do with the relationship existing between two sets of data which vary together in linear fashion. Consider, for example, Chart 6.1, on which are

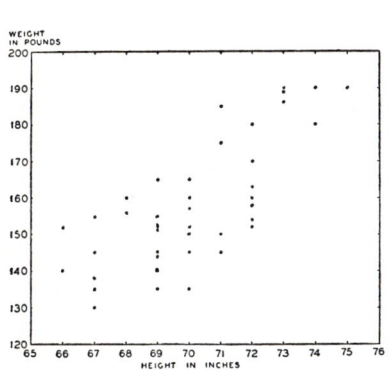

Chart 6.1. Heights and Weights of 41 Male Students. The vertical and horizontal alignment of the dots is not characteristic of all scatter plots, but is due to the fact that the students reported their heights in whole inches and their weights in whole pounds.

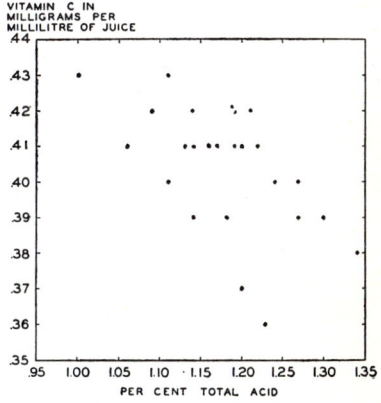

Chart 6.2. Total Acid and Vitamin C in the Expressed Juice of Stylar Halves of 25 Marsh Grapefruit. Data from Paul L. Harding, Plant Pathologist, Division of Fruit and Vegetable Crops and Diseases, Bureau of Plant Industry, Soils and Agricultural Engineering, Agricultural Research Administration, U. S. Department of Agriculture.

plotted the heights (horizontal axis) and the weights (vertical axis) of 41 male students who were registered in a course in statistics. It is clear from the chart, which we call a *scatter plot*, that correlation is present and that the relationship is linear rather than curvilinear. Only linear relationships are dealt with in this chapter.

110   LINEAR CORRELATION OF TWO VARIABLES   [Chap. 6

Curvilinear correlation is discussed in the following chapter, and a non-linear relationship may be observed in Chart 7.1.

The correlation shown in Chart 6.1 is positive; that is, small values of one series are, in general, associated with small values of the other series, and large values of one series are, in general, associated with large values of the other series. Negative correlation is illustrated in Chart 6.2, which shows total acid (as a per-

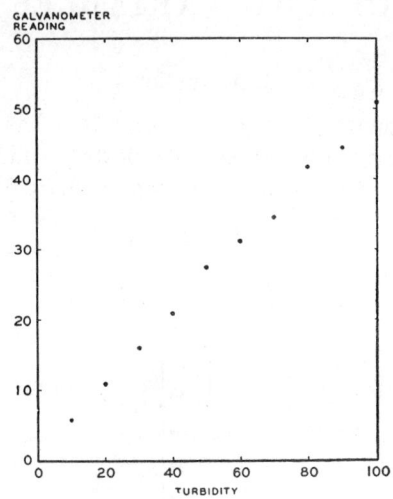

Chart 6.3. **Turbidity and Galvanometer Readings in a Photronreflectometer.** Redrawn from a chart in "A Modified Photronreflectometer for Use with Test Tubes," by Raymond L. Libby, *Science*, Vol. 93, No. 2419, May 9, 1941, pp. 459–460. Turbidity is expressed as a percentage dilution of a bacterial suspension.

centage of expressed juice) and vitamin C (in milligrams per millilitre of expressed juice) in the stylar halves of 25 Marsh grapefruit. In this chart, small values of one series tend to be associated with large values of the other series, and large values of one series tend to be associated with small values of the other series.

Correlation may be high, as in Chart 6.3, or low,[1] as in Chart 6.4. The correlation shown in Chart 6.1 is "moderately high," while that shown in Chart 6.2 is also "moderately high." Perfect

---

[1] Correlation may be low but significantly greater than zero if the sample is large. Correlation may be high but not significantly greater than zero if the sample is small. This is discussed in Chapter 12.

CHAP. 6] LINEAR CORRELATION OF TWO VARIABLES 111

linear correlation would be indicated by a series of dots all lying on a sloping straight line.[2] Chart 6.5 shows perfect linear correlation, which is positive because the line on which the dots lie slopes upward

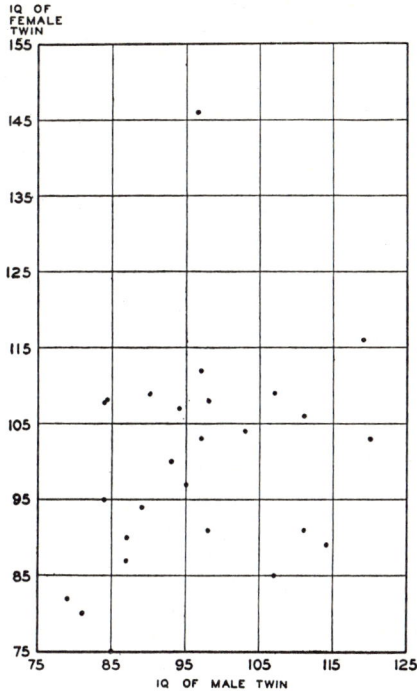

Chart 6.4. Intelligence Quotients of 26 Fraternal Twins of Different Sex. Data from Alex H. Wingfield, *Twins and Orphans*, J. M. Dent and Sons, Ltd., London and Toronto, 1928, pp. 121–123. The 26 pairs of items have a correlation coefficient of +0.290. If the pair of values represented by the one dot far removed from the others is omitted, the remaining 25 pairs of items have a correlation coefficient of +0.348. Both coefficients are low.

from left to right. Perfect negative linear correlation would be indicated by a series of dots lying on a straight line which slopes downward from left to right. No correlation is present in the scatter plot of Chart 6.6.

---

[2] The angle of the line does not affect the degree of correlations, since the angle is largely determined by the scales chosen for the scatter plot. However, if the straight line is either horizontal or vertical, the correlation is zero. This should be clear after reading the paragraphs on pages 120–126 explaining the coefficient of determination.

Although correlation is clearly present between the height and weight data of Chart 6.1, the correlation is not especially high. One reason for this is that the data are not homogeneous. They are for students of various ages some of whom were as young as 18 while others were as old as 36. If we were to make a scatter plot of the heights and weights of male students all aged 20, it would be reasonable to expect a slightly higher correlation than that shown in Chart 6.1, since one source of variation would have been eliminated. Another procedure, which will be examined in the

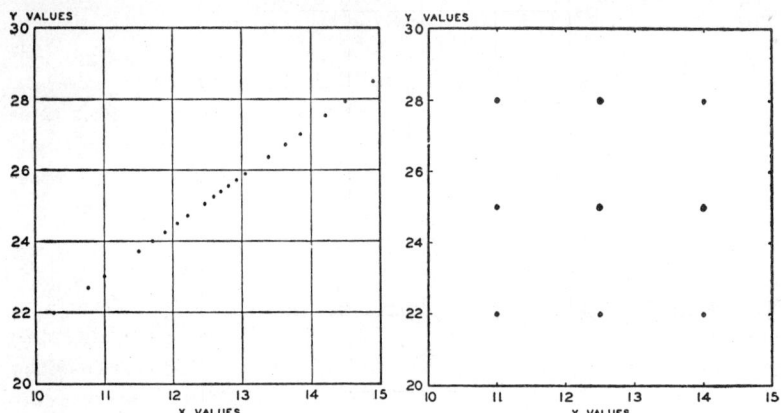

Chart 6.5. Scatter Plot Illustrating Perfect Linear Correlation. The correlation would also be perfect if the line on which the dots lie had a negative instead of a positive slope.

Chart 6.6. Scatter Plot Illustrating No Correlation. Various other arrangements of dots are possible which will also show no correlation.

following chapter, consists of setting up a three-variable multiple-correlation problem involving height, age, and weight, Multiple correlation enables us to consider any number of variables. We are limited only by our ability to obtain the necessary quantitative data, to measure a variable (it is difficult if not impossible, for example, to express hair color quantitatively), and to perform the necessary computations, which increase in complexity as the number of variables is increased.

Correlation of Ungrouped Data

The scatter plot. The initial step in any correlation problem should be the construction of a scatter plot. Such a chart gives prompt visual evidence of the presence or absence of correlation,

Chap. 6] LINEAR CORRELATION OF TWO VARIABLES 113

indicating also whether the relationship is positive or negative and linear or non-linear. Occasionally, an investigator may find that a scatter plot is all that is necessary and that the measures described in the following sections of this chapter are not required in order to make his point. This is true particularly when the investigator wishes merely to point out the presence or absence of correlation and when the scatter plot shows very high or very low correlation. Again, if one is searching for series which may be related to one particular series, he may use the scatter plot as a probing tool. This is accomplished by making many scatter plots, each with the particular series on one axis (preferably the vertical axis) and with one of the presumably related series on the other axis. The two or three series most closely related to the particular series may then be selected for further study and the others discarded.

It is perhaps desirable to point out, at the outset, that correlation cannot exist without pairing. The data plotted in Chart 6.1 are the heights and weights for each of a group of male students. Any given height figure is paired with one, and only one, of the weight figures, the two figures referring to the same student. This is an elementary but very important point. It is stressed here because of the occasional occurrence of statements such as the one that the "grades of a group of girls taking American History I may be correlated with the grades of a group of boys taking the same course." Unless each girl is a sister of one of the boys (possibly the entire class consists of fraternal twins of unlike sex!), there is no pairing of the grades. Lacking pairing, the grades of the girls and boys may be compared by use of the techniques described in Chapters 9 and 12, but they cannot be correlated.

As will be seen by referring to the preceding charts in this chapter, the scatter plot is designed so that it will be *approximately* square. This arrangement makes the relationship easier to see; if either dimension of the chart were to be unduly expanded (or compressed) in relation to the other, the existing correlation would not be so readily observed.

It is not necessary, and in fact it is often undesirable, to begin the scales of a scatter plot at zero. Zero should be shown on a scatter-plot scale only if the values of the variable concerned are negative as well as positive or if one or more of the values is zero or very small. The disadvantage of showing zeros, when not needed, on the two scales may be seen by referring to Chart 6.1, in which the smallest height figure is 66 inches and the smallest weight figure is 130 pounds. If Chart 6.1 had been made with both scales beginning at zero, and if it were allowed to occupy the same space as at present, the entire 41 dots would be merely a small smudge in the upper right corner of the chart.

It is often one purpose of a correlation analysis to estimate, by the use of an estimating equation, the values of one variable, referred to as the *dependent variable*, from the values of another variable, referred to as the *independent variable*. The terms *independent* and *dependent* carry no necessary implication concerning cause and effect. Ordinarily, the values of the independent variable are shown on the horizontal axis of the scatter plot, while the values of the dependent variable are on the vertical axis. If one variable is believed to be the cause of the other, the causal series is usually (but not necessarily) placed on the horizontal axis. If the values of one variable are controlled by the investigator while the values of the other variable are free to vary, according to the changes in the controlled variable, the values of the controlled variable should be on the horizontal axis of the scatter plot. Such a situation exists when an investigator studies the relationship of the blood sugar and the body temperature of a group of laboratory animals, the body temperature being brought to selected readings by the use of ice packs and heat.

Another objective of correlation analysis is the determination of the relationship existing between the two variables. The degree of association may be measured by the use of the coefficient of determination, which may have a value as low as zero (indicating no correlation) or as high as 1.0 (indicating perfect correlation). Alternatively, we may use the coefficient of correlation, which is the square root of the coefficient of determination and which varies from 0 to ±1.0. Although the correlation coefficient indicates whether the association is positive or negative, while the coefficient of determination does not, we shall see later that it is easier to put into words the meaning of a given value of the coefficient of determination.

The Estimating Equation[3]

The data of Table 6.1 show the amount of glucose injected intravenously and the amount retained for each of 18 hospital

---
[3] The term "estimating equation" is used throughout this volume in preference to the older and less descriptive term "regression equation."

patients. The scatter plot of Chart 6.7 indicates the presence of high positive linear correlation. Since we are interested in estimating the amount of glucose retained when a specified amount has been injected, the amount injected is the independent variable and we have placed it on the horizontal or X axis. The amount

TABLE 6.1

COMPUTATION OF SUMS FOR CORRELATION OF INTRAVENOUS INJECTIONS OF GLUCOSE (X) AND GLUCOSE RETAINED (Y), BOTH IN GRAMS PER KILOGRAM OF BODY WEIGHT PER HOUR, FOR 18 HOSPITAL PATIENTS

Case	X	Y	X^2	Y^2	XY
1	0.073	0.072	0.005329	0.005184	0.005256
2	.159	.154	.025281	.023716	.024486
3	.222	.217	.049284	.047089	.048174
4	.390	.290	.152100	.084100	.113100
5	.463	.458	.214369	.209764	.212054
6	.512	.500	.262144	.250000	.256000
7	.753	.686	.567009	.470596	.516558
8	.926	.832	.857476	.692224	.770432
9	1.13	.82	1.2769	.6724	.9266
10	1.16	1.04	1.3456	1.0816	1.2064
11	1.193	.871	1.423249	.758641	1.039103
12	1.301	1.065	1.692601	1.134225	1.385565
13	1.323	1.132	1.750329	1.281424	1.497636
14	1.46	1.43	2.1316	2.0449	2.0878
15	1.59	1.44	2.5281	2.0736	2.2896
16	1.824	1.307	3.326976	1.708249	2.383968
17	1.960	1.953	3.841600	3.814209	3.827880
18	2.216	1.565	4.910656	2.449225	3.468040
Total	18.655	15.832	26.360603	18.801146	22.058652

Data from James C. Cain and William P. Belk, "The Assimilation Rate of Intravenously Injected Glucose in Hospital Patients," *American Journal of the Medical Sciences*, Vol. 203, No. 3, March 1942, pp. 359–363. The authors present a total of 22 cases, one of which they reject because the patient was found, on autopsy, to have a carcinoma of the pancreas and was believed to be diabetic. For purpose of illustration, only cases 1–18 are used in this text. Cases 19, 20, and 21 were given (and retained) much more glucose than those shown above. Computations made by the writer gave $r = +0.9653$ for cases 1–18; $r = +0.9777$ for cases 1–19; $r = +0.9920$ for cases 1–20; $r = +0.9991$ for cases 1–21. All relationships were linear.

retained is the dependent variable and it appears on the vertical or Y axis. An unusual feature of our illustration, which is shown clearly in Chart 6.7, is that each value of the Y variable is numerically smaller than the associated value of the X variable.

To estimate the amount of glucose retained, we use the estimating equation

$$Y_c = a + bX,$$

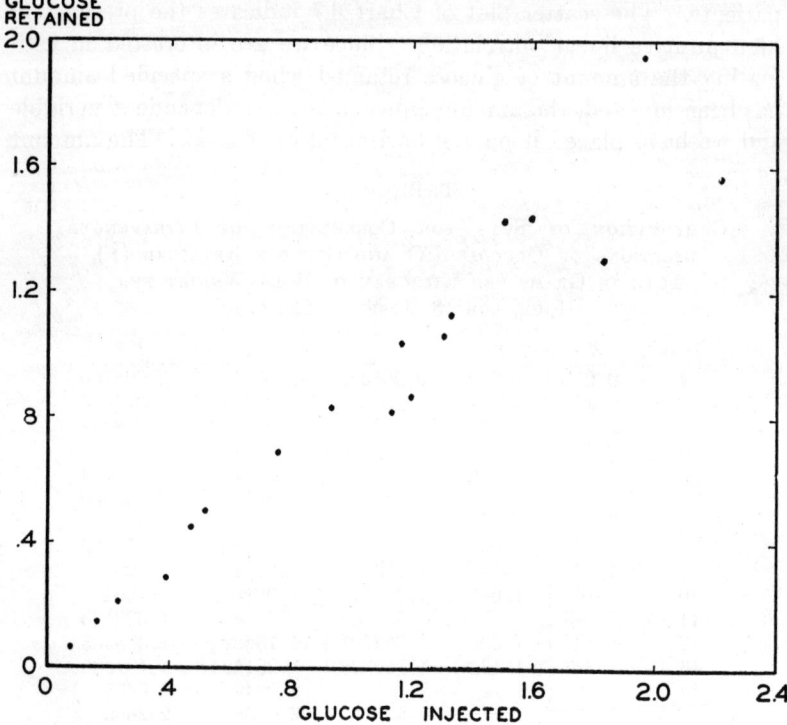

Chart 6.7. Intravenous Injections of Glucose and Glucose Retained, both in Grams per Kilogram of Body Weight per Hour, for 18 Hospital Patients. Data of Table 6.1.

where

Y_c is the estimated amount of glucose retained,
X is the amount of glucose injected,
a is the "Y intercept," that is, the value where the estimating equation intersects the Y axis when X is zero, and
b is the slope of the estimating equation, indicating by its sign the direction of slope (and also whether the correlation is positive or negative) and by its value the amount of change in the Y series for each unit change of the X series.

It is necessary to determine the value of the two unknowns a and b in the estimating equation. This is accomplished by the method of least squares and involves solving the two "normal equations,"

CHAP. 6] LINEAR CORRELATION OF TWO VARIABLES 117

$$\text{I.} \quad \Sigma Y = Na + b\Sigma X.$$
$$\text{II.} \quad \Sigma XY = a\Sigma X + b\Sigma X^2.$$

There are two normal equations because there are two unknowns. If there were three (or more) unknowns, as there are in some types of non-linear correlation and in multiple correlation, three (or more) normal equations would be required. The method of least squares gives values for a and b which so locate the estimating equation $Y_c = a + bX$ that the sum of the squared vertical deviations of each Y-value from the estimating equation [that is, $\Sigma(Y - Y_c)^2$] is less than from any other straight line.[4]

The values which we wish to substitute in the two normal equations are found in Table 6.1, giving:

$$\text{I.} \quad 15.832 \quad = 18a + 18.655b.$$
$$\text{II.} \quad 22.058652 = 18.655a + 26.360603b.$$

If normal equation I is multiplied by 1.036389, and if the resulting equation is subtracted from normal equation II, we cancel out a and can obtain the value of b, thus:

$$\text{II.} \quad 22.058652 = 18.655a + 26.360603b,$$
$$(\text{I} \times 1.036389). \quad 16.408111 = 18.655a + 19.333837b,$$
$$\overline{ 5.650541 = 7.026766b,}$$
$$b = +0.804145.$$

If this value of b is substituted in either normal equation I or normal equation II, we obtain the value of a. Substituting in I,

$$15.832 = 18a + (18.655)(0.804145),$$
$$18a = 0.830675,$$
$$a = 0.046149.$$

---

[4] For a more complete treatment of the normal equations and for mathematical developments, see F. E. Croxton and D. J. Cowden, *Applied General Statistics*, Prentice-Hall, Inc., New York, 1939, pp. 399–404 and 850–852.

Occasionally it may be desired to estimate X values from known Y values, minimizing the squared horizontal deviations $\Sigma(X - X_c)^2$. For this the estimating equation would be

$$X_c = a' + b'Y,$$

and the two normal equations would be written

$$\Sigma X = Na' + b'\Sigma Y;$$
$$\Sigma XY = a'\Sigma Y + b'\Sigma Y^2.$$

118 LINEAR CORRELATION OF TWO VARIABLES [Chap. 6

As a check on our computations, we may substitute the values just obtained for a and for b in normal equation II, giving

$$22.058652 = (18.655)(0.046149) + (26.360603)(0.804145),$$
$$= 22.058657.$$

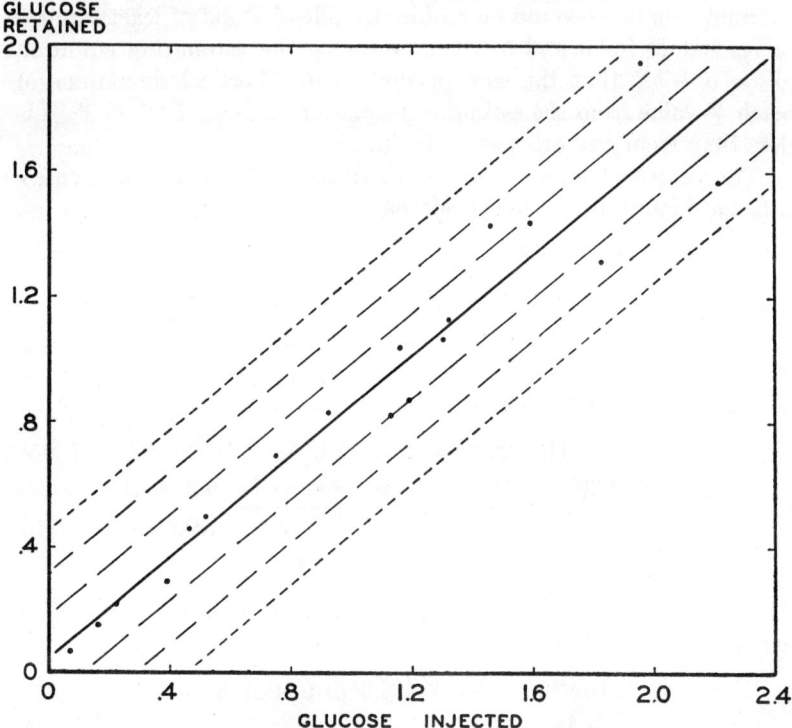

Chart 6.8. Scatter Plot, Estimating Equation (Solid Line), and Zones of $\pm s_{Y.X}$ (Long Dashes), $\pm 2s_{Y.X}$ (Medium Dashes), and $\pm 3s_{Y.X}$ (Short Dashes) for Data of Intravenous Injections of Glucose and Glucose Retained, both in Grams per Kilogram of Body Weight per Hour, for 18 Hospital Patients. Data of Table 6.1.

The estimating equation is

$$Y_c = 0.046 + 0.804X,$$

and it is shown, together with the scatter plot, in Chart 6.8. As an illustration of the use of this equation, suppose that a patient has been given 1.5 grams of glucose per kilogram per hour. What is the estimated amount that will be retained? Since $X = 1.5$, we have

$$Y_c = 0.046 + (0.804)(1.5),$$
$$= 1.252 \text{ grams per kilogram per hour.}$$

It must be recognized that this is an average estimate, and that if a number of patients had actually been given 1.5 grams per kilogram per hour of glucose intravenously, some would retain more than 1.252 grams and some would retain less. As an over-all measure of the accuracy of our estimates, we compute a measure which is very similar to the standard deviation discussed in Chapter 5. This measure is called the *scatter* or the *standard error of estimate* and is based on the difference between each Y value and the Y_c value determined from the paired X value. Symbolically,

$$s_{Y.X} = \sqrt{\frac{\Sigma(Y - Y_c)^2}{N}}$$

and it is apparent that this measure[5] differs from the standard deviation of the Y values $s_Y = \sqrt{\dfrac{\Sigma(Y - \bar{Y})^2}{N}}$ only in that Y_c appears in place of $\bar{Y}$.

If we were to compute $s_{Y.X}$ from the formula just given, it would be necessary to compute Y_c, from the expression $Y_c = a + bX$, eighteen times. In general, for any problem, the value of Y_c would have to be computed N times. To obviate the necessity of repeatedly solving the estimating equation, we rewrite the formula for $s_{Y.X}$, putting $a + bX$ in place of Y_c, giving,

$$s_{Y.X} = \sqrt{\frac{\Sigma[Y - (a + bX)]^2}{N}},$$

which simplifies to

$$s_{Y.X} = \sqrt{\frac{\Sigma Y^2 - (a\Sigma Y + b\Sigma XY)}{N}}.$$

This is a longer expression, but all of the values called for under the radical have already been obtained, and we have

---

[5] Note that $s_{Y.X}$ is analogous to s_Y rather than to $\hat{\sigma}_Y$. That is to say, it is not actually a "standard error" but a "standard deviation."

$$s_{Y.x} = \sqrt{\frac{18.801146 - [(0.046149)(15.832) + (0.804145)(22.058652)]}{18}},$$

$$= 0.136.$$

This measure of the general reliableness of estimates tells us that, if the scatter plot is normal around the estimating equation, we can expect about 68 per cent of the actual values to be within $\pm 1 s_{Y.x}$ (vertically) of the estimating equation, about 95 per cent to be within $\pm 2 s_{Y.x}$, and about 99.7 per cent to be within $\pm 3 s_{Y.x}$. For a set of data such as in our illustration, we need not expect very close agreement with these percentages, first, because the dots of the scatter plot are not normally distributed and, second, because each dot accounts for $\frac{1}{18}$, or 5.6 per cent, of all the dots, and the occurrence of one dot too few or too many in a zone would result in an appreciable departure from the expected percentages. The zone of $\pm 1 s_{Y.x}$ around the estimating equation, shown in Chart 6.8, includes 14, or 77.8 per cent, of the dots in the scatter plot. The two dots which appear to be on the $-s_{Y.x}$ line are actually within the zone of $\pm s_{Y.x}$.

Although $s_{Y.x}$ is, as already noted, a measure of the general reliableness of estimates rather than a specific measure applicable to a particular estimate, it is nevertheless customary to state individual estimates $\pm 1 s_{Y.x}$. Thus, when $X = 1.5$ grams, we would write $Y_c = 1.252 \pm 0.136$.

The coefficient of determination and the coefficient of correlation. Chart 6.9 shows the estimating equation which was just obtained. It also shows one of the dots of the scatter plot, the dot representing case number 15 in Table 6.1, and the value of $\bar{Y}$. For case number 15, $X = 1.59$ grams and $Y = 1.44$ grams. The Y value for the dot shown in Chart 6.9 deviates from $\bar{Y}$ by 0.56 grams, that is, $Y - \bar{Y} = 1.44 - 0.88 = 0.56$ grams. We shall use the term "total deviation" to refer to $Y - \bar{Y}$ for this, or any other, Y value.

By use of the estimating equation $Y_c = 0.046 + 0.804X$ we are able to determine that, when $X = 1.59$ grams, $Y_c = 0.046 + 0.804 (1.59) = 1.32$ grams. This value of Y_c differs from $\bar{Y}$ by 0.44 grams, that is, $Y_c - \bar{Y} = 1.32 - 0.88 = 0.44$ grams. Our estimating equation has enabled us to explain[6] statistically part of the deviation of Y from $\bar{Y}$. Consequently, we shall refer to $Y_c - \bar{Y}$,

---

[6] Note that we are not using *explain* in the sense of "to make plain" or "to expound"; we mean explained statistically or computed. More specifically, "explained deviation" is a label for the $Y_c - \bar{Y}$ line of Chart 6.9.

for this or any other item, as the "explained deviation." Obviously, part of the deviation of Y from $\bar{Y}$ remains unexplained, and that

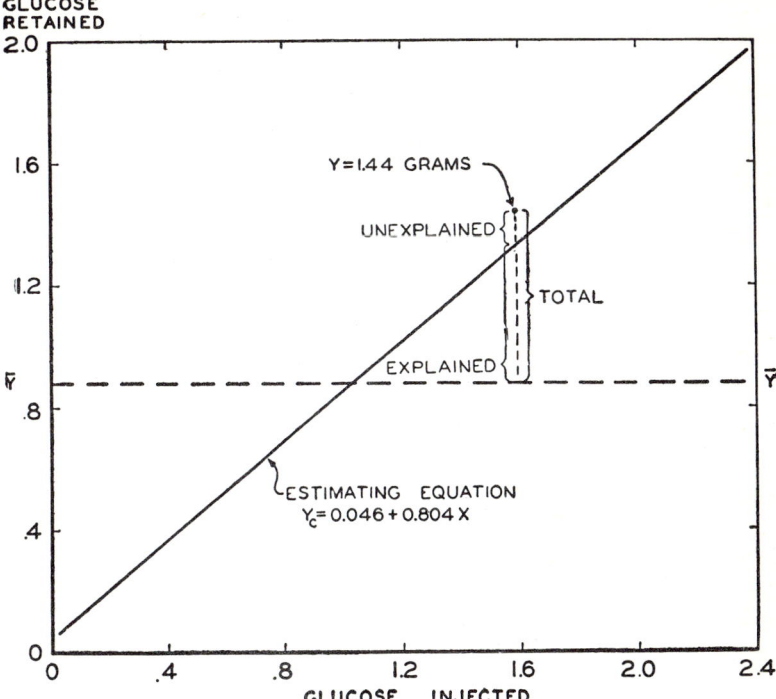

Chart 6.9. Total Deviation, Explained Deviation, and Unexplained Deviation for Case 15 of Table 6.1. For simplicity, this chart shows only the situation in which the explained deviation is less than the total deviation and is in the same direction. There are two other possible situations which are likely to occur in nearly every correlation problem: (1) the explained deviation may be greater than the total deviation, the dot being between the $\bar{Y}$ line and the estimating equation, and (2) the explained deviation may be in the opposite direction from the total deviation, the dot being above the $\bar{Y}$ line if the estimating equation is below the $\bar{Y}$ line, or below the $\bar{Y}$ line if the estimating equation is above the $\bar{Y}$ line.

portion, which is $Y - Y_c$, will be called the "unexplained deviation." It should be noted that, for Case 15:

Explained deviation + unexplained deviation = total deviation,

$$(Y_c - \bar{Y}) \quad + \quad (Y - Y_c) \quad = \quad Y - \bar{Y},$$
$$(1.32 - 0.88) \quad + \quad (1.44 - 1.32) \quad = \quad 1.44 - 0.88,$$
$$0.44 \quad + \quad 0.12 \quad = \quad 0.56.$$

The same would be true for any other case.

Since the estimating equation was fitted by least squares, a process which minimized the sum of the squares of the vertical deviations from the estimating equation, and since we are concerned with all of the dots of the scatter plot rather than with just one, we shall square the deviations and total them for all of the cases concerned. Now, using the term *variation* instead of *deviation*, the resulting sums are:

$$\text{Explained variation, } \Sigma(Y_c - \overline{Y})^2;$$
$$\text{Unexplained variation, } \Sigma(Y - Y_c)^2;$$
$$\text{Total variation, } \Sigma(Y - \overline{Y})^2.$$

For the data of Table 6.1, it is found (by methods described on pages 123–125) that

$$\text{Explained variation} = 4.543862,$$
$$\text{Unexplained variation} = 0.332160,$$
$$\text{Total variation} = 4.876022.$$

Note that explained variation + unexplained variation = total variation,[7] and that we have explained $\dfrac{4.543862}{4.876022}$ of the variation that was present in the Y series. Since $4.543862 \div 4.876022 = 0.9319$, we have explained 93 per cent of the variation in the Y series, and 0.93 is the *coefficient of determination*, r^2. The coefficient of correlation, r, is the square root of the *coefficient of determination* and takes the sign of b in the estimating equation. For our problem, $r = +0.9653$.

The foregoing explanation gives real meaning to a value obtained for a correlation coefficient, since, if we square the correlation coefficient, we obtain the coefficient of determination, which is

$$\frac{\text{explained variation}}{\text{total variation}}.$$

This basic idea holds true for two-variable linear or non-linear correlation and for multiple correlation. For all of these procedures, the coefficient of determination tells us the proportion of the variation present in the dependent variable which has been explained by the use of the estimating equation.

---

[7] A more general demonstration of this equality is given on page 124.

Suppose that the results of a test, designed to measure the ability of prospective employees, correlate +0.60 with the actual performance of employees. This means that $r^2 = 0.36$ and that *only 36 per cent* of the variation in the performance of the employees has been explained.

To return to the data of Table 6.1, if 93 per cent of the variation in the Y series has been explained, then 7 per cent is unexplained. This is the coefficient of non-determination, k^2, and may also be obtained from the expression

$$k^2 = \frac{\text{unexplained variation}}{\text{total variation}} = \frac{\Sigma(Y - Y_c)^2}{\Sigma(Y - \overline{Y})^2} = \frac{0.332160}{4.876022} = 0.07.$$

It must be obvious that, for any set of data, $r^2 + k^2 = 1.0$. However, $r + k \geq 1.0$, being equal to 1.0 only when r or k (the coefficient of alienation) is 1.0 or 0, and under all other conditions greater than 1.0. By now it must also be clear (1) that r^2, and therefore r, can never be greater than 1.0, since we can never explain more than the total variation present in the dependent variable, which would be the situation if the estimating equation passed through all of the dots of the scatter plot, as in Chart 6.5, and (2) that r^2, and therefore r, has zero as its lower limit, since we might explain none of the variation present in the dependent variable, as in Chart 6.6, where the estimating equation would coincide with and therefore be no better than $\overline{Y}$.

The expressions previously given for explained variation, unexplained variation, and total variation were for the purpose of elucidating a concept and not for purposes of computation. The symbol Y_c appears in two of the expressions and (as was pointed out in connection with the discussion of $s_{Y.X}$) would necessitate solving the estimating equation N times in any correlation problem. By substituting $a + bX$ for Y_c and by simplifying, we obtain:

$$\begin{aligned}\text{Explained variation} &= \Sigma(Y_c - \overline{Y})^2, \\ &= \Sigma[(a + bX) - \overline{Y}]^2, \\ &= a\Sigma Y + b\Sigma XY - \frac{(\Sigma Y)^2}{N}.\end{aligned}$$

$$\begin{aligned}\text{Unexplained variation} &= \Sigma(Y - Y_c)^2, \\ &= \Sigma[Y - (a + bX)]^2, \\ &= \Sigma Y^2 - (a\Sigma Y + b\Sigma XY).\end{aligned}$$

An expression for total variation which facilitates computation is obtained as follows:

$$\begin{aligned}
\text{Total variation} &= \Sigma(Y - \bar{Y})^2, \\
&= \Sigma(Y^2 - 2Y\bar{Y} + \bar{Y}^2), \\
&= \Sigma Y^2 - 2\bar{Y}\Sigma Y + N\bar{Y}^2, \\
&= \Sigma Y^2 - 2\frac{\Sigma Y}{N}\Sigma Y + N\left(\frac{\Sigma Y}{N}\right)^2, \\
&= \Sigma Y^2 - \frac{(\Sigma Y)^2}{N}.
\end{aligned}$$

If these three expressions are brought together, it will be clear that explained variation + unexplained variation = total variation, thus:

$$\begin{aligned}
\text{Explained variation} &= a\Sigma Y + b\Sigma XY - \frac{(\Sigma Y)^2}{N}, \\
\text{Unexplained variation} &= \underline{\Sigma Y^2 - (a\Sigma Y + b\Sigma XY),} \\
\text{Total variation} &= \Sigma Y^2 - \frac{(\Sigma Y)^2}{N}.
\end{aligned}$$

In order to avoid needless repetition of the phrases "explained variation," "unexplained variation," and "total variation," we shall henceforth use the symbol Σy_c^2 for explained variation, Σy_s^2 for unexplained variation, and Σy^2 for total variation. Using these symbols, the statement at the end of the preceding paragraph becomes $\Sigma y_c^2 + \Sigma y_s^2 = \Sigma y^2$.

Note that all of the values called for in the three expressions have already been computed; thus, it is a simple matter to obtain the three desired numerical values. These are:

$$\begin{aligned}
\Sigma y_c^2 &= a\Sigma Y + b\Sigma XY - \frac{(\Sigma Y)^2}{N}, \\
&= (0.046149)(15.832) + (0.804145)(22.058652) - \frac{(15.832)^2}{18}, \\
&= 18.468986 - 13.925122, \\
&= 4.543862.
\end{aligned}$$

$$\begin{aligned}
\Sigma y_s^2 &= \Sigma Y^2 - (a\Sigma Y + b\Sigma XY), \\
&= 18.801146 - [(0.046149)(15.832) + (0.804145)(22.058652)], \\
&= 0.332160.
\end{aligned}$$

CHAP. 6] LINEAR CORRELATION OF TWO VARIABLES 125

$$\Sigma y^2 = \Sigma Y^2 - \frac{(\Sigma Y)^2}{N},$$

$$= 18.801146 - \frac{(15.832)^2}{18},$$

$$= 18.801146 - 13.925124,$$

$$= 4.876022.$$

From these we obtain:

$$r^2 = \frac{\Sigma y_c^2}{\Sigma y^2} = \frac{4.543862}{4.876022} = 0.9319 \text{ and}$$

$$r = +0.9653$$

Upon occasion it is desirable to be able to determine the value of r without first ascertaining a and b, since there are times when the value of r may be all that is needed. To do this, we make use of the "Pearson product-moment[8] formula":

$$r = \frac{\Sigma xy}{N s_X s_Y}$$

---

[8] The term "product-moment" is used because the xy products appear in the numerator of the formula and the second moments $\frac{\Sigma x^2}{N}$ and $\frac{\Sigma y^2}{N}$ are used in the denominator.

Although the product-moment formula, which is sometimes written

$$\frac{\Sigma xy}{\sqrt{\Sigma x^2 \Sigma y^2}},$$

is the algebraic equivalent of the square root of the expression previously given for r^2, it can also be explained on a logical basis of its own as follows: The slope of the estimating equation $Y_c = a + bX$ is a measure of the relationship existing between the two variables telling us the number of *units* of change in Y occurring with each change of *one unit* in X. If all of the X values are divided by s_X, if all of the Y values are divided by s_Y, and if the resulting paired $\frac{x}{s_X}$ and $\frac{y}{s_Y}$ values are correlated, the slope of the new estimating equation is the same as r obtained from either the X and Y values or the $\frac{x}{s_X}$ and $\frac{y}{s_Y}$ values. This may be stated another way by saying:

$$b \div \frac{s_Y}{s_X} = r.$$

If now we write our estimating equation $y_c = a + bx$ (using x and y, devia-

but substitute $X - \bar{X}$ for x and $Y - \bar{Y}$ for y, giving

$$r = \frac{\Sigma[(X - \bar{X})(Y - \bar{Y})]}{N s_X s_Y},$$

$$= \frac{\dfrac{\Sigma XY}{N} - \dfrac{\Sigma X}{N} \dfrac{\Sigma Y}{N}}{\sqrt{\dfrac{\Sigma X^2}{N} - \left(\dfrac{\Sigma X}{N}\right)^2} \sqrt{\dfrac{\Sigma Y^2}{N} - \left(\dfrac{\Sigma Y}{N}\right)^2}},$$

$$= \frac{N\Sigma XY - \Sigma X \Sigma Y}{\sqrt{[N\Sigma X^2 - (\Sigma X)^2][N\Sigma Y^2 - (\Sigma Y)^2]}}.$$

This expression calls only for summations already obtained in Table 6.1. These give

$$r = \frac{18(22.058652) - (18.655)(15.832)}{\sqrt{[18(26.360603) - (18.655)^2][18(18.801146) - (15.832)^2]}},$$
$$= +0.9653.$$

When negative correlation is present, the sign will appear in the numerator either because $\Sigma X \Sigma Y$ exceeds $N\Sigma XY$ or (rarely) because ΣXY is negative. ΣXY can be negative only if one or both of the series includes negative values.

---

tions from $\bar{X}$ and $\bar{Y}$, in place of X and Y), we obtain the two normal equations:

I. $\Sigma y = Na + b\Sigma x.$
II. $\Sigma xy = a\Sigma x + b\Sigma x^2.$

But $\Sigma x = 0$ and $\Sigma y = 0$; therefore, these become:

I. $a = 0.$
II. $b = \dfrac{\Sigma xy}{\Sigma x^2}.$

Now, dividing b by $\dfrac{s_Y}{s_X}$, we have:

$$b \div \frac{s_Y}{s_X} = \frac{\Sigma xy}{\Sigma x^2} \div \frac{s_Y}{s_X} = \frac{(\Sigma xy)(s_X)}{(\Sigma x^2)(s_Y)},$$
$$= \frac{(\Sigma xy)(s_X)}{N s_X^2 s_Y} = \frac{\Sigma xy}{N s_X s_Y},$$

which is the product-moment formula.

Some Cautions

Correlation and causation. The presence of correlation between two sets of data does not necessarily mean that causation is present even though the correlation may be high. A high positive correlation coefficient merely tells us that low and high values of one series are, respectively, associated with low and high values of the other series; a high negative correlation coefficient indicates that low and high values of one series are, respectively, associated with high and low values of the other series. Correlation may be present as the result of any one of several conditions.

1. *Correlation may be fortuitous.* The situation pictured in Chart 6.6 shows no correlation. If samples of three pairs of values were to be drawn from the nine pairs of values shown in the chart, one might obtain those represented by the dot in the lower left corner, the central dot, and the dot in the upper right corner. These three would have $r = +1.0$! If, for a group of male students, one were to record the height and the amount of change in the pockets of each, a high positive or negative correlation might be found. There is no reason to believe that these two variables should be correlated, but occasionally, by chance, a sizeable correlation would appear. In Chapter 12 we shall consider a method of ascertaining whether an observed correlation coefficient differs significantly from zero.

2. *One variable is the cause, although not necessarily the sole cause, of the other.* Such a situation is present in the data of Chart 6.7; although the correlation is not perfect (that is, not $+1.0$), the amount of glucose retained is a direct result of the amount injected by the physician.

3. *The two variables may be interdependent.* There may be a reciprocal cause-and-effect relationship present, so that each series is to some extent the cause of the other. Such a situation is common in business, where price changes bring about production changes and these in turn result in further price changes.

4. *The two variables may be affected by the same cause.* One underlying cause, or several such causes, may influence the two variables similarly, or the effect may be such as to increase one variable but to decrease the other. Although the correlation shown in Chart 6.4 is low, it is nevertheless attributable to the fact that each pair of twins had the same parents and, therefore, in a very crude sense,

the same general inheritance pattern. If we were to correlate the IQ's of a group of identical male twins (letting the X values be the IQ's of the first-born[9] and the Y values the IQ's of the second-born), we would expect to obtain a high positive r. Now, each pair of twins not only had the same parents but, being monozygotic, had the same inheritance pattern and would be expected to be much alike in regard to IQ as well as in regard to other characteristics.

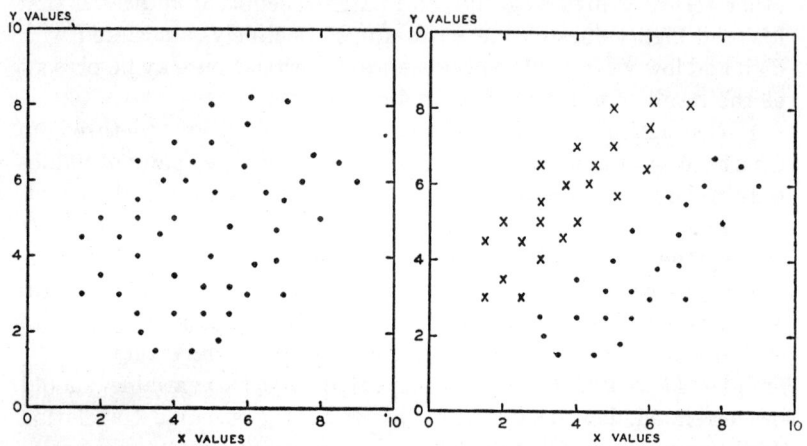

Chart 6.10A. Illustrative Scatter Plot Showing Low Correlation: Two Dissimilar Groups Not Identified.

Chart 6.10B. Same Scatter Plot as in Chart 6.10A, but Indicating Fairly High Correlation for Each of Two Dissimilar Groups shown by Crosses and Dots.

Heterogeneity. The data which are to be correlated should always be homogeneous. Heterogeneity may be present because the data include two or more groups, such as males and females, healthy persons and sick persons, or children and adults. These are some of the most obvious sources of heterogeneity; there are many others. Chart 6.10A shows an illustrative scatter plot indicating low correlation. In Chart 6.10B the two component groups are shown by means of different symbols, and it is seen that two fairly high correlations are present. It is also possible that two different groups, each having little or no correlation, could be so located on a scatter

---

[9] Often we do not know which twin was first-born and which second-born. A method of correlating paired values when we are unable to say which of each pair belongs in the X series and which in the Y series is given on pages 138-140.

CHAP. 6] LINEAR CORRELATION OF TWO VARIABLES 129

plot that, if they were combined, moderate positive (or negative) correlation would appear to be present.

Another sort of heterogeneity is shown in Chart 6.11. In this chart the nature of the data and the source are omitted in order to avoid possible embarrassment to the person responsible. There are nine clustered dots in Chart 6.11 which show low correlation, $r = +0.32$, and one dot far removed from the others. For all ten dots, $r = +0.79$. The presence of a single, almost certainly non-homogeneous (or, at least, non-comparable) observation such as this may result in an even higher correlation coefficient when little or no correlation exists for the other observations. It is altogether possible that Chart 6.11 illustrates also the sort of heterogeneity mentioned in the preceding paragraph; the upper four dots of the cluster of nine may represent a category different from that represented by the lower five dots. In any event, the investigator should look into that possibility.

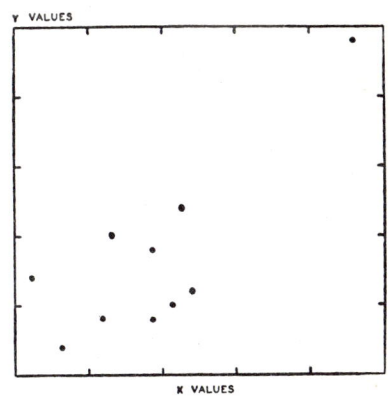

Chart 6.11. Scatter Plot Illustrating a Type of Heterogeneity. Source and nature of data withheld.

It should be fairly obvious that the reverse of the situation shown in Chart 6.11 might also occur. That is to say, a cluster of dots might show high correlation, but one extreme dot might be so located that its inclusion with the others would result in low correlation. Chart 6.4 shows a situation in which a low correlation is made even lower through the inclusion of an extreme pair of values. The values of r are given below Chart 6.4.

Use of averages. Chart 6.12 shows data of the coagulation time of plasma in relation to temperature. From 19° to 28° centigrade, the correlation appears to be high and non-linear. However, each figure of coagulation time is an average of a varying number of readings, so that the closeness of the relationship is more apparent than real. The use of averages of Y values results in decreasing the unexplained variation, $\Sigma(Y - Y_c)^2$, and therefore increases the value of r. It has not been possible to obtain the 180 individual

130 LINEAR CORRELATION OF TWO VARIABLES [Chap. 6

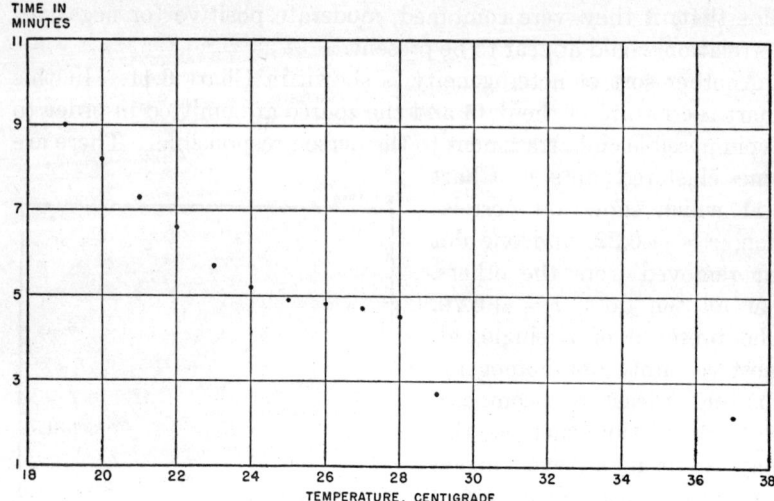

Chart 6.12. Temperature and Average Coagulation Time. Source and exact nature of data withheld.

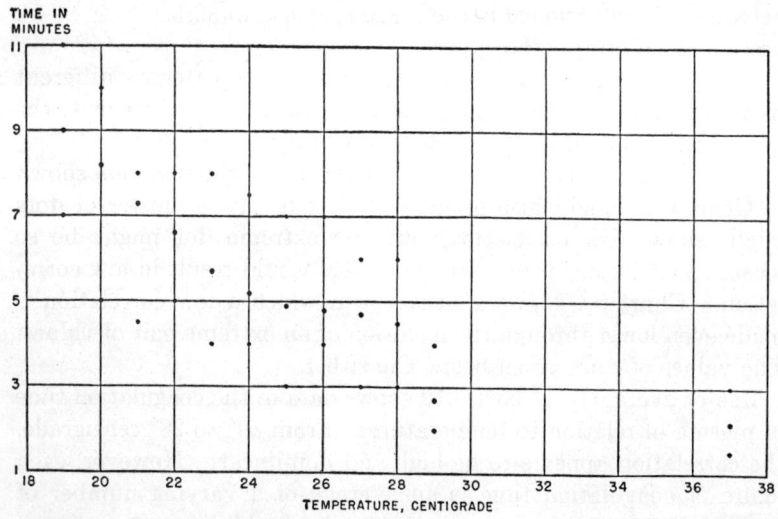

Chart 6.13. Average, Maximum, and Minimum Coagulation Times at Specified Temperatures. Source and exact nature of data withheld.

CHAP. 6] LINEAR CORRELATION OF TWO VARIABLES 131

observations from which the 12 averages were computed, but we do know the shortest and longest coagulation time for each temperature. These are shown, together with the averages, in Chart 6.13, and it is clear that the correlation is not nearly as high as it appeared to be in Chart 6.12, where only the averages were given. Furthermore, the limited additional information given by the high and low values causes the non-linearity to be less pronounced, although one would expect a non-linear relationship for these variables.

If averages of X values are correlated with individual Y values, the result is the same: to increase the value of r over what it would be for the individual X and Y values. Similarly, if averages of subgroups are used for both the X and the Y series, the value of r will be increased, but the difference decreases as the number of subgroups increases.

Correlation of Grouped Data

The illustrative problem of Table 6.1 and Chart 6.7 involved but 18 pairs of values. If we had had, say, 1800 pairs, the computations necessary to obtain the sums, sums of squares, and sums of products would have been extensive and time-consuming. We would have had to compute 1800 products, look up[10] or compute 3600 squares, and obtain 5 totals each consisting of 1800 items. After the five totals were obtained, the work would be no more arduous than for a problem involving fewer pairs of values.

In Chapter 3 we compressed raw data into a frequency distribution. We shall adopt a similar procedure here, using what is sometimes called a "two-way frequency distribution." We shall correlate the hip-girth (X) and weight (Y) for 9,941 white women. The *correlation table* or two-way frequency distribution for these data is shown as Table 6.2. Perhaps it is well to make clear at this point that a correlation table does not come "ready-made." It may be constructed by hand-scoring of the information from record forms to a tally sheet similar to, but larger than, Table 6.2; it may be obtained by hand-sorting of record cards; it may be gotten

---

[10] In Appendix XI, which gives squares of numbers from 1 to 1,000, or in *Barlow's Tables of Squares, Cubes, Square Roots, Cube Roots, and Reciprocals of all Integer Numbers up to 12,500*, Chemical Publishing Co., Inc., Brooklyn, N. Y., 1941.

132 LINEAR CORRELATION OF TWO VARIABLES [Chap. 6

TABLE 6.2

Correlation Table of Hip Girth and Weight for 9,941 White Women

Hip Girth in Inches

Weight in Pounds	32.5	34.5	36.5	38.5	40.5	42.5	44.5	46.5	48.5	50.5
220						1	9	13	20	10
210						3	15	30	18	6
200					3	13	36	33	20	2
190					8	51	74	55	14	1
180			1	1	29	112	126	37	7	1
170				1	11	111	204	81	10	
160				2	63	286	257	61	6	
150			1	21	242	450	135	16		
140			5	134	683	434	48	1		
130			29	565	936	156	9			
120		10	252	1,225	390	14				
110		30	786	636	70	2				
100		169	445	63	2					
90		102	38							

Data from U. S. Department of Agriculture, Miscellaneous Publication #454, *Women's Measurements for Garment and Pattern Construction*, by Ruth O'Brien and William C. Shelton, p. 67. Not included in the above table are 57 women having hip girth of less than 31.5 inches and/or weighing less than 85 pounds and 44 women having hip girth of 51.5 inches or more and/or weighing 230 pounds or more. In the weight class having a mid-value of 220 pounds, the above table includes a very small number of women weighing 225–230 pounds. The exact number could not be ascertained and therefore could not be eliminated.

mechanically from punched cards.[11] The data of Table 6.2, together with many other women's measurements, were assembled in this manner.

When a correlation analysis is being made from grouped data, we must do without a scatter plot. We can have only the correlation table, which is a very inadequate substitute for a scatter plot. From the correlation table one can get an idea whether positive or negative correlation is present, but it is often difficult to say from visual inspection of a correlation table whether the correlation is moderate or high. Note that the classes along the vertical edge of the correlation table increase from bottom to top rather than from top to bottom. Although this is the reverse of the usual arrangement of a frequency distribution (used in Chapters 3, 4, and 5), it is customary in order that positive correlation may show

---

[11] When punch-card equipment is available, or when it may be made use of at moderate cost, one has the alternative of using the procedure for ungrouped data, described earlier in this chapter.

an upward slope from left to right and negative correlation a downward slope from left to right as on a scatter plot.

It is possible, working from Table 6.2, to set up and solve the two normal equations[12] as was done for ungrouped data, but that procedure is not recommended, since it is too laborious. It is much better first to obtain r, then the estimating equation, and then $s_{Y.X}$.

The expression previously used to obtain the correlation coefficient for ungrouped data was

$$r = \frac{N\Sigma XY - \Sigma X \Sigma Y}{\sqrt{[N\Sigma X^2 - (\Sigma X)^2][N\Sigma Y^2 - (\Sigma Y)^2]}}.$$

It is possible to introduce the symbol f (meaning frequency, as heretofore) into this expression, giving

$$r = \frac{\Sigma fXY - \Sigma f_X X \Sigma f_Y Y}{\sqrt{[N\Sigma f_X X^2 - (\Sigma f_X X)^2][N\Sigma f_Y Y^2 - (\Sigma f_Y Y)^2]}},$$

where:

X and Y are class mid-values,
f is the frequency in a box or cell,
f_X is a column frequency, and
f_Y is a row frequency.

However, the use of this expression would involve rather large numbers and, consequently, the expenditure of more time than necessary. When computing the arithmetic mean, the standard deviation, and the moments of a frequency distribution, we found it advantageous to make use of an arbitrary origin. We shall do the same thing here, using arbitrary origins (or assumed means) for the X series and the Y series. The expression for r then becomes

$$r = \frac{N\Sigma f d'_X d'_Y - \Sigma f_X d'_X \Sigma f_Y d'_Y}{\sqrt{[N\Sigma f_X (d'_X)^2 - (\Sigma f_X d'_X)^2][N\Sigma f_Y (d'_Y)^2 - (\Sigma f_Y d'_Y)^2]}},$$

where d'_X and d'_Y are deviations in terms of classes from $\overline{X}_d$ and $\overline{Y}_d$, respectively, as shown in Table 6.3. Observe that all computations are in terms of class intervals, the numerator and denominator both

---

[12] See F. E. Croxton and D. J. Cowden, *Applied General Statistics*, Prentice-Hall, Inc., New York, 1939, p. 675, note 18.

TABLE 6.3

COMPUTATION OF VALUES FOR CORRELATION OF HIP GIRTH AND WEIGHT FOR 9,941 WHITE WOMEN

Hip Girth in Inches (columns); Weight in Pounds (rows)

Weight in Pounds	32.5	34.5	36.5	38.5	40.5	42.5	44.5	46.5	48.5	50.5	f_Y	d'_Y	$f_Y d'_Y$	$f_Y (d'_Y)^2$
220						1 *+8* **8**	9 *+16* **144**	13 *+24* **312**	20 *+32* **640**	10 *+40* **400**	53	+8	+424	3,392
210						3 *+7* **21**	15 *+14* **210**	30 *+21* **630**	18 *+28* **504**	6 *+35* **210**	72	+7	+504	3,528
200					3	13 *+6* **78**	36 *+12* **432**	33 *+18* **594**	20 *+24* **480**	2 *+30* **60**	107	+6	+642	3,852
190					8	51 *+5* **255**	74 *+10* **740**	55 *+15* **825**	14 *+20* **280**	1 *+25* **25**	203	+5	+1,015	5,075
180			1 *−8* **−8**	1 *−4* **−4**	29	112 *+4* **448**	126 *+8* **1,008**	37 *+12* **444**	7 *+16* **112**	1 *+20* **20**	314	+4	+1,256	5,024
170			1 *−6* **−6**	11 *−3* **−33**	111	204 *+3* **612**	81 *+6* **486**	10 *+9* **90**			418	+3	+1,254	3,762
160			2 *−4* **−8**	63 *−2* **−126**	286	257 *+2* **514**	61 *+4* **244**	6 *+6* **36**			675	+2	+1,350	2,700
150		1 *−3* **−3**	21 *−2* **−42**	242 *−1* **−242**	450	135 *+1* **135**	16 *+2* **32**				865	+1	+865	865
140		5	134	683	434	48	1				1,305	+0		
130		29 *+3* **87**	565 *+2* **1,130**	936 *+1* **936**	156	9 *−1* **−9**					1,695	−1	−1,695	1,695
120	10 *+8* **80**	252 *+6* **1,512**	1,225 *+4* **4,900**	390 *+2* **780**	14						1,891	−2	−3,782	7,564
110	30 *+12* **360**	786 *+9* **7,074**	636 *+6* **3,816**	70 *+3* **210**	2						1,524	−3	−4,572	13,716
100	169 *+16* **2,704**	445 *+12* **5,340**	63 *+8* **504**	2 *÷4* **8**							679	−4	−2,716	10,864
90	102 *+20* **2,040**	38 *+15* **570**									140	−5	−700	3,500
f_X	311	1,556	2,648	2,398	1,493	833	419	184	79	20	$N = 9{,}941$		$\Sigma f_Y d'_Y = -6{,}155$	$\Sigma f_Y (d'_Y)^2 = 65{,}537$
d'_X	−4	−3	−2	−1	0	+1	+2	+3	+4	+5				
$f_X d'_X$	−1,244	−4,668	−5,296	−2,398		+833	+838	+552	+316	+100	$\Sigma f_X d'_X = -10{,}967$		$\Sigma f d'_X d'_Y = +42{,}599$	
$f_X (d'_X)^2$	4,976	14,004	10,592	2,398		833	1,676	1,656	1,264	500	$\Sigma f_X (d'_X)^2 = 37{,}899$			

being in terms of $i_X i_Y$, that is, the product of the class interval on the X axis and the class interval on the Y axis.

In order to work with as small figures as possible, the origin on each axis has been taken near the center, as indicated by the pairs of double lines in Table 6.3. The various summations called for in the formula for r are all rather obvious if reference is made to Table 6.3. All, that is, except, perhaps, $\Sigma f d'_X d'_Y$. This is a summation obtained from individual computations for each of the various cells. Consider the cell in the upper right corner of Table 6.3, which has $f = 10$. This cell has $d'_X = +5$ and $d'_Y = +8$, so that $d'_X d'_Y = +40$, the value shown in italics at the top of the cell. Since $f = 10$, $f d'_X d'_Y = +400$, the value shown in boldface at the bottom of the cell. In similar fashion, $f d'_X d'_Y$ is obtained for the other cells and their sum $\Sigma f d'_X d'_Y$ obtained as shown in the lower right corner of Table 6.3. It takes a little time to obtain this summation, but it, with the rest of the numerator in our expression for r, takes the place of 9,941 multiplications. Substituting the values shown in the lower right portion of the table in the formula for r gives

$$r = \frac{N \Sigma f d'_X d'_Y - \Sigma f_X d'_X \Sigma f_Y d'_Y}{\sqrt{[N \Sigma f_X (d'_X)^2 - (\Sigma f_X d'_X)^2][N \Sigma f_Y (d'_Y)^2 - (\Sigma f_Y d'_Y)^2]}},$$

$$= \frac{9{,}941(+42{,}599) - (-10{,}967)(-6{,}155)}{\sqrt{[9{,}941(37{,}899) - (-10{,}967)^2][9{,}941(65{,}537) - (-6{,}155)^2]}},$$

$$= \frac{423{,}476{,}659 - 67{,}501{,}885}{\sqrt{(256{,}478{,}870)(613{,}619{,}292)}},$$

$$= \frac{355{,}974{,}774}{396{,}712{,}019} = +0.8973.$$

The value of r obtained from a correlation table will, of course, not be exactly the same as if the correlation coefficient had been computed from the ungrouped data. The value of r computed from the grouped data will tend to be slightly smaller. Referring to the expression

$$r = \frac{\Sigma xy}{N s_X s_Y}$$

may help to clarify this point. Because of grouping errors (see Chapter 5), s_X and s_Y computed from grouped data will tend to be too large. On the other hand, the grouping errors involved in the

xy-products will tend to cancel out. Satisfactory results will be obtained from the grouped correlation formula only if N is large and if a reasonably large number of cells is used in the correlation table. In the publication from which the hip girth and weight data were taken, hip girths were given in one-inch classes and weights were presented in 5-pound classes. The data were compressed into 2-inch and 10-pound classes for our illustration in order that Table 6.3 might fit on a single printed page. A correlation coefficient computed from the ungrouped data of hip girth and weight, but including also the 101 very small and very large women omitted from Table 6.2, was found[13] to be +0.9190.

To obtain the estimating equation, we refer to footnote 8 in this chapter, where it was indicated (1) that if the estimating equation is written $y_c = a + bx$, the value of a is zero, and (2) that $b \div \dfrac{s_Y}{s_X} = r$. From the first of these equations we may write $y_c = bx$, from the second $b = r\dfrac{s_Y}{s_X}$, and, bringing the two together,

$$y_c = r\frac{s_Y}{s_X} x.$$

Since $y_c = Y_c - \bar{Y}$ and $x = X - \bar{X}$, the estimating equation becomes

$$Y_c - \bar{Y} = r\frac{s_Y}{s_X}(X - \bar{X}).$$

From the computations already made in Table 6.3, we obtain

$$\bar{X} = \bar{X}_d + \frac{\Sigma f_x d'_x}{N} i_x,$$

$$= 40.5 - \frac{10{,}967}{9{,}941} 2,$$

$$= 38.29 \text{ inches, and}$$

---

[13] See Table 5 of the reference cited below Table 6.2.

CHAP. 6] LINEAR CORRELATION OF TWO VARIABLES 137

$$\bar{Y} = \bar{Y}_d + \frac{\Sigma f_Y d'_Y}{N} i_Y,$$

$$= 140 - \frac{6{,}155}{9{,}941} 10,$$

$$= 133.81 \text{ pounds.}$$

We use the expressions

$$s_X = i_X \sqrt{\frac{\Sigma f_X (d'_X)^2}{N} - \left(\frac{\Sigma f_X d'_X}{N}\right)^2} \text{ and}$$

$$s_Y = i_Y \sqrt{\frac{\Sigma f_Y (d'_Y)^2}{N} - \left(\frac{\Sigma f_Y d'_Y}{N}\right)^2}$$

to determine the values of s_X and s_Y. These are the same as used in Chapter 5 for computing the standard deviation of a frequency distribution. Here, however, we use the subscripts "$_X$" and "$_Y$" to identify the two series. Substituting gives

$$s_X = 2 \sqrt{\frac{37{,}899}{9{,}941} - \left(\frac{10{,}967}{9{,}941}\right)^2},$$

$$= 3.2220 \text{ inches, and}$$

$$s_Y = 10 \sqrt{\frac{65{,}537}{9{,}941} - \left(\frac{6{,}155}{9{,}941}\right)^2},$$

$$= 24.918 \text{ pounds.}$$

We may now obtain the estimating equation:

$$Y_c - \bar{Y} = r \frac{s_Y}{s_X}(X - \bar{X}),$$

$$Y_c - 133.81 = +0.8973 \frac{24.918}{3.2220}(X - 38.29),$$

$$Y_c = +6.9395(X - 38.29) + 133.81,$$
$$= -131.90 + 6.9395X.$$

To obtain the value of $s_{Y \cdot X}$, we make use of the expression[14]

$$s_{Y \cdot X} = s_Y \sqrt{1 - r^2}.$$

---

[14] In an earlier part of this chapter it was noted that $\Sigma y_c^2 + \Sigma y_s^2 = \Sigma y^2$ and

Substituting the values of s_Y and r, which have already been computed, gives

$$s_{Y \cdot X} = 24.918 \sqrt{1 - (0.8973)^2},$$
$$= 10.99 \text{ pounds.}$$

Suppose that a woman has a hip girth of 39 inches. What is the estimate of her weight? It is

$$Y_c = -131.90 + 6.9395\,(39),$$
$$= -131.90 + 270.64,$$
$$= 138.7 \text{ pounds.}$$

Using the standard error of estimate, the estimate would be written 138.7 ± 11.0 pounds.

If it occurs to the reader that he could make a more exact estimate of the weight of the lady by looking at her, the answer is that he has no opportunity to look at her. The only available information is her hip girth. If he could look at her, he might possibly make a better estimate of her weight, but it is interesting to note that he would (unconsciously) be using multiple correlation.

Intraclass Correlation

Instances occur in which there are two sets of paired values but where it is not possible to say in which set each item of a pair belongs. Data of this type are shown in Table 6.4, which gives the IQ's of a group of 13 identical (monozygotic) male twins. The first pair of twins had IQ's of 97 and 96, but the assignment of one

---

that $r^2 = \dfrac{\Sigma y_c^2}{\Sigma y^2}$. Therefore,

$$r^2 = \frac{\Sigma y^2 - \Sigma y_s^2}{\Sigma y^2},$$

$$= 1 - \frac{\Sigma y_s^2}{\Sigma y^2}.$$

$$\frac{\Sigma y_s^2}{\Sigma y^2} = 1 - r^2.$$

$$\Sigma y_s^2 = \Sigma y^2 (1 - r^2).$$

Dividing by N,

$$s_{Y \cdot X}^2 = s_Y^2 (1 - r^2).$$
$$s_{Y \cdot X} = s_Y \sqrt{1 - r^2}.$$

LINEAR CORRELATION OF TWO VARIABLES

TABLE 6.4

INTELLIGENCE QUOTIENTS OF 13 PAIRS OF IDENTICAL MALE TWINS

Pair number*	X	Y	XY	X^2	Y^2
2	97	96	9,312	9,409	9,216
3	116	113	13,108	13,456	12,769
8	77	83	6,391	5,929	6,889
10	126	127	16,002	15,876	16,129
12	91	93	8,463	8,281	8,649
13	93	95	8,835	8,649	9,025
20	76	81	6,156	5,776	6,561
23	99	103	10,197	9,801	10,609
24	92	99	9,108	8,464	9,801
33	84	84	7,056	7,056	7,056
41	97	97	9,409	9,409	9,409
43	107	100	10,700	11,449	10,000
44	117	105	12,285	13,689	11,025
Total	1,272	1,276	127,022	127,244	127,138

* Missing numbers from 1 to 45 were identical female twins.
Data from A. H. Wingfield, *Twins and Orphans*, pp. 119–121, J. M. Dent and Sons, Ltd., London and Toronto, 1928.

of the IQ values to the X column and the other to the Y column of the table is strictly arbitrary. (We do not know which twin of any pair was born first.) In spite of the fact that the two separate sets of data cannot be identified, it may be desirable to know the amount of correlation present. Correlation of data of this sort is referred to as *intraclass correlation* to distinguish it from the type of correlation discussed in earlier pages and termed *interclass correlation*. The intraclass correlation coefficient r' is not affected by transposition of one or more pairs between columns X and Y. It is

$$r' = \frac{\Sigma[(X - \overline{XY})(Y - \overline{XY})]}{Ns^2},$$

where:

N is the number of pairs of items,

$\overline{XY}$ is the arithmetic mean of all the $2N$ values $\dfrac{\Sigma X + \Sigma Y}{2N}$, and

s^2 is the standard deviation squared of all the $2N$ values

$$\frac{\Sigma(X - \overline{XY})^2 + \Sigma(Y - \overline{XY})^2}{2N}.$$

140 LINEAR CORRELATION OF TWO VARIABLES [Chap. 6]

Substituting the expressions for $\overline{XY}$ and s^2 in the formula for r', the value of the intraclass correlation coefficient may be computed from

$$r' = \frac{2\Sigma XY - \frac{(\Sigma X + \Sigma Y)^2}{2N}}{\Sigma X^2 + \Sigma Y^2 - \frac{(\Sigma X + \Sigma Y)^2}{2N}}.$$

For the data of Table 6.4, we have

$$r' = \frac{2(127{,}022) - \frac{(1{,}272 + 1{,}276)^2}{26}}{127{,}244 + 127{,}138 - \frac{(1{,}272 + 1{,}276)^2}{26}}$$

$$= \frac{254{,}044 - 249{,}704}{254{,}382 - 249{,}704} = \frac{4{,}340}{4{,}678} = +0.9277.$$

Since there is no way of assigning either one of a pair of items to the X or Y series, it follows that we can have no scatter plot and no estimating equation.

Rank Correlation

Sometimes we wish to correlate data which are available only in terms of ranks, as in Table 6.5. If the actual frequency rates and severity rates were available, it would, of course, be preferable to correlate those rates. However, we have only the ranks given in Table 6.5.

We could obtain the correlation coefficient for the data of Table 6.5 by using the product-moment formula

$$r = \frac{\Sigma xy}{N s_X s_Y}$$

or any of the various modifications of it which were given earlier. However, when the two series to be correlated consist of ranks (none of which are tied, for example, 7 and 8 not being replaced by $7\frac{1}{2}$ and $7\frac{1}{2}$), this expression may be reduced to

$$r_{\text{rank}} = 1 - \frac{6\Sigma D^2}{N(N^2 - 1)},$$

TABLE 6.5

Rank, According to Frequency and Severity Rates, of Accidents in Identical Establishments in 30 Manufacturing Industries, 1935

Industry	Frequency	Severity	D	D^2
Agricultural implements	25	21	4	16
Automobiles	3	5	− 2	4
Automobile tires and rubber goods	12	4	8	64
Boots and shoes	2	1	1	1
Brick, tile, and terra cotta	26	24	2	4
Carpets and rugs	5	9	− 4	16
Chemicals	7	25	−18	324
Cotton goods	6	3	3	9
Electrical machinery, apparatus, and supplies	1	7	− 6	36
Fertilizers	28	28	0	0
Flour, feed, and other grain-mill products	20	26	− 6	36
Foundry and machine-shop products	23	22	1	1
Furniture	15	20	− 5	25
Glass	17	9	8	64
Hardware	19	6	13	169
Iron and steel	8	11	− 3	9
Leather	18	14	4	16
Logging	30	30	0	0
Lumber:				
Planing mills	27	27	0	0
Sawmills	29	29	0	0
Machine tools	13	13	0	0
Paper and pulp	22	23	− 1	1
Petroleum refining	4	16	−12	144
Pottery	9	2	7	49
Shipbuilding, steel and wood	10	18	− 8	64
Slaughtering and meat packing	21	15	6	36
Stamped and enameled ware	14	17	− 3	9
Steam fittings, apparatus, and supplies	16	12	4	16
Stoves	24	19	5	25
Woolen goods	11	9	2	4
Total	...	...	0	1,142

The lowest rate is ranked first, the second lowest second, and so forth. The injury frequency rate is the average number of disabling injuries for each million man-hours worked. The injury severity rate is the average number of days lost for each thousand man-hours worked. The term "injury" connotes a disability which involves loss of time beyond the day or shift on which the injury occurred, or a permanent impairment of some member of the body, even if not accompanied by lost time.

Data from *Monthly Labor Review*, March 1938, p. 680.

where D is the difference between the ranks of paired values. The correlation of the ranks will yield the same value for r as the correlation of the data from which the ranks were obtained only if the actual differences underlying any two adjacent ranks are constant. This, of course, is rarely true,[15] and r_{rank} must ordinarily be considered as merely an approximation of the value which would have been obtained if we could have had the underlying data. For the ranks of Table 6.5,

$$r_{\text{rank}} = 1 - \frac{6(1142)}{30(900-1)},$$
$$= +0.746.$$

It is possible to make a scatter plot of ranked data, the scales on the two axes being the ranks applicable to the problem, in this case the ranks 1–30. The equation for estimating values of Y from known values of X is very simply written:

$$Y_c - \overline{Y} = r_{\text{rank}}(X - \overline{X})$$

because the two standard deviations are the same. The standard error of estimate could be obtained as for grouped data:

$$s_{Y.X} = s_Y \sqrt{1 - r_{\text{rank}}^2}.$$

In using these last two expressions, it should be remembered that the ranks with which we are concerned are discrete and (except when tied ranks occur) will always be integers. These two formulas will not often yield integers when they are used.

The rank correlation coefficient is sometimes used as a probing tool, to obtain an approximation of the correlation coefficient for data *which are not expressed in ranks*. To the writer, this seems an undesirable practice, first, because time is wasted in obtaining the

---

[15] It would be rather surprising if the first differences of the values of each series, from which the ranks were obtained or which the ranks stand in place of, were a constant. One possibility (there are many others) is that the gaps between the adjacent ranks of the series are wider at the ends of the series and narrower in the middle, so that a normal distribution is present. On this assumption, a correction has been devised to correct r_{rank} to the value that would have been obtained by correlating the underlying data. The correction always increases r_{rank}, but never as much as 0.02. Tables of corrected values of r_{rank} are to be found in various textbooks.

CHAP. 6] LINEAR CORRELATION OF TWO VARIABLES 143

ranks for the two series and, second, because a scatter plot of the data before ranking is at least as good, and sometimes better,[16] for the purpose.

Correlation measures have been devised for numerous other arrangements of data. For example, when one variable is divided into two categories while the other variable is quantitative, bi-serial r may be employed; when both variables are classified into several categories, the coefficient of mean square contingency may be used. These measures are not discussed in this volume, but we shall proceed in Chapter 7 to consider non-linear and multiple correlation.

---

[16] For instance, r_{rank} could have a value of $+1.0$ while the data from which the ranks were made could have $r < +1.0$. This is true of the data of Chart 6.3.

Symbols Used in

CHAPTER 7

Each listed coefficient of determination, r^2 or R^2, has an associated coefficient of correlation, r or R, and vice versa.

Non-Linear Correlation

a: value of Y_c when $X = 0$ in the estimating equations $Y_c = a + bX$ and $Y_c = a + bX + cX^2$; value of Y_c when $X = 1$ in the estimating equation $Y_c = a + b \log X$. Log a is the value of log Y_c when $X = 0$ in the estimating equation $\log Y_c = \log a + X \log b$ and when $X = 1$ in the estimating equation $\log Y_c = \log a + b \log X$.

b: a constant in the estimating equations $Y_c = a + bX$, $Y_c = a + b \log X$, $\log Y_c = \log a + b \log X$, and $Y_c = a + bX + cX^2$. Log b is a constant in the estimating equation $\log Y_c = \log a + X \log b$.

c: a constant in the estimating equation $Y_c = a + bX + cX^2$.

N: the number of items in a sample. In two-variable non-linear correlation, N is the number of pairs of items.

$r^2_{Y.X}$: coefficient of determination for X and Y.

$r^2_{Y.X,X^2}$: coefficient of determination for X and Y, the estimating equation $Y_c = a + bX + cX^2$ having been used.

$r^2_{Y.\log X}$: coefficient of determination for log X and Y.

$r^2_{\log Y.X}$: coefficient of determination for X and log Y.

$r^2_{\log Y.\log X}$: coefficient of determination for log X and log Y.

$s_{Y.X}$: standard error of estimate for the estimating equation $Y_c = a + bX$.

$s_{Y.X,X^2}$: standard error of estimate for the estimating equation $Y_c = a + bX + cX^2$.

$s_{Y.\log X}$: standard error of estimate for the estimating equation $Y_c = a + b \log X$.

$s_{\log Y.X}$: standard error of estimate for the estimating equation $\log Y_c = \log a + X \log b$.

$s_{\log Y.\log X}$: standard error of estimate for the estimating equation $\log Y_c = \log a + b \log X$.

SYMBOLS USED IN CHAPTER 7

Σ: upper-case Greek sigma, meaning "take the sum of."
X: the X series, also an observed value in the X series. Thus, we refer to correlating X and Y, but ΣX means "sum the values in the X series."
Y: the Y series, also an observed value in the Y series. Thus, we refer to correlating X and Y, but ΣY means "sum the values in the Y series."
Y_c: a computed Y value.

Multiple and Partial Correlation

$a_{1.2}$: value of $X_{c1.2}$ when $X_2 = 0$ in the estimating equation $X_{c1.2} = a_{1.2} + b_{12}X_2$. Same as a in the estimating equation $Y_c = a + bX$.

$a_{1.3}$: value of $X_{c1.3}$ when $X_3 = 0$ in the estimating equation $X_{c1.3} = a_{1.3} + b_{13}X_3$.

$a_{1.23}$: value of $X_{c1.23}$ when $X_2 = 0$ and $X_3 = 0$ in the estimating equation $X_{c1.23} = a_{1.23} + b_{12.3}X_2 + b_{13.2}X_3$.

$a_{1.234}$: value of $X_{c1.234}$ when $X_2 = 0$, $X_3 = 0$, and $X_4 = 0$ in the estimating equation $X_{c1.234} = a_{1.234} + b_{12.34}X_2 + b_{13.24}X_3 + b_{14.23}X_4$.

b_{12}: coefficient of X_2 in the estimating equation $X_{c1.2} = a_{1.2} + b_{12}X_2$. Same as b in Chapter 6.

b_{13}: coefficient of X_3 in the estimating equation $X_{c1.3} = a_{1.3} + b_{13}X_3$.

$b_{12.3}$: coefficient of X_2 in the estimating equation $X_{c1.23} = a_{1.23} + b_{12.3}X_2 + b_{13.2}X_3$.

$b_{13.2}$: coefficient of X_3 in the estimating equation $X_{c1.23} = a_{1.23} + b_{12.3}X_2 + b_{13.2}X_3$.

$b_{12.34}$: coefficient of X_2 in the estimating equation $X_{c1.234} = a_{1.234} + b_{12.34}X_2 + b_{13.24}X_3 + b_{14.23}X_4$.

$b_{13.24}$: coefficient of X_3 in the estimating equation $X_{c1.234} = a_{1.234} + b_{12.34}X_2 + b_{13.24}X_3 + b_{14.23}X_4$.

$b_{14.23}$: coefficient of X_4 in the estimating equation $X_{c1.234} = a_{1.234} + b_{12.34}X_2 + b_{13.24}X_3 + b_{14.23}X_4$.

N: the number of items in a sample. In multiple or partial correlation, N is the number of sets of observations.

r_{12}^2: coefficient of determination for X_1 and X_2.
r_{13}^2: coefficient of determination for X_1 and X_3.
r_{14}^2: coefficient of determination for X_1 and X_4.
r_{23}^2: coefficient of determination for X_2 and X_3.
r_{24}^2: coefficient of determination for X_2 and X_4.
r_{34}^2: coefficient of determination for X_3 and X_4.

SYMBOLS USED IN CHAPTER 7

$r_{12.3}^2$: coefficient of partial determination; the *additional* variation in X_1 explained by X_2, expressed as a proportion of the variation in X_1 which was *unexplained* by X_3.

$r_{13.2}^2$: coefficient of partial determination; the *additional* variation in X_1 explained by X_3, expressed as a proportion of the variation in X_1 which was *unexplained* by X_2.

$r_{12.34}^2$: coefficient of partial determination; the *additional* variation in X_1 explained by X_2, expressed as a proportion of the variation in X_1 which was *unexplained* by X_3 and X_4.

$r_{13.24}^2$: coefficient of partial determination; the *additional* variation in X_1 explained by X_3, expressed as a proportion of the variation in X_1 which was *unexplained* by X_2 and X_4.

$r_{14.23}^2$: coefficient of partial determination; the *additional* variation in X_1, explained by X_4, expressed as a proportion of the variation in X_1 which was *unexplained* by X_2 and X_3.

$r_{13.4}, r_{14.2}, r_{14.3}, r_{24.3}, r_{34.2}$: coefficients of partial correlation, used in this chapter to assist in computing various other measures.

$R_{1.23}^2$: coefficient of multiple determination; the proportion of variation in X_1 which was explained by X_2 and X_3.

$R_{1.234}^2$: coefficient of multiple determination; the proportion of variation in X_1 which was explained by X_2, X_3, and X_4.

$s_1, s_2, s_3, s_4, \cdots$: respectively, the standard deviations of the $X_1, X_2, X_3, X_4, \cdots$ series.

$s_{1.2}$: standard error of estimate for the estimating equation $X_{c1.2} = a_{1.2} + b_{12}X_2$. Same as $s_{Y.X}$ in Chapter 6.

$s_{1.3}$: standard error of estimate for the estimating equation $X_{c1.3} = a_{1.3} + b_{13}X_3$.

$s_{1.23}$: standard error of estimate for the estimating equation $X_{c1.23} = a_{1.23} + b_{12.3}X_2 + b_{13.2}X_3$.

$s_{1.234}$: standard error of estimate for the estimating equation $X_{c1.234} = a_{1.234} + b_{12.34}X_2 + b_{13.24}X_3 + b_{14.23}X_4$.

$s_{2.13}, s_{3.12}$: standard errors of estimate used in this chapter to assist in computing other measures.

Σ: upper-case Greek sigma, meaning "take the sum of."

$x_1, x_2, x_3, x_4, \cdots$: values in the $X_1, X_2, X_3, X_4, \cdots$ series expressed as deviations from their respective arithmetic means.

$x_{c1.23}$: a computed deviation of the X_1 series when the estimating equation $x_{c1.23} = b_{12.3}x_2 + b_{13.2}x_3$ is used.

$x_{c1.234}$: a computed deviation of the X_1 series when the estimating equation $x_{c1.234} = b_{12.34}x_2 + b_{13.24}x_3 + b_{14.23}x_4$ is used.

SYMBOLS USED IN CHAPTER 7

X_1: the X_1 series, also an observed value in the X_1 series. Thus, we refer to correlating X_1 with X_2, X_3, and X_4, but ΣX_1 means "take the sum of the values in the X_1 series."

X_2, X_3, X_4, $\cdots$: respectively, the X_2, X_3, X_4, $\cdots$ series, also observed values in those series. See X_1.

$\bar{X}_1$, $\bar{X}_2$, $\bar{X}_3$, $\bar{X}_4$, $\cdots$: respectively, the arithmetic means of the X_1, X_2, X_3, X_4, $\cdots$ series.

$X_{c1.2}$: a computed value of the X_1 series when the estimating equation $X_{c1.2} = a_{1.2} + b_{12}X_2$ is used. Same as Y_c in Chapter 6.

$X_{c1.3}$: a computed value of the X_1 series when the estimating equation $X_{c1.3} = a_{1.3} + b_{13}X_3$ is used.

$X_{c1.23}$: a computed value of the X_1 series when the estimating equation $X_{c1.23} = a_{1.23} + b_{12.3}X_2 + b_{13.2}X_3$ is used.

$X_{c1.234}$: a computed value of the X_1 series when the estimating equation $X_{c1.234} = a_{1.234} + b_{12.34}X_2 + b_{13.24}X_3 + b_{14.23}X_4$ is used.

Chapter 7

NON-LINEAR AND MULTIPLE CORRELATION

In the preceding chapter it was noted that correlation may be linear or non-linear. Linear relationships were considered first because they involve the more simple procedures and thus gave a useful introduction to the more general problem involving non-linear relationships as well as linear. In the first part of this chapter we shall examine a few of the numerous curvilinear formulas.

In Chapter 6 attention was given only to two-variable correlation, but it was mentioned that more than two variables could be correlated. In the second part of the present chapter we shall consider a three-variable correlation problem and indicate how to proceed if it is desired to correlate four variables.

Non-linear Correlation

An apparently non-linear relationship was indicated in Charts 6.12 and 6.13, which showed temperature and coagulation time. Chart 7.1, showing light transmission in a photoelectric colorimeter and mg. per cent of iron in blood specimens, and Chart 7.2, depicting concentration of pitocinase and weeks of pregnancy, are also curvilinear. Note that in Chart 7.1 one series decreases as the other increases, and that in Chart 7.2 both series increase together. Nonlinear relationships are occasionally of such a nature that in one part of the scatter plot the two series move together but in another part move inversely. Such a situation would occur, for example, if the scatter plot were U-shaped. For this reason it is customary not to prefix a sign to a non-linear correlation coefficient.

As an illustration of non-linear correlation, we shall use the data of concentration of pitocinase and weeks of pregnancy shown in Chart 7.2 and Table 7.1. It is obvious that a linear estimating equation is inappropriate; but for purposes of comparison with the non-linear analysis, the results of linear correlation are recorded:

CHAP. 7] NON-LINEAR AND MULTIPLE CORRELATION 149

$$Y_c = 6.39 + 1.10X.$$
$$s_{Y.x} = 2.6 \text{ weeks}.$$
$$r_{Y.x}^2 = 0.668.$$
$$r_{Y.x} = +0.818.$$

The estimating equation and the zones of $\pm 1 s_{Y.x}$ are shown in Chart 7.3. The subscript "$_{Y.x}$" is used to identify the linear standard error of estimate and the linear coefficients so that they may be distinguished from the various non-linear measures given later.

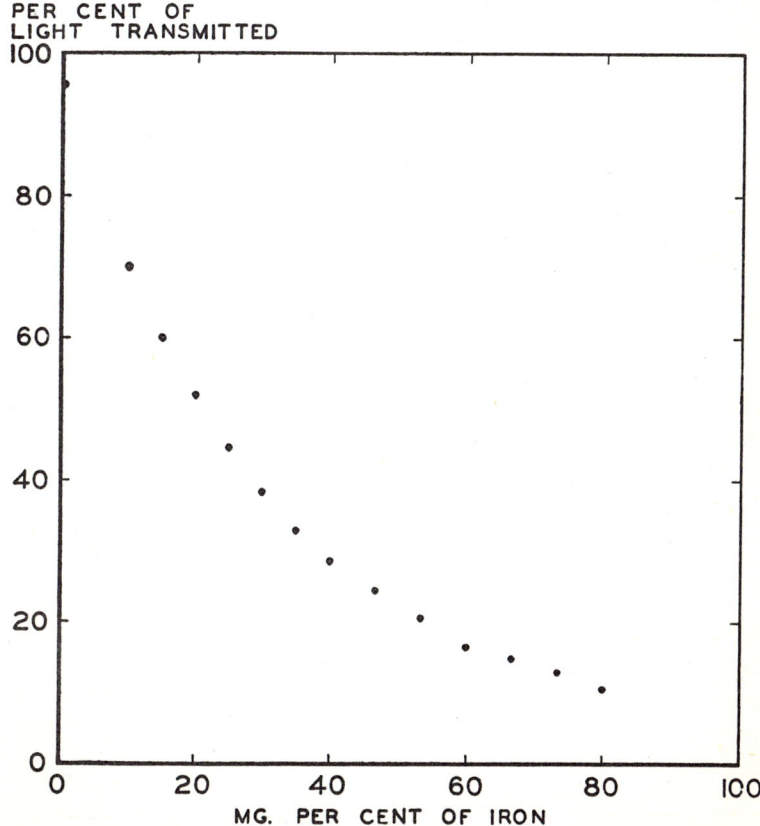

Chart 7.1. **Per cent of Light Transmitted in a Photoelectric Colorimeter and Mg. Per cent of Iron in Blood Specimens.** Data from Dr. Aldula J. Meyers, Child Research Council, University of Colorado School of Medicine, Denver, Colorado.

150 NON-LINEAR AND MULTIPLE CORRELATION [Chap. 7

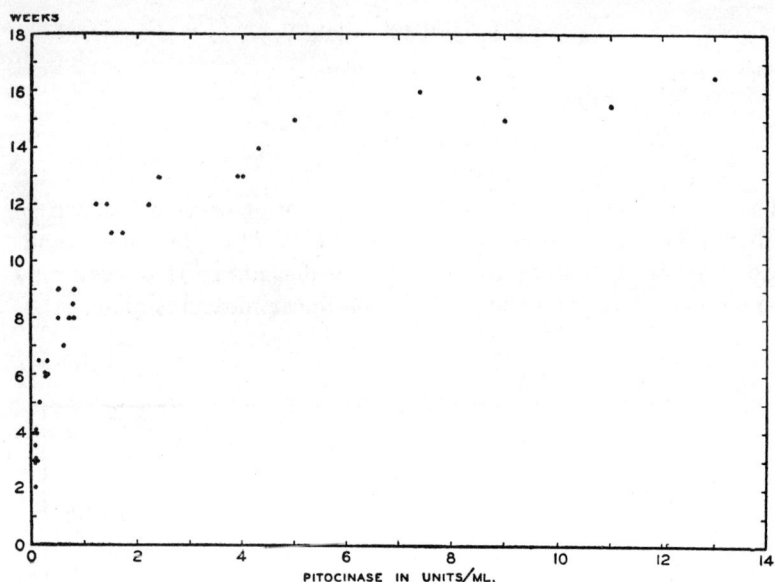

Chart 7.2. Pitocinase and Weeks of Pregnancy. Data of Table 7.1.

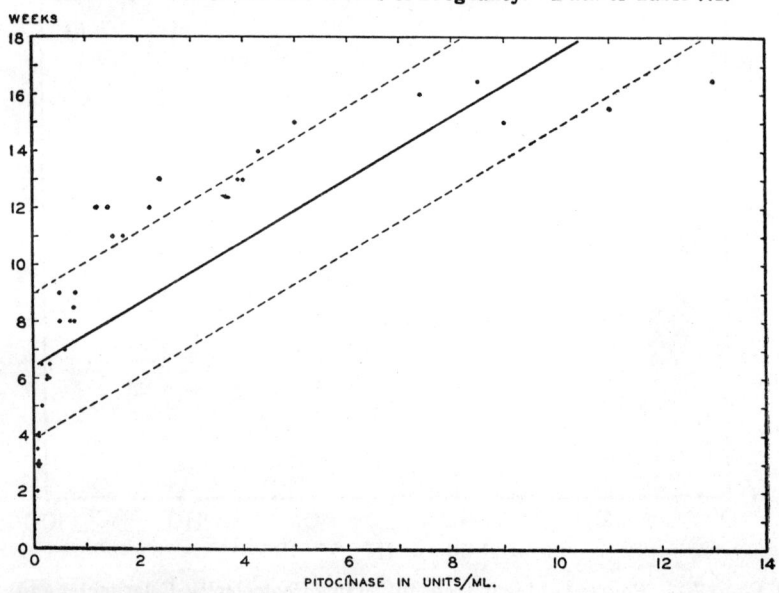

Chart 7.3. Pitocinase and Weeks of Pregnancy, Including Inappropriate Linear Estimating Equation and Zone of $\pm s_{Y.X}$. Data of Table 7.1. The estimating equation, shown by the solid line, is $Y_c = 6.39 + 1.10X$. The value of $s_{Y.X}$ is 2.6 weeks.

Chap. 7] NON-LINEAR AND MULTIPLE CORRELATION

TABLE 7.1
Computation of Sums for Correlation of Concentration of Pitocinase in Units/ml. of Plasma (X) and Weeks of Pregnancy (Y) for 37 Women

Case	X Amount of pitocinase	Y Weeks	Log X	(Log X)(Y)	(Log X)^2	Y^2
1	0.06	2	−1.221849	−2.443698	1.492915	4
2	0.05	3	−1.301030	−3.903090	1.692679	9
3	0.10	3	−1.000000	−3.000000	1.000000	9
4	0.07	3	−1.154902	−3.464706	1.333799	9
5	0.064	3	−1.193820	−3.581460	1.425206	9
6	0.07	3.5	−1.154902	−4.042157	1.333799	12.25
7	0.09	4	−1.045757	−4.183028	1.093608	16
8	0.10	4	−1.000000	−4.000000	1.000000	16
9	0.066	4	−1.180456	−4.721824	1.393476	16
10	0.14	5	−0.853872	−4.269360	0.729097	25
11	0.28	6	−0.552842	−3.317052	0.305634	36
12	0.30	6	−0.522879	−3.137274	0.273402	36
13	0.26	6	−0.585027	−3.510162	0.342257	36
14	0.15	6.5	−0.823909	−5.355408	0.678826	42.25
15	0.30	6.5	−0.522879	−3.398714	0.273402	42.25
16	0.60	7	−0.221849	−1.552943	0.049217	49
17	0.70	8	−0.154902	−1.239216	0.023995	64
18	0.50	8	−0.301030	−2.408240	0.090619	64
19	0.77	8	−0.113509	−0.908072	0.012884	64
20	0.77	8.5	−0.113509	−0.964826	0.012884	72.25
21	0.50	9	−0.301030	−2.709270	0.090619	81
22	0.80	9	−0.096910	−0.872190	0.009392	81
23	1.5	11	0.176091	1.937001	0.031008	121
24	1.7	11	0.230449	2.534939	0.053107	121
25	2.2	12	0.342423	4.109076	0.117254	144
26	1.2	12	0.079181	0.950172	0.006270	144
27	1.4	12	0.146128	1.753536	0.021353	144
28	3.9	13	0.591065	7.683845	0.349358	169
29	2.4	13	0.380211	4.942743	0.144560	169
30	4.0	13	0.602060	7.826780	0.362476	169
31	4.3	14	0.633468	8.868552	0.401282	196
32	9.0	15	0.954243	14.313645	0.910580	225
33	5.0	15	0.698970	10.484550	0.488559	225
34	11.0	15.5	1.041393	16.141592	1.084499	240.25
35	7.4	16	0.869232	13.907712	0.755564	256
36	8.5	16.5	0.929419	15.335414	0.863820	272.25
37	13.0	16.5	1.113943	18.380060	1.240869	272.25
Total	83.24	328.5	−6.628587	62.186927	21.488269	3,660.75

Data from Ernest W. Page, M.D., Division of Obstetrics and Gynecology, University of California Medical School. For definition of units and description of methods, see Ernest W. Page, "A Blood Test for Estimating the Week of Pregnancy," *Science*, Vol. 105, No. 2724, March 14, 1947, pp. 292–293.

152 NON-LINEAR AND MULTIPLE CORRELATION [Chap. 7

The estimating equation. There are many possible equations which might be used to describe a curvilinear relationship. One procedure would be to try several equations and employ the one for which r was largest. Of course, the equation should be a relatively simple one, designed to describe the general tendency shown in the scatter plot. Another procedure consists of plotting the data on specially ruled paper in order to produce a scatter plot which shows a linear relationship. For example, if graph paper having a logarithmic vertical scale and an arithmetic horizontal scale were employed (or if log Y values and X values were plotted on ordinary coordinate paper) and a linear relationship appeared, one would use the equation

$$\log Y_c = \log a + X \log b.$$

Another possibility consists of plotting the data in relation to an arithmetic vertical scale and a logarithmic horizontal scale (or plotting Y values and log X values on an arithmetic grid). If the resulting scatter plot shows a linear relationship, the equation to use is

$$Y_c = a + b \log X.$$

If neither of the two scatter plots just mentioned shows a straight-line relationship, use may be made of graph paper having logarithmic vertical and horizontal scales (or log Y and log X values may be plotted on ordinary coordinate paper). The appearance of a linear relationship would indicate that the equation

$$\log Y_c = \log a + b \log X$$

should be used.

Not all equation types may be handled in this fashion. For example, there is no simple graphic device for ascertaining the suitability of the equation

$$Y_c = a + bX + cX^2.$$

Reference to Chart 7.2 will make it clear to the reader that the use of a logarithmic vertical scale would not serve to give us a scatter plot showing a linear relationship. However, a linear relationship appears in Chart 7.4, which uses an arithmetic scale for the Y values and a logarithmic scale for the X values. Apparently the equation type

$$Y_c = a + b \log X$$

CHAP. 7] NON-LINEAR AND MULTIPLE CORRELATION 153

should be satisfactory. The normal equations are

I. $\Sigma Y = Na + b\Sigma \log X.$
II. $\Sigma(\log X \cdot Y) = a\Sigma \log X + b\Sigma(\log X)^2.$

Before writing the two normal equations with the numerical values of the summations obtained from Table 7.1, it is desirable to

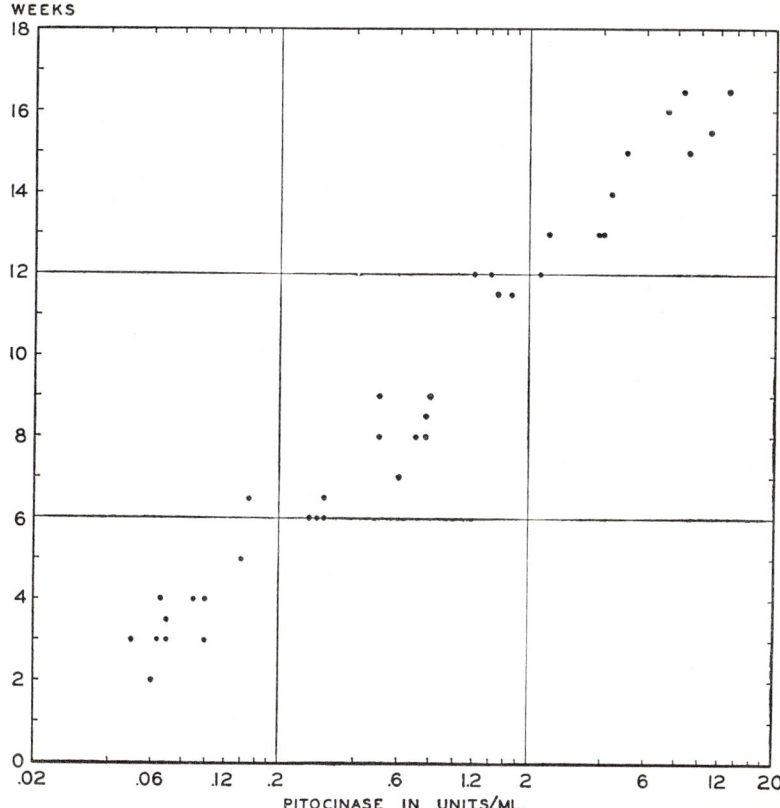

Chart 7.4. **Pitocinase and Weeks of Pregnancy.** Logarithmic horizontal scale. Data of Table 7.1.

note a peculiarity of our problem. Twenty-two of the X values are less than 1.0 and therefore have logarithms which are negative; for example, $\log 0.06 = 8.778151 - 10$, when written in the usual manner with positive mantissa (.778151) and negative characteristic $(8 - 10)$. If we proceed to square the logarithm of 0.06, when written in this form, we have

$$(\log 0.06)^2 = (8.778151 - 10)^2$$
$$= (8.778151)^2 - 2(8.778151)(10) + (10)^2,$$
$$= 1.492915.$$

This is a rather awkward manner of obtaining $(\log 0.06)^2$, and, in order to avoid the necessity of 22 such time-consuming computations, Table 7.1 uses the logarithms of the 22 numbers which are less than 1.0 as negative logarithms. Thus,

$$\log 0.06 = 8.778151 - 10 = -1.221849;$$
$$\log 0.05 = 8.698970 - 10 = -1.301030;$$
$$\log 0.10 = 9.000000 - 10 = -1.000000;$$

and so forth.

With values substituted from Table 7.1, the two normal equations are

I. $\quad 328.5 = 37a - 6.628587b;$
II. $\quad 62.186927 = -6.628587a + 21.488269b.$

$(I \times 0.179151).\quad 58.851104 = 6.628587a - 1.187518b;$
$\text{II.}\quad \underline{62.186927 = -6.628587a + 21.488269b.}$
$\phantom{(I \times 0.179151).\text{II.}\quad}121.038031 = 20.300751b.$
$\phantom{(I \times 0.179151).\text{II.}\quad}b = 5.962244.$

Substituting in I,

$$328.5 = 37a - (6.628587)(5.962244).$$
$$37a = 328.5 + 39.521253,$$
$$= 368.021253.$$
$$a = 9.946520.$$

Check, using II:

$$62.186927 = (-6.628587)(9.946520) + (21.488269)(5.962244),$$
$$= 62.186930.$$

The equation (shown in Chart 7.5) for estimating weeks of pregnancy from amount of pitocinase is, therefore,

$$Y_c = 9.95 + 5.96 \log X.$$

CHAP. 7] NON-LINEAR AND MULTIPLE CORRELATION

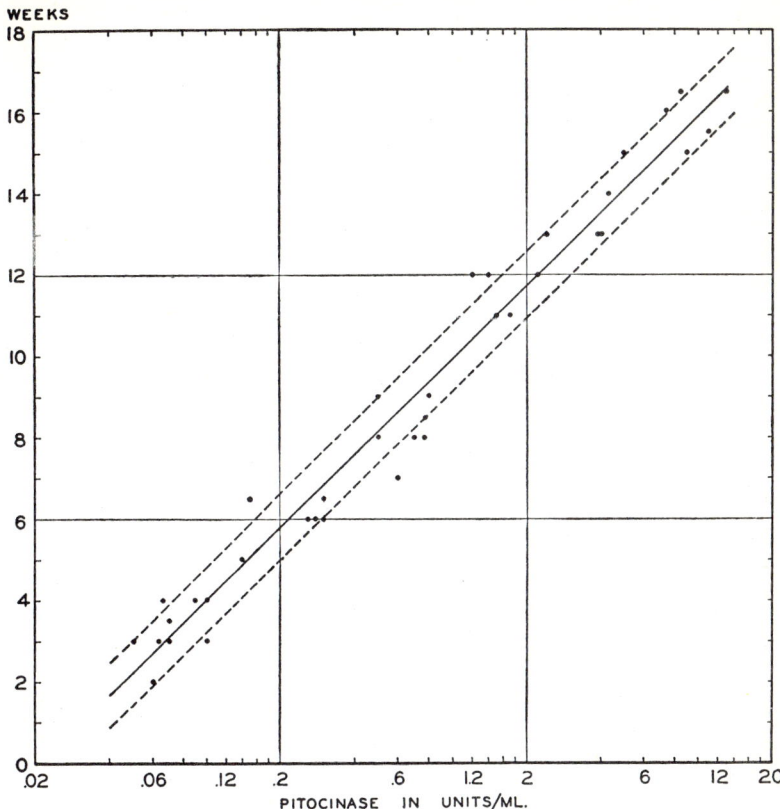

Chart 7.5. Pitocinase and Weeks of Pregnancy, Including Estimating Equation of Type $Y_c = a + b \log X$ and Zone of $\pm s_{Y.\log X}$. Logarithmic horizontal scale. Data of Table 7.1. The estimating equation, shown by the solid line, is $Y_c = 9.95 + 5.96 \log X$. The value of $s_{Y.\log X}$ is 0.8 week.

For a woman whose plasma showed 0.85 units/millilitre of pitocinase the estimate of weeks of pregnancy is given by

$$Y_c = 9.95 + (5.96)(\log 0.85),$$
$$= 9.95 - 0.42,$$
$$= 9.53 \text{ weeks.}$$

As in the case of nearly all correlation problems, the relationship shown by the estimating equation should not be expected to hold beyond the limits of the scatter plot.

156 NON-LINEAR AND MULTIPLE CORRELATION [Chap. 7]

The standard error of estimate is obtained from

$$s_{Y.\log X} = \sqrt{\frac{\Sigma Y^2 - [a\Sigma Y + b\Sigma(\log X \cdot Y)]}{N}},$$

$$= \sqrt{\frac{3660.75 - [(9.946520)(328.5) + (5.962244)(62.186927)]}{37}},$$

$$= \sqrt{\frac{3660.75 - 3638.21}{37}},$$

$$= \sqrt{0.6092},$$

$$= 0.8 \text{ week.}$$

We may say, then, that in general about 68 per cent of the actual figures for week of pregnancy may be expected to fall within ± 0.8 week of the figures obtained by means of the estimating equation. The zone of $\pm s_{Y.\log X}$ around the estimating equation is shown in Chart 7.5.

The coefficient of determination for the data of pitocinase and week of pregnancy is given by the usual expression, where

$$r^2 = \frac{\text{explained variation}}{\text{total variation}}.$$

That is,

$$r^2_{Y.\log X} = \frac{[a\Sigma Y + b\Sigma(\log X \cdot Y)] - \frac{(\Sigma Y)^2}{N}}{\Sigma Y^2 - \frac{(\Sigma Y)^2}{N}},$$

$$= \frac{(9.946520)(328.5) + (5.962244)(62.186927) - \frac{(328.5)^2}{37}}{3660.75 - \frac{(328.5)^2}{37}},$$

$$= \frac{3638.21 - 2916.55}{3660.75 - 2916.55} = \frac{721.66}{744.20},$$

$$= 0.970.$$

$$r_{Y.\log X} = 0.985.$$

In spite of the fact that it is not customary to use a sign with a non-linear correlation coefficient, it would not be incorrect, in this

Chap. 7] NON-LINEAR AND MULTIPLE CORRELATION 157

instance, to write $r_{Y \cdot \log X} = +0.985$, since the relationship between Y and $\log X$ is linear. For the same reason, it is possible to compute $r_{Y \cdot \log X}$ by means of the expression

$$r_{Y \cdot \log X} = \frac{N\Sigma(\log X \cdot Y) - (\Sigma \log X)(\Sigma Y)}{\sqrt{[N\Sigma(\log X)^2 - (\Sigma \log X)^2][N\Sigma Y^2 - (\Sigma Y)^2]}},$$

$$= \frac{(37)(62.186927) - (-6.628587)(328.5)}{\sqrt{[37(21.488269) - (-6.628587)^2][37(3660.75) - (328.5)^2]}},$$

$$= \frac{4{,}478.407}{4{,}547.821},$$

$$= 0.985.$$

This, of course, would be the expression to use if one desired only the value of $r_{Y \cdot \log X}$ and were not concerned with the estimating equation or standard error of estimate.

A comparison of Charts 7.3 and 7.5 shows clearly that the estimating equation $Y_c = a + b \log X$ is much more suitable than $Y_c = a + bX$. The use of $\log X$ instead of X results in a much smaller standard error of estimate, $s_{Y \cdot \log X} = 0.8$ week while $s_{Y \cdot X} = 2.6$ weeks, and a much larger coefficient of determination, $r^2_{Y \cdot \log X} = 0.970$ while $r^2_{Y \cdot X} = 0.668$.

Formulas for other non-linear relationships. Only one of the four curvilinear equation types mentioned earlier in this chapter has been fully considered with formulas and a numerical illustration. For the other three equation types, the formulas only will be given.

For $\log Y_c = \log a + X \log b$, the normal equations are:

I. $\quad \Sigma \log Y = N \log a + \log b \Sigma X;$

II. $\quad \Sigma(X \cdot \log Y) = \log a \Sigma X + \log b \Sigma X^2.$

The standard error of estimate is obtained from the expression

$$s_{\log Y \cdot X} = \sqrt{\frac{\Sigma(\log Y)^2 - [\log a \Sigma \log Y + \log b \Sigma(X \cdot \log Y)]}{N}}$$

and the coefficient of determination may be computed by using

$$r^2_{\log Y \cdot X} = \frac{\log a \Sigma \log Y + \log b \Sigma(X \cdot \log Y) - \dfrac{(\Sigma \log Y)^2}{N}}{\Sigma(\log Y)^2 - \dfrac{(\Sigma \log Y)^2}{N}}.$$

The coefficient of correlation is, of course, the square root of the above expression. However, if only $r_{\log Y \cdot X}$ is desired, it is quicker to avoid solving the two normal equations by using

$$r_{\log Y \cdot X} = \frac{N \Sigma (X \cdot \log Y) - (\Sigma X)(\Sigma \log Y)}{\sqrt{[N \Sigma X^2 - (\Sigma X)^2][N \Sigma (\log Y)^2 - (\Sigma \log Y)^2]}}.$$

One caution, applicable to this equation type and also to the one to be described next, has to do with the computation of estimated values plus and minus the standard error of estimate. These must be obtained from $\log Y_c \pm s_{\log Y \cdot X}$, after which the two antilogarithms are looked up. It is incorrect to look up the antilogarithms of $\log Y_c$ and $s_{\log Y \cdot X}$ first and then combine these antilogarithms. This is an elementary consideration, but one that is sometimes overlooked.

For $\log Y_c = \log a + b \log X$, the normal equations are

I. $\quad\quad\quad \Sigma \log Y = N \log a + b \Sigma \log X;$
II. $\quad \Sigma(\log X \cdot \log Y) = \log a \Sigma \log X + b \Sigma (\log X)^2.$

The standard error of estimate is

$$s_{\log Y \cdot \log X} = \sqrt{\frac{\Sigma (\log Y)^2 - [\log a \Sigma \log Y + b \Sigma (\log X \cdot \log Y)]}{N}}.$$

The coefficient of determination may be obtained from

$$r^2_{\log Y \cdot \log X} = \frac{\log a \Sigma \log Y + b \Sigma (\log X \cdot \log Y) - \dfrac{(\Sigma \log Y)^2}{N}}{\Sigma (\log Y)^2 - \dfrac{(\Sigma \log Y)^2}{N}}.$$

The coefficient of correlation may be computed by taking the square root of the coefficient of determination, or, if only $r_{\log Y \cdot \log X}$ (and not the estimating equation) is wanted, use

$$r_{\log Y \cdot \log X} = \frac{N \Sigma (\log X \cdot \log Y) - (\Sigma \log X)(\Sigma \log Y)}{\sqrt{[N \Sigma (\log X)^2 - (\Sigma \log X)^2][N \Sigma (\log Y)^2 - (\Sigma \log Y)^2]}}.$$

If an estimating equation of the type $Y_c = a + bX + cX^2$, which has one point of inflection, is used, the normal equations are three in number because there are three unknowns. The normal equations are

I. $\quad \Sigma Y = Na + b\Sigma X + c\Sigma X^2;$
II. $\quad \Sigma XY = a\Sigma X + b\Sigma X^2 + c\Sigma X^3;$
III. $\quad \Sigma X^2 Y = a\Sigma X^2 + b\Sigma X^3 + c\Sigma X^4.$

For the standard error of estimate, the expression is

$$s_{Y \cdot X, X^2} = \sqrt{\frac{\Sigma Y^2 - (a\Sigma Y + b\Sigma XY + c\Sigma X^2 Y)}{N}}$$

and for the coefficient of determination

$$r^2_{Y \cdot X, X^2} = \frac{a\Sigma Y + b\Sigma XY + c\Sigma X^2 Y - \dfrac{(\Sigma Y)^2}{N}}{\Sigma Y^2 - \dfrac{(\Sigma Y)^2}{N}}.$$

The correlation coefficient is obtained by taking the square root of the coefficient of determination. Note that, except for the inclusion of the term "$c\Sigma X^2 Y$," the expressions for the standard error of estimate and the coefficient of determination are the same as the corresponding expressions used with equation type $Y_c = a + bX$, which was discussed in Chapter 6.

Multiple Correlation

Three variables. The preceding discussion has dealt with situations in which there was a dependent variable (Y) and one independent variable (X). We shall now consider the use of two independent variables for estimating the values of a dependent variable. The data of Table 7.2 refer to the height, the femur length, and the length of the radius for each of 18 young adult females. All measurements were in centimeters, the lengths of the two long bones having been obtained from radiographs. It is desired to estimate height from a knowledge of femur length and radius length. Height is, therefore, the dependent variable, and femur length and radius length are the two independent variables. If we were to follow the notation previously employed, we might use Y for the dependent variable and X and Z for the two independent variables. Such a system could be used, but its difficulty would increase if we had a larger number of independent variables. It is preferable, therefore, to adopt a slightly different system in which X_1 represents the dependent variable, while X_2, X_3, and so forth, represent the inde-

TABLE 7.2

COMPUTATION OF SUMS FOR CORRELATION OF HEIGHT (X_1), FEMUR LENGTH (X_2), AND RADIUS LENGTH (X_3) FOR 18 YOUNG ADULT FEMALES

(All measurements are in centimeters.)

Case	X_1 Height	X_2 Femur length	X_3 Radius length	X_1X_2	X_1X_3	X_2X_3	X_1^2	X_2^2	X_3^2
1	157.6	44.15	23.65	6,958.040	3,727.240	1,044.1475	24,837.76	1,949.2225	559.3225
2	175.8	48.30	25.25	8,491.140	4,438.950	1,219.5750	30,905.64	2,332.8900	637.5625
3	167.4	47.20	24.20	7,901.280	4,051.080	1,142.2400	28,022.76	2,227.8400	585.6400
4	164.4	45.30	23.00	7,447.320	3,781.200	1,041.9000	27,027.36	2,052.0900	529.0000
5	172.8	49.30	24.30	8,519.040	4,199.040	1,197.9900	29,859.84	2,430.4900	590.4900
6	161.8	47.50	23.60	7,685.500	3,818.480	1,121.0000	26,179.24	2,256.2500	556.9600
7	166.8	47.10	23.00	7,856.280	3,836.400	1,083.3000	27,822.24	2,218.4100	529.0000
8	164.1	46.70	25.00	7,663.470	4,102.500	1,167.5000	26,928.81	2,180.8900	625.0000
9	172.9	48.10	23.70	8,316.490	4,097.730	1,139.9700	29,894.41	2,313.6100	561.6900
10	170.0	48.50	24.40	8,245.000	4,148.000	1,183.4000	28,900.00	2,352.2500	595.3600
11	170.0	47.10	24.00	8,007.000	4,080.000	1,130.4000	28,900.00	2,218.4100	576.0000
12	168.2	47.45	24.60	7,981.090	4,137.720	1,167.2700	28,291.24	2,251.5025	605.1600
13	177.0	52.00	25.20	9,204.000	4,460.400	1,310.4000	31,329.00	2,704.0000	635.0400
14	166.1	47.90	23.90	7,956.190	3,969.790	1,144.8100	27,589.21	2,294.4100	571.2100
15	165.3	46.30	24.20	7,653.390	4,000.260	1,120.4600	27,324.09	2,143.6900	585.6400
16	164.0	47.40	23.10	7,773.600	3,788.400	1,094.9400	26,896.00	2,246.7600	533.6100
17	172.2	50.15	24.50	8,635.830	4,218.900	1,228.6750	29,652.84	2,515.0225	600.2500
18	157.4	45.20	22.95	7,114.480	3,612.330	1,037.3400	24,774.76	2,043.0400	526.7025
Total	3,013.8	855.65	432.55	143,409.140	72,468.420	20,575.3175	505,135.20	40,730.7775	10,403.6375

Data from Marion M. Maresh, M.D., Child Research Council, University of Colorado School of Medicine.

Chap. 7] NON-LINEAR AND MULTIPLE CORRELATION 161

pendent variables. For the data of the three-variable problem which is being used as an illustration, X_1 is height, X_2 is femur length, and X_3 is radius length.

Simple correlation of X_1 and X_2, and of X_1 and X_3. Before proceeding with the three-variable correlation analysis, it will be worth while to make two two-variable analyses, one involving X_1 and X_2 and the other making use of X_1 and X_3. The purpose of this step is partly to familiarize ourselves with the new symbols but, what is more important, to obtain certain values from the two-variable analyses in order that we may compare with them the values obtained later from the three-variable analysis. Two-variable correlation is often referred to as "simple correlation," to distinguish it from the more complex multiple and partial correlation.

Simple correlation of X_1 and X_2. From the data of Table 7.2, we obtain the summations which are to be substituted in the two normal equations necessary to determine the estimating equation:

$$X_{c1.2} = a_{1.2} + b_{12}X_2.$$

The normal equations are:

I. $\Sigma X_1 = Na_{1.2} + b_{12}\Sigma X_2;$
II. $\Sigma X_1 X_2 = a_{1.2}\Sigma X_2 + b_{12}\Sigma X_2^2.$

Substituting the numerical values, we have:

I. $3{,}013.8 = 18a_{1.2} + 855.65b_{12};$
II. $143{,}409.140 = 855.65a_{1.2} + 40{,}730.7775b_{12}.$

When these two equations are solved simultaneously, we obtain

$$a_{1.2} = 45.6078;$$
$$b_{12} = 2.5628; \text{ and}$$
$$X_{c1.2} = 45.61 + 2.56X_2.$$

The standard error of estimate is

$$s_{1.2} = \sqrt{\frac{\Sigma X_1^2 - (a_{1.2}\Sigma X_1 + b_{12}\Sigma X_1 X_2)}{N}},$$

$$= \sqrt{\frac{505{,}135.20 - [(45.6078)(3{,}013.8) + (2.5628)(143{,}409.140)]}{18}},$$

$$= \sqrt{\frac{505{,}135.20 - 504{,}981.73}{18}} = \sqrt{8.53},$$

$$= 2.9 \text{ cm.}$$

162 NON-LINEAR AND MULTIPLE CORRELATION [CHAP. 7

and the coefficient of determination is

$$r_{12}^2 = \frac{a_{1.2}\Sigma X_1 + b_{12}\Sigma X_1 X_2 - \frac{(\Sigma X_1)^2}{N}}{\Sigma X_1^2 - \frac{(\Sigma X_1)^2}{N}},$$

$$= \frac{(45.6078)(3,013.8) + (2.5628)(143,409.130) - \frac{(3,013.8)^2}{18}}{505,135.20 - \frac{(3,013.8)^2}{18}},$$

$$= \frac{504,981.73 - 504,610.58}{505,135.20 - 504,610.58} = \frac{371.15}{524.62},$$

$$= 0.707.$$

Taking the square root of this figure gives $r_{12} = +0.841$.

Simple correlation of X_1 and X_3. The estimating equation is

$$X_{c1.3} = a_{1.3} + b_{13}X_3.$$

Substituting the summations from Table 7.2 in the normal equations,

I. $\Sigma X_1 = Na_{1.3} + b_{13}\Sigma X_3;$
II. $\Sigma X_1 X_3 = a_{1.3}\Sigma X_3 + b_{13}\Sigma X_3^2;$

gives

I. $3,013.8 = 18a_{1.3} + 432.55b_{13};$
II. $72,468.420 = 432.55a_{1.3} + 10,403.6375b_{13}.$

When these are solved simultaneously, it is found that

$$a_{1.3} = 49.8134,$$
$$b_{13} = 4.8946, \text{ and}$$
$$X_{c1.3} = 49.81 + 4.89X_3.$$

The standard error of estimate is

$$s_{1.3} = \sqrt{\frac{\Sigma X_1^2 - (a_{1.3}\Sigma X_1 + b_{13}\Sigma X_1 X_3)}{N}},$$

$$= \sqrt{\frac{505,135.20 - [(49.8134)(3,013.8) + (4.8946)(72,468.420)]}{18}},$$

$$= \sqrt{\frac{505,135.20 - 504,831.55}{18}} = \sqrt{16.87},$$

$$= 4.1 \text{ cm}.$$

CHAP. 7] NON-LINEAR AND MULTIPLE CORRELATION 163

and the coefficient of determination is

$$r_{13}^2 = \frac{a_{1.3}\Sigma X_1 + b_{13}\Sigma X_1 X_3 - \frac{(\Sigma X_1)^2}{N}}{\Sigma X_1^2 - \frac{(\Sigma X_1)^2}{N}},$$

$$= \frac{(49.8134)(3{,}013.8) + (4.8946)(72{,}468.420) - \frac{(3{,}013.8)^2}{18}}{505{,}135.20 - \frac{(3{,}013.8)^2}{18}},$$

$$= \frac{504{,}831.55 - 504{,}610.58}{505{,}135.20 - 504{,}610.58} = \frac{220.97}{524.62},$$

$$= 0.421.$$

$r_{13} = +0.649.$

It is of interest to note that 71 per cent of the variation in height is explained by referring to the length of the femur, and that 42 per cent of the variation in height is explained by referring to the length of the radius. Of course, these two percentages must not be added, because femur length and radius length do not provide mutually independent bases for estimating height. In other words, femur length and radius length are correlated, as indicated by their coefficient of determination, which is $r_{23}^2 = 0.595$. Estimates of height made from femur length involve a standard error of estimate of 2.9 cm., while estimates made from radius length are subject to a standard error of estimate of 4.1 cm. We shall proceed to correlate height with *both* femur length and radius length and shall see that the multiple coefficient of determination $R_{1.23}^2$ is *larger* than either r_{12}^2 or r_{13}^2 and that the multiple standard error of estimate $s_{1.23}$ is *smaller* than either $s_{1.2}$ or $s_{1.3}$.

Estimating equation for three variables. For a three-variable multiple correlation problem, the estimating equation is of the type:[1]

$$X_{c1.23} = a_{1.23} + b_{12.3}X_2 + b_{13.2}X_3,$$

---

[1] We are considering only linear multiple correlation. If the relationship between X_1 and X_2 were linear but the relationship between X_1 and X_3 non-linear, one possible equation type would be

$$X_{c1.233'} = a_{1.233'} + b_{12.33'}X_2 + b_{13.23'}X_3 + b_{13'.23}X_3^2.$$

For further discussion, see F. E. Croxton and D. J. Cowden, *Applied General Statistics*, Prentice-Hall, Inc., New York, 1939, pp. 779–784.

where $X_{c1.23}$ is the computed value of X_1 obtained from given values of X_2 and X_3,

$a_{1.23}$ is the constant in the equation in which X_1 is being estimated by use of X_2 and X_3,

$b_{12.3}$ indicates the amount of change in the computed value of X_1 which accompanies a change of one unit in X_2 when the effect of X_3 is also being considered, and

$b_{13.2}$ indicates the amount of change in the computed value of X_1 which accompanies a change of one unit in X_3 when the effect of X_2 is also being considered.

From the foregoing it should be obvious that a multiple correlation symbol tells one quite explicitly what it means. For example, $a_{1.2345}$ is the constant in the equation which undertakes to estimate X_1 from known values of $X_2, X_3, X_4,$ and X_5. Also, $b_{13.245}$ indicates, for the same sort of equation, the change in the computed value of X_1 which accompanies a change of one unit in X_3 when the effects of $X_2, X_4,$ and X_5 are also being considered.

Three normal equations are necessary to determine the three unknowns in the estimating equation

They are:
$$X_{c1.23} = a_{1.23} + b_{12.3}X_2 + b_{13.2}X_3.$$

I. $\quad \Sigma X_1 = Na_{1.23} + b_{12.3}\Sigma X_2 + b_{13.2}\Sigma X_3;$
II. $\quad \Sigma X_1 X_2 = a_{1.23}\Sigma X_2 + b_{12.3}\Sigma X_2^2 + b_{13.2}\Sigma X_2 X_3;$
III. $\quad \Sigma X_1 X_3 = a_{1.23}\Sigma X_3 + b_{12.3}\Sigma X_2 X_3 + b_{13.2}\Sigma X_3^2.$

The sums of squares and sums of products required for these three equations (and also ΣX_1^2, which will be needed later) are obtained from Table 7.2, giving

I. $\quad 3{,}013.8 = 18a_{1.23} + 855.65b_{12.3} + 432.55b_{13.2};$
II. $\quad 143{,}409.140 = 855.65a_{1.23} + 40{,}730.7775b_{12.3}$
$\qquad\qquad\qquad\qquad\qquad\qquad\qquad + 20{,}575.3175b_{13.2};$
III. $\quad 72{,}468.420 = 432.55a_{1.23} + 20{,}575.3175b_{12.3}$
$\qquad\qquad\qquad\qquad\qquad\qquad\qquad + 10{,}403.6375b_{13.2}.$

To obtain the values of $a_{1.23}, b_{12.3},$ and $b_{13.2}$ from these equations, it would be necessary to solve the three equations simultaneously. However, it is possible to put the estimating equation in terms of deviations from the mean of each series. That is, instead of using

CHAP. 7] NON-LINEAR AND MULTIPLE CORRELATION 165

X_1, X_2, and X_3, we may use x_1, x_2, and x_3, where x_1, x_2, and x_3 are, respectively, deviations from $\bar{X}_1$, $\bar{X}_2$, and $\bar{X}_3$. The estimating equation now is

$$x_{c1.23} = a_{1.23} + b_{12.3}x_2 + b_{13.2}x_3.$$

However, if we write the first normal equation in deviation form,

I. $\Sigma x_1 = Na_{1.23} + b_{12.3}\Sigma x_2 + b_{13.2}\Sigma X_3$,

it is apparent that $a_{1.23} = 0$, since $\Sigma x_1 = 0$, $\Sigma x_2 = 0$, and $\Sigma x_3 = 0$. This makes it possible to write the estimating equation

$$x_{c1.23} = b_{12.3}x_2 + b_{13.2}x_3$$

and makes it necessary to use only the two normal equations II and III to obtain $b_{12.3}$ and $b_{13.2}$. In deviation form, the normal equations are:

II. $\Sigma x_1 x_2 = b_{12.3}\Sigma x_2^2 + b_{13.2}\Sigma x_2 x_3$;
III. $\Sigma x_1 x_3 = b_{12.3}\Sigma x_2 x_3 + b_{13.2}\Sigma x_3^2$.

The sums of the squared deviations and the sums of the products of the deviations are obtained from the sums of squares and sums of products given in Table 7.2 by means of the following expressions:[2]

$$\Sigma x_1^2 = \Sigma X_1^2 - \frac{(\Sigma X_1)^2}{N};$$

---

[2] Using Σx_1^2 and $\Sigma x_1 x_2$ to demonstrate how these expressions are obtained, we have:

$$\Sigma x_1^2 = \Sigma(X_1 - \bar{X}_1)^2,$$
$$= \Sigma(X_1^2 - 2X_1\bar{X}_1 + \bar{X}_1^2),$$
$$= \Sigma X_1^2 - 2\bar{X}_1\Sigma X_1 + N\bar{X}_1^2,$$
$$= \Sigma X_1^2 - 2\frac{\Sigma X_1}{N}\Sigma X_1 + \frac{\Sigma X_1}{N}\Sigma X_1,$$
$$= \Sigma X_1^2 - \frac{(\Sigma X_1)^2}{N}.$$

$$\Sigma x_1 x_2 = \Sigma(X_1 - \bar{X}_1)(X_2 - \bar{X}_2),$$
$$= \Sigma(X_1 X_2 - X_2\bar{X}_1 - X_1\bar{X}_2 + \bar{X}_1\bar{X}_2),$$
$$= \Sigma X_1 X_2 - \bar{X}_1\Sigma X_2 - \bar{X}_2\Sigma X_1 + N\bar{X}_1\bar{X}_2,$$
$$= \Sigma X_1 X_2 - \frac{\Sigma X_1 \Sigma X_2}{N} - \frac{\Sigma X_1 \Sigma X_2}{N} + \frac{\Sigma X_1 \Sigma X_2}{N},$$
$$= \Sigma X_1 X_2 - \frac{\Sigma X_1 \Sigma X_2}{N}.$$

166 NON-LINEAR AND MULTIPLE CORRELATION [CHAP. 7

$$\Sigma x_2^2 = \Sigma X_2^2 - \frac{(\Sigma X_2)^2}{N};$$

$$\Sigma x_3^2 = \Sigma X_3^2 - \frac{(\Sigma X_3)^2}{N};$$

$$\Sigma x_1 x_2 = \Sigma X_1 X_2 - \frac{\Sigma X_1 \Sigma X_2}{N};$$

$$\Sigma x_1 x_3 = \Sigma X_1 X_3 - \frac{\Sigma X_1 \Sigma X_3}{N};$$

$$\Sigma x_2 x_3 = \Sigma X_2 X_3 - \frac{\Sigma X_2 \Sigma X_3}{N}.$$

The numerical value of each of these six sums is:

$$\Sigma x_1^2 = 505{,}135.20 - \frac{(3{,}013.8)^2}{18},$$

$$= 524.62.$$

$$\Sigma x_2^2 = 40{,}730.7775 - \frac{(855.65)^2}{18},$$

$$= 56.5040.$$

$$\Sigma x_3^2 = 10{,}403.6375 - \frac{(432.55)^2}{18},$$

$$= 9.2207.$$

$$\Sigma x_1 x_2 = 143{,}409.140 - \frac{(3{,}013.8)(855.65)}{18},$$

$$= 144.808.$$

$$\Sigma x_1 x_3 = 72{,}468.420 - \frac{(3{,}013.8)(432.55)}{18},$$

$$= 45.132.$$

$$\Sigma x_2 x_3 = 20{,}575.3175 - \frac{(855.65)(432.55)}{18},$$

$$= 13.5726.$$

We are now in a position to substitute the required values in normal equations II and III, expressed in deviation form, and to ascertain the values of $b_{12.3}$ and $b_{13.2}$.

II. $144.808 = 56.5040 b_{12.3} + 13.5726 b_{13.2}$;
III. $45.132 = 13.5726 b_{12.3} + 9.2207 b_{13.2}.$

CHAP. 7] NON-LINEAR AND MULTIPLE CORRELATION 167

To solve these simultaneously, we may multiply II by 0.240206 and subtract the result from III, giving

$$\text{III.} \quad 45.132 = 13.5726 b_{12.3} + 9.2207 b_{13.2};$$
$$(\text{II} \times 0.240206). \quad 34.784 = 13.5726 b_{12.3} + 3.2602 b_{13.2};$$
$$\overline{10.348 = \phantom{13.5726 b_{12.3} + {}} 5.9605 b_{13.2}.}$$
$$b_{13.2} = 1.7361.$$

Substituting the value of $b_{13.2}$ in II, we have

$$144.808 = 56.5040 b_{12.3} + (13.5726)(1.7361),$$
$$= 56.5040 b_{12.3} + 23.5634.$$
$$56.5040 b_{12.3} = 121.2446.$$
$$b_{12.3} = 2.1458.$$

Checking by using the values of $b_{12.3}$ and $b_{13.2}$ in III gives

$$45.132 = (13.5726)(2.1458) + (9.2207)(1.7361),$$
$$= 29.124 + 16.008,$$
$$= 45.132.$$

We now have the values of $b_{12.3}$ and $b_{13.2}$, and can write the estimating equation

$$x_{c1.23} = 2.1458 x_2 + 1.7361 x_3;$$

but we do not know the value of $a_{1.23}$, and without that we are unable to write the estimating equation in the form

$$X_{c1.23} = a_{1.23} + b_{12.3} X_2 + b_{13.2} X_3.$$

It is possible to obtain the value of $a_{1.23}$ from the expression

$$a_{1.23} = \frac{\Sigma X_1 - b_{12.3} \Sigma X_2 - b_{13.2} \Sigma X_3}{N},$$

which is a modified form[3] of normal equation I. Using the sum-

---

[3] Normal equation I is

$$\Sigma X_1 = N a_{1.23} + b_{12.3} \Sigma X_2 + b_{13.2} \Sigma X_3, \text{ or}$$
$$N a_{1.23} = \Sigma X_1 - b_{12.3} \Sigma X_2 - b_{13.2} \Sigma X_3, \text{ and}$$
$$a_{1.23} = \frac{\Sigma X_1 - b_{12.3} \Sigma X_2 - b_{13.2} \Sigma X_3}{N}.$$

mations from Table 7.2 and the b values just obtained, we have

$$a_{1.23} = \frac{3,013.8 - (2.1458)(855.65) - (1.7361)(432.55)}{18},$$

$$= 23.71.$$

The complete estimating equation may now be written:

$$X_{c1.23} = 23.71 + 2.146X_2 + 1.736X_3.$$

To illustrate the application of this estimating equation, suppose that for one individual the femur length (X_2) was 48.2 cm. and the radius length (X_3) was 25.0 cm. The estimate of height would then be

$$X_{c1.23} = 23.71 + (2.146)(48.2) + (1.736)(25.0),$$
$$= 23.71 + 103.44 + 43.40,$$
$$= 170.6 \text{ cm}.$$

Standard error of estimate. The expression[4] for the standard error of estimate is similar to those previously used for linear and non-linear relationships:

$$s_{1.23} = \sqrt{\frac{\Sigma X_1^2 - (a_{1.23}\Sigma X_1 + b_{12.3}\Sigma X_1 X_2 + b_{13.2}\Sigma X_1 X_3)}{N}},$$

and for our illustration,

$$s_{1.23} = \sqrt{\frac{505,135.20 - [(23.711)(3,013.8) + (2.1458)(143,409.140) + (1.7361)(72,468.420)]}{18}}$$

$$= \sqrt{\frac{505,135.20 - 504,999.96}{18}},$$

$$= \sqrt{7.51} = 2.7 \text{ cm}.$$

This means that about 68 per cent of actual height values could be expected to fall with ± 2.7 cm. of those obtained from the estimating equation. Note that $s_{1.23} = 2.7$ cm. is *smaller* than either $s_{1.2} = 2.9$ cm. or $s_{1.3} = 4.1$ cm. This will always be true if the inde-

---

[4] It is also possible to use the shorter expression

$$s_{1.23} = \sqrt{\frac{\Sigma x_1^2 - (b_{12.3}\Sigma x_1 x_2 + b_{13.2}\Sigma x_1 x_3)}{N}}.$$

Chap. 7] NON-LINEAR AND MULTIPLE CORRELATION 169

pendent variables are germane. If a variable, say X_3, is not relevant, then $s_{1.23}$ will have the same value as $s_{1.2}$. $s_{1.23}$ cannot be larger than $s_{1.2}$ or $s_{1.3}$.

Coefficient of multiple determination and coefficient of multiple correlation. The coefficient of multiple determination involves the same basic idea as that first discussed for 2-variable linear correlation. It is the proportion of total variation that has been explained by use of the multiple estimating equation. Symbolically,[5]

$$R^2_{1.23} = \frac{a_{1.23}\Sigma X_1 + b_{12.3}\Sigma X_1 X_2 + b_{13.2}\Sigma X_1 X_3 - \frac{(\Sigma X_1)^2}{N}}{\Sigma X_1^2 - \frac{(\Sigma X_1)^2}{N}}.$$

Using values already computed, we have

$$R^2_{1.23} = \frac{(23.711)(3{,}013.8) + (2.1458)(143{,}409.140) + (1.7361)(72{,}468.420) - \frac{(3{,}013.8)^2}{18}}{505{,}135.20 - \frac{(3{,}013.8)^2}{18}},$$

$$= \frac{504{,}999.96 - 504{,}610.58}{505{,}135.20 - 504{,}610.58} = \frac{389.38}{524.62},$$

$$= 0.742.$$

$R_{1.23} = 0.861.$

The reader is urged to compare the symbolic expression for $R^2_{1.23}$ with those for r^2_{12} and r^2_{13}, given earlier in the chapter, and to note (1) that the denominator is the same in all three cases, (2) that the term $\frac{(\Sigma X_1)^2}{N}$ in the numerator is the same for all three expressions, and (3) that the formulas differ from each other only in regard to the two or three additive terms at the left in the numerator. It may also be of interest to compare the expression for $s_{1.23}$ with those for $s_{1.2}$ and $s_{1.3}$.

By using both femur length and radius length as independent

---

[5] It is also possible to use the shorter expression

$$R^2_{1.23} = \frac{b_{12.3}\Sigma x_1 x_2 + b_{13.2}\Sigma x_1 x_3}{\Sigma x_1^2}.$$

variables, we have explained 74 per cent of the variation in height. This compares with 71 per cent ($r_{12}^2 = 0.707$) explained when femur length alone was used and 42 per cent ($r_{13}^2 = 0.421$) when radius length only was considered. $R_{1.23}^2$ will always be larger than either r_{12}^2 or r_{13}^2 unless one of the independent variables is not relevant. If one variable, say, X_3, has no relevancy, then $R_{1.23}^2$ will be the same as r_{12}^2. $R_{1.23}^2$ cannot be smaller than r_{12}^2 or r_{13}^2.

Partial correlation. The value obtained earlier for r_{12}^2 was 0.707, meaning that we had succeeded in explaining 70.7 per cent of the variation in X_1 by use of the estimating equation involving X_2. When we employed X_3 also in the estimating equation, it was found that $R_{1.23}^2 = 0.742$, indicating that the use of both X_2 and X_3 explained 74.2 per cent of the variation in X_1. The improvement in our ability to explain the variation present in X_1 may be seen as follows. Using X_2 only, we explained 0.707 of the variation in X_1, but failed to explain $1 - 0.707 = 0.293$ or 29.3 per cent. It is this unexplained portion which we seek to decrease by introducing another independent variable X_3. By use of X_3 in addition to X_2, we increased the proportion of explained variation from 0.707 to 0.742, an increase of 0.035. Or, to state it in another way, *by using X_3 in addition to X_2, we have explained* $\dfrac{0.035}{0.293} = 0.119$, *or 11.9 per cent of the variation which X_2 alone had failed to explain.* This is the coefficient of partial or net determination $r_{13.2}^2$. What has just been said may be written

$$r_{13.2}^2 = \frac{R_{1.23}^2 - r_{12}^2}{1 - r_{12}^2},$$

$$= \frac{0.742 - 0.707}{1 - 0.707} = \frac{0.035}{0.293},$$

$$= 0.119.$$

The coefficient of partial correlation is $r_{13.2} = +0.335$, its sign always being the same as that of $b_{13.2}$. A more customary alternative, but longer, method of computing $r_{13.2}^2$ is based upon the concept[6]

---

[6] Use may also be made of the expression

$$r_{13.2}^2 = \frac{b_{12.3}\Sigma x_1 x_2 + b_{13.2}\Sigma x_1 x_3 - b_{12}\Sigma x_1 x_2}{\Sigma x_1^2 - b_{12}\Sigma x_1 x_2}.$$

CHAP. 7] NON-LINEAR AND MULTIPLE CORRELATION 171

$$r^2_{13.2} = \frac{\text{additional variation explained by } X_3}{\text{variation unexplained by } X_2},$$

$$= \frac{\left[a_{1.23}\Sigma X_1 + b_{12.3}\Sigma X_1 X_2 + b_{13.2}\Sigma X_1 X_3 - \frac{(\Sigma X_1)^2}{N} \right] - \left[a_{1.2}\Sigma X_1 + b_{12}\Sigma X_1 X_2 - \frac{(\Sigma X_1)^2}{N} \right]}{\left[\Sigma X_1^2 - \frac{(\Sigma X_1)^2}{N} \right] - \left[a_{1.2}\Sigma X_1 + b_{12}\Sigma X_1 X_2 - \frac{(\Sigma X_1)^2}{N} \right]},$$

$$= \frac{(a_{1.23}\Sigma X_1 + b_{12.3}\Sigma X_1 X_2 + b_{13.2}\Sigma X_1 X_3) - (a_{1.2}\Sigma X_1 + b_{12}\Sigma X_1 X_2)}{\Sigma X_1^2 - (a_{1.2}\Sigma X_1 + b_{12}\Sigma X_1 X_2)},$$

$$= \frac{504{,}999.96 - 504{,}981.73}{505{,}135.20 - 504{,}981.73} = \frac{18.23}{153.47},$$

$$= 0.119.$$

The reader may well ask: If X_3 has explained only 11.9 per cent of the variation which X_2 failed to explain, is the use of X_3 warranted? We shall answer this question in the latter part of Chapter 12 when we undertake to ascertain whether $r^2_{13.2}$ is significantly greater than zero.

We may use formulas similar to those just given[7] if we wish the value of $r^2_{12.3}$. Thus,

$$r^2_{12.3} = \frac{R^2_{1.23} - r^2_{13}}{1 - r^2_{13}},$$

$$= \frac{0.742 - 0.421}{1 - 0.421} = \frac{0.321}{0.579},$$

$$= 0.554.$$

---

[7] Paralleling the expression shown in footnote 6, we may use

$$r^2_{12.3} = \frac{b_{12.3}\Sigma x_1 x_2 + b_{13.2}\Sigma x_1 x_3 - b_{13}\Sigma x_1 x_3}{\Sigma x_1^2 - b_{13}\Sigma x_1 x_3}.$$

$$r_{12.3}^2 = \frac{(a_{1.23}\Sigma X_1 + b_{12.3}\Sigma X_1 X_2 + b_{13.2}\Sigma X_1 X_3)}{\Sigma X_1^2 - (a_{1.3}\Sigma X_1 + b_{13}\Sigma X_1 X_3)},$$

$$= \frac{504{,}999.96 - 504{,}831.55}{505{,}135.20 - 504{,}831.55} = \frac{168.41}{303.65},$$

$$= 0.555.$$

$$r_{12.3} = +0.744.$$

The two values shown for $r_{12.3}^2$ actually differ by only 0.0002, since one is 0.5544 and the other 0.5546.

Computation of multiple and partial coefficients from simple coefficients. Occasionally a published study is encountered which gives simple correlation coefficients but which does not give multiple or partial correlation coefficients which may be desired by the reader. As an illustration, we shall use a few of the results from an extensive study[8] which, although it gave more than just the simple correlation coefficients for some series, did not give multiple and partial coefficients for the series to which we shall refer. Measurements were made of 32,165 boys 4–14 years of age and included, among many other physical characteristics, weight (which we shall call X_1), stature (X_2), and upper-arm girth (X_3). The simple correlation coefficients were given, and they and the simple coefficients of determination were:

$$r_{12} = +0.927, \qquad r_{12}^2 = 0.859329,$$
$$r_{13} = +0.912, \qquad r_{13}^2 = 0.831744,$$
$$r_{23} = +0.776, \qquad r_{23}^2 = 0.602176.$$

To compute the coefficient of multiple determination, we use the expression

$$R_{1.23}^2 = \frac{r_{12}^2 + r_{13}^2 - 2r_{12}r_{13}r_{23}}{1 - r_{23}^2},$$

$$= \frac{0.859329 + 0.831744 - 2(0.927)(0.912)(0.776)}{1 - 0.602176},$$

$$= \frac{0.378975}{0.397824} = 0.953,$$

---

[8] Ruth O'Brien and Meyer A. Girshick, *Children's Body Measurements for Sizing Garments and Patterns*, United States Department of Agriculture, Miscellaneous Publication No. 365.

CHAP. 7] NON-LINEAR AND MULTIPLE CORRELATION 173

which is, of course, larger than either r_{12}^2 or r_{13}^2. Although 86 per cent of the variation in weight was explained by referring to stature and 83 per cent was explained by referring to upper-arm girth, 95 per cent was explained by referring to *both* stature and upper-arm girth.

If the coefficient of partial determination, $r_{13.2}^2$, is desired, it may be ascertained from the expression previously used:

$$r_{13.2}^2 = \frac{R_{1.23}^2 - r_{12}^2}{1 - r_{12}^2}.$$

Alternatively, we may obtain the coefficient of partial correlation $r_{13.2}$ (which, of course, we can square to get $r_{13.2}^2$) from

$$r_{13.2} = \frac{r_{13} - r_{12}r_{23}}{\sqrt{1 - r_{12}^2}\sqrt{1 - r_{23}^2}}.$$

Using both of these expressions to demonstrate their equivalence, we have

$$r_{13.2}^2 = \frac{R_{1.23}^2 - r_{12}^2}{1 - r_{12}^2},$$

$$= \frac{0.953 - 0.859}{1 - 0.859} = \frac{0.094}{0.141} = 0.667,$$

$$r_{13.2} = \frac{r_{13} - r_{12}r_{23}}{\sqrt{1 - r_{12}^2}\sqrt{1 - r_{23}^2}},$$

$$= \frac{0.912 - (0.927)(0.776)}{\sqrt{1 - 0.859329}\sqrt{1 - 0.602176}} = \frac{0.193}{0.2365} = 0.816,$$

and

$$r_{13.2}^2 = (0.816)^2 = 0.666.$$

Upper-arm girth has, therefore, explained 67 per cent of the variation in weight which stature alone had failed to explain.

If we wish the value of $r_{12.3}^2$, we may use either

$$r_{12.3}^2 = \frac{R_{1.23}^2 - r_{13}^2}{1 - r_{13}^2} \quad \text{or}$$

$$r_{12.3} = \frac{r_{12} - r_{13}r_{23}}{\sqrt{1 - r_{13}^2}\sqrt{1 - r_{23}^2}}.$$

Since the first is easier to compute, we shall use it, obtaining

$$r_{12.3}^2 = \frac{0.953 - 0.832}{1 - 0.832} = \frac{0.121}{0.168} = 0.720,$$

indicating that stature explained 72 per cent of the variation in weight which upper-arm girth alone had failed to explain.

From the information available it is not possible to obtain the multiple estimating equation

$$X_{c1.23} = a_{1.23} + b_{12.3}X_2 + b_{13.2}X_3.$$

This equation could, however, be gotten if the arithmetic means and standard deviations of the three series were available. The expressions to use would be:

$$b_{12.3} = r_{12.3}\frac{s_{1.23}}{s_{2.13}},$$

$$b_{13.2} = r_{13.2}\frac{s_{1.23}}{s_{3.12}},$$

$$s_{1.23} = \sqrt{s_1^2(1 - r_{13}^2)(1 - r_{12.3}^2)},$$
$$s_{2.13} = \sqrt{s_2^2(1 - r_{23}^2)(1 - r_{12.3}^2)},$$
$$s_{3.12} = \sqrt{s_3^2(1 - r_{23}^2)(1 - r_{13.2}^2)}, \text{ and}$$

$$a_{1.23} = \frac{\Sigma X_1 - b_{12.3}\Sigma X_2 - b_{13.2}\Sigma X_3}{N},$$
$$= \bar{X}_1 - b_{12.3}\bar{X}_2 - b_{13.2}\bar{X}_3.$$

Returning to our illustration, it is interesting to note that, if a third independent variable, age (X_4), is introduced, there is not much improvement in our ability to explain the variation in weight. The reader may wish to verify this for himself, using formulas given on the following pages. The needed additional simple correlation coefficients are:

$$r_{14} = +0.822,$$
$$r_{24} = +0.897,$$
$$r_{34} = +0.688.$$

Multiple and partial correlation formulas for four variables. Any number of independent variables may be employed to explain the variation of a dependent variable. With the addition of each *germane* independent variable,[9] the coefficient of multiple determina-

---

[9] However, the introduction of another variable also causes us to lose an additional degree of freedom, so that, if N is small, the increase in explained variation may not be significant (see pages 317–318).

tion (or correlation) will increase and the multiple standard error of estimate will decrease. In other words, we shall be able to make better estimates of X_1. Increasing the number of variables in a correlation problem also increases, more than proportionally, the amount of computational work involved. A four-variable correlation problem, compared with a three-variable problem, for example, involves more than one-third as much additional labor. Since most readers of this book will not have occasion to handle problems involving more than four variables, we shall list the formulas for four-variable multiple and partial correlation only. Those who encounter more complicated problems may refer to other publications[10] or may wish to make use of the services of a commercial computing organization.

For four-variable multiple correlation, the estimating equation is

$$X_{c1.234} = a_{1.234} + b_{12.34}X_2 + b_{13.24}X_3 + b_{14.23}X_4.$$

Four normal equations are required. In terms of the X-values, they are

I. $\quad \Sigma X_1 = Na_{1.234} + b_{12.34}\Sigma X_2 + b_{13.24}\Sigma X_3 + b_{14.23}\Sigma X_4.$

II. $\quad \Sigma X_1 X_2 = a_{1.234}\Sigma X_2 + b_{12.34}\Sigma X_2^2 + b_{13.24}\Sigma X_2 X_3$
$\qquad\qquad\qquad\qquad\qquad\qquad\qquad + b_{14.23}\Sigma X_2 X_4.$

III. $\quad \Sigma X_1 X_3 = a_{1.234}\Sigma X_3 + b_{12.34}\Sigma X_2 X_3 + b_{13.24}\Sigma X_3^2$
$\qquad\qquad\qquad\qquad\qquad\qquad\qquad + b_{14.23}\Sigma X_3 X_4.$

IV. $\quad \Sigma X_1 X_4 = a_{1.234}\Sigma X_4 + b_{12.34}\Sigma X_2 X_4 + b_{13.24}\Sigma X_3 X_4$
$\qquad\qquad\qquad\qquad\qquad\qquad\qquad + b_{14.23}\Sigma X_4^2.$

As before, an appreciable amount of time can be saved by writing the normal equations in terms of deviations. For a four-variable problem, this enables us to obtain the three b-values by solving normal equations II, III, and IV simultaneously. In deviation form, normal equations II, III, and IV are:

II. $\quad \Sigma x_1 x_2 = b_{12.34}\Sigma x_2^2 + b_{13.24}\Sigma x_2 x_3 + b_{14.23}\Sigma x_2 x_4.$

III. $\quad \Sigma x_1 x_3 = b_{12.34}\Sigma x_2 x_3 + b_{13.24}\Sigma x_3^2 + b_{14.23}\Sigma x_3 x_4.$

IV. $\quad \Sigma x_1 x_4 = b_{12.34}\Sigma x_2 x_4 + b_{13.24}\Sigma x_3 x_4 + b_{14.23}\Sigma x_4^2.$

---

[10] For example, Mordecai Ezekiel, *Methods of Correlation Analysis*. New York: John Wiley and Sons, 2nd ed., 1941. See particularly pages 203–205, 209–213, and Table 91.

176 NON-LINEAR AND MULTIPLE CORRELATION [Chap. 7

The sums of squared deviations and the sums of products of deviations are obtained as shown for three-variable multiple correlation, with four additional expressions also being used:

$$\Sigma x_4^2 = \Sigma X_4^2 - \frac{(\Sigma X_4)^2}{N},$$

$$\Sigma x_1 x_4 = \Sigma X_1 X_4 - \frac{\Sigma X_1 \Sigma X_4}{N},$$

and similarly for $\Sigma x_2 x_4$ and $\Sigma x_3 x_4$.

Normal equations II, III, and IV may be solved simultaneously as follows:

(1) Multiply normal equation II by the numerical value of $\Sigma x_2 x_3 \div \Sigma x_2^2$, obtaining normal equation II'.

(2) Subtract normal equation III from II' (or vice versa, if more convenient), thus eliminating $b_{12.34}$ and obtaining a new equation "A" in terms of $b_{13.24}$ and $b_{14.23}$.

(3) Multiply normal equation III by the numerical value of $\Sigma x_2 x_4 \div \Sigma x_2 x_3$, obtaining normal equation III'.

(4) Subtract normal equation IV from III' (or vice versa, if more convenient), thus again eliminating $b_{12.34}$ and obtaining another new eqution "B" in terms of $b_{13.24}$ and $b_{14.23}$.

(5) Solve equations A and B simultaneously, as described on pages 166 and 167, to obtain the value of $b_{14.23}$.

(6) Substitute the value of $b_{14.23}$ in equation A or equation B to obtain the value of $b_{13.24}$, after which the values of the two b's may be substituted in equation B or equation A as a check.

(7) Substitute the values of $b_{13.24}$ and $b_{14.23}$ in normal equation II, III, or IV to obtain the value of $b_{12.34}$.

(8) Substitute the values of $b_{12.34}$, $b_{13.24}$, and $b_{14.23}$ in a normal equation not used in step (7) in order to check the computations.

After the three b-values have been obtained, the value of $a_{1.234}$ is computed from normal equation I written

$$a_{1.234} = \frac{\Sigma X_1 - b_{12.34} \Sigma X_2 - b_{13.24} \Sigma X_3 - b_{14.23} \Sigma X_4}{N}.$$

CHAP. 7] NON-LINEAR AND MULTIPLE CORRELATION 177

The standard error of estimate is

$$s_{1.234} = \sqrt{\frac{\Sigma X_1^2 - (a_{1.234}\Sigma X_1 + b_{12.34}\Sigma X_1 X_2 + b_{13.24}\Sigma X_1 X_3 + b_{14.23}\Sigma X_1 X_4)}{N}}.$$

Several alternative expressions are available for obtaining the value of the standard error of estimate. Among them are

$$s_{1.234} = \sqrt{\frac{\Sigma x_1^2 - (b_{12.34}\Sigma x_1 x_2 + b_{13.24}\Sigma x_1 x_3 + b_{14.23}\Sigma x_1 x_4)}{N}},$$

$$s_{1.234} = \sqrt{s_1^2(1 - r_{12}^2)(1 - r_{13.2}^2)(1 - r_{14.23}^2)},$$

$$s_{1.234} = \sqrt{s_1^2(1 - r_{12}^2)(1 - r_{14.2}^2)(1 - r_{13.24}^2)},$$

and four other expressions similar to the last two. Use may also be made of

$$s_{1.234} = \sqrt{s_1^2(1 - R_{1.234}^2)}.$$

The coefficient of multiple determination may be computed from

$$R_{1.234}^2 = \frac{a_{1.234}\Sigma X_1 + b_{12.34}\Sigma X_1 X_2 + b_{13.24}\Sigma X_1 X_3 + b_{14.23}\Sigma X_1 X_4 - \frac{(\Sigma X_1)^2}{N}}{\Sigma X_1^2 - \frac{(\Sigma X_1)^2}{N}}.$$

Some of the alternative expressions are

$$R_{1.234}^2 = \frac{b_{12.34}\Sigma x_1 x_2 + b_{13.24}\Sigma x_1 x_3 + b_{14.23}\Sigma x_1 x_4}{\Sigma x_1^2},$$

$$R_{1.234}^2 = 1 - \frac{s_{1.234}^2}{s_1^2},$$

$$R_{1.234}^2 = 1 - [(1 - r_{12}^2)(1 - r_{13.2}^2)(1 - r_{14.23}^2)],$$

$$= 1 - [(1 - r_{14}^2)(1 - r_{13.4}^2)(1 - r_{12.34}^2)],$$

and four other expressions similar to the last two.

The coefficient of partial determination $r_{14.23}^2$ may be obtained from

$$r_{14.23}^2 = \frac{R_{1.234}^2 - R_{1.23}^2}{1 - R_{1.23}^2}.$$

178 NON-LINEAR AND MULTIPLE CORRELATION [Chap. 7

There are a number of alternative formulas for $r_{14.23}^2$ or $r_{14.23}$, such as

$$r_{14.23} = \frac{r_{14.2} - (r_{13.2})(r_{34.2})}{\sqrt{1 - r_{13.2}^2}\sqrt{1 - r_{34.2}^2}},$$

$$r_{14.23} = \frac{r_{14.3} - (r_{12.3})(r_{24.3})}{\sqrt{1 - r_{12.3}^2}\sqrt{1 - r_{24.3}^2}},$$

$$r_{14.23}^2 = 1 - \frac{s_{1.234}^2}{s_{1.23}^2}.$$

Parallel expressions would be used for $r_{12.34}^2$ or $r_{12.34}$ and for $r_{13.24}^2$ or $r_{13.24}$.

SYMBOLS USED IN

CHAPTER 8

a: the number of occurrences in a sample.
$C_0, C_1, C_2, \cdots$: the binomial coefficients.
e: 2.71828.
h: in coin tossing, the occurrence of a head.
i: the class interval.
k: the number of samples.
N: the number of items in a sample.
p: the proportion of occurrences in a sample.
$\mathcal{P}$: the number of items in a population. As a subscript, in later chapters, $\mathcal{P}$ means "population"; thus, $\bar{X}_\mathcal{P}$ is the arithmetic mean of a population.
π: lower-case Greek pi, the proportion of occurrences in a population.
q: the proportion of non-occurrences in a sample.
s: the standard deviation of a sample.
σ: lower-case Greek sigma, the standard deviation of a population.
t: in coin tossing, the occurrence of a tail or non-occurrence of a head.
τ: lower-case Greek tau, the proportion of non-occurrences in a population.
x: $X - \bar{X}$.
X: an observed value in a sample.
$\bar{X}$: the arithmetic mean. For a Poisson distribution, $\bar{X} = pN$.
χ^2: chi-square, the subject matter of Chapter 11. The symbol is a lower-case Greek chi.
Y_c: a computed ordinate of the normal curve.
Y_0: the computed ordinate of the normal curve at $\bar{X}$.
!: factorial. $4! = 1 \times 2 \times 3 \times 4$.

Chapter 8

THE NORMAL CURVE, THE BINOMIAL, AND THE POISSON DISTRIBUTION

In this chapter we shall consider, in order, the normal curve, the binomial, and the Poisson distribution. The normal curve and the Poisson are both limiting forms of the binomial, and it would therefore be logical to discuss the binomial first. However, many readers will have occasion to make use of the normal curve, but fewer are likely to encounter problems involving the binomial. For this reason, consideration of the fitting of a binomial will be deferred until after the discussion of the normal curve.

The Normal Curve

The equation. The shape of the normal curve is shown in Chart 8.1. When a normal curve is to be fitted to a sample distribution,

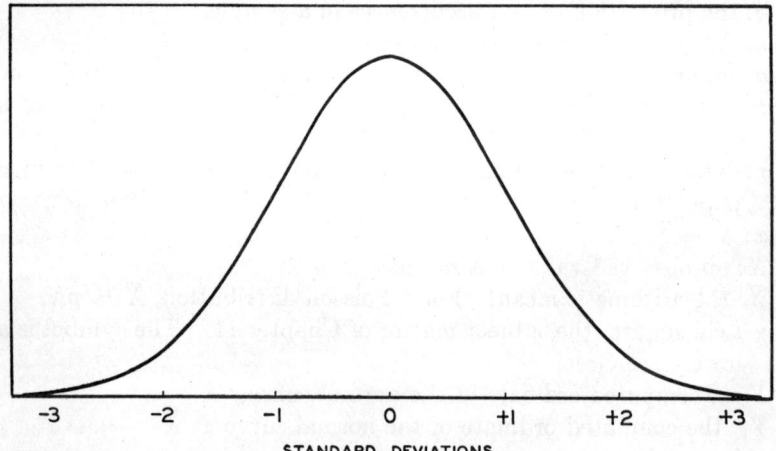

Chart 8.1. The Normal Curve.

the equation of the curve is written

$$Y_c = \frac{Ni}{2.5066s} 2.71828^{\frac{-x^2}{2s^2}},$$

where Y_c is the height of an ordinate at distance x from the arithmetic mean,
N is the number of observations in the sample to which the curve is to be fitted,
i is the class interval of the sample distribution,
s is the standard deviation of the sample, and
x is a selected deviation from $\bar{X}$.

The normal curve of Chart 8.1 may be approximated if we consider the results of tossing a number of "perfect" coins. Such a coin will not stand on edge and is equally likely to show a tail or a

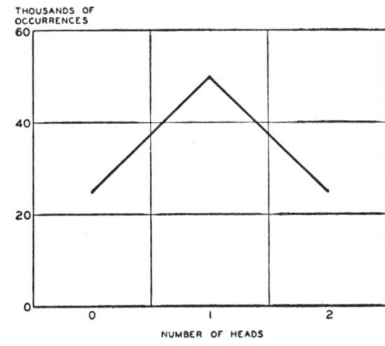

Chart 8.2. Expected Results of 100,000 Tosses of Two Coins.

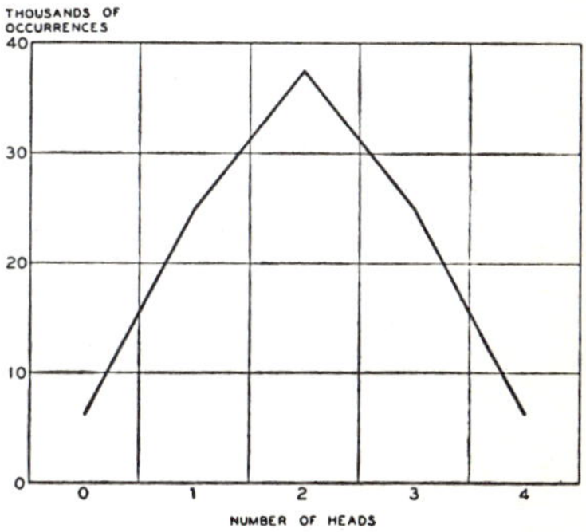

Chart 8.3. Expected Results of 100,000 Tosses of Four Coins.

head when tossed. For a single coin, the chances of throwing a tail or a head are given by $\frac{1}{2}t + \frac{1}{2}h$, the sum of the two probabilities being 1.0. For two coins, the probabilities are given by

$$(\tfrac{1}{2}t + \tfrac{1}{2}h)^2 = \tfrac{1}{4}t^2 + \tfrac{1}{2}ht + \tfrac{1}{4}h^2.$$

We may interpret this by saying that if 100,000 throws were to be made, we should expect to obtain no heads (indicated by t^2, which means "two tails") 25,000 times, one head (ht) 50,000 times, and two heads (h^2) 25,000 times. These results are shown in Chart 8.2.

If four coins are tossed repeatedly, the probabilities are given by

$$(\tfrac{1}{2}t + \tfrac{1}{2}h)^4 = \tfrac{1}{16}t^4 + \tfrac{4}{16}ht^3 + \tfrac{6}{16}h^2t^2 + \tfrac{4}{16}h^3t + \tfrac{1}{16}h^4,$$

and are shown in Chart 8.3. There is not much difference in the appearance of Charts 8.2 and 8.3, and neither looks like the normal curve of Chart 8.1. However, if we consider six coins, represented by

$$(\tfrac{1}{2}t + \tfrac{1}{2}h)^6 = \tfrac{1}{64}t^6 + \tfrac{6}{64}ht^5 + \tfrac{15}{64}h^2t^4 + \tfrac{20}{64}h^3t^3 + \tfrac{15}{64}h^4t^2 + \tfrac{6}{64}h^5t + \tfrac{1}{64}h^6,$$

the resulting curve, shown in Chart 8.4, begins vaguely to resemble the smooth normal curve of Chart 8.1.

As a final step, suppose that twelve coins be tossed. We then have

$$(\tfrac{1}{2}t + \tfrac{1}{2}h)^{12} = \tfrac{1}{4096}t^{12} + \tfrac{12}{4096}ht^{11} + \tfrac{66}{4096}h^2t^{10} + \tfrac{220}{4096}h^3t^9 + \tfrac{495}{4096}h^4t^8 + \tfrac{792}{4096}h^5t^7 + \tfrac{924}{4096}h^6t^6 + \tfrac{792}{4096}h^7t^5 + \tfrac{495}{4096}h^8t^4 + \tfrac{220}{4096}h^9t^3 + \tfrac{66}{4096}h^{10}t^2 + \tfrac{12}{4096}h^{11}t + \tfrac{1}{4096}h^{12},$$

and Chart 8.5 shows the curve of this expansion. This curve is much smoother than the preceding one and clearly begins to resem-

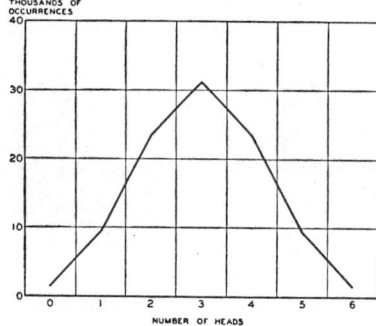

Chart 8.4. Expected Results of 100,000 Tosses of Six Coins.

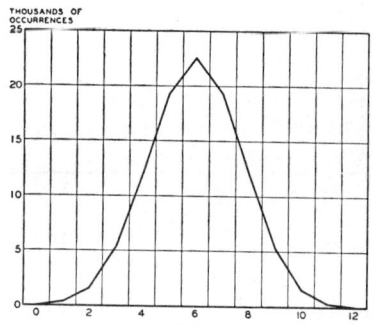

Chart 8.5. Expected Results of 100,000 Tosses of Twelve Coins.

ble the normal curve of Chart 8.1. It must be apparent that, if the exponent of the expression $(\tfrac{1}{2}t + \tfrac{1}{2}h)$ is increased from 12 to some larger number, the curve will become still smoother. It can be shown that, as the exponent approaches infinity, the entire expression approaches, as a limit, the expression for the normal curve,[1]

---

[1] For a development, see C. H. Richardson, *An Introduction to Statistical Analysis*, Harcourt, Brace and Co., New York, 1944, rev. ed., pp. 397–401. Another proof, which considers also the case where the two probabilities are not equal, is given in G. U. Yule and M. G. Kendall, *An Introduction to the Theory of Statistics*. Charles Griffin and Co., Ltd., London, 1940, 12th ed., pp. 177–180.

$$Y_c = \frac{1}{2.5066\sigma}\, 2.71828^{\frac{-x^2}{2\sigma^2}},$$

where σ is the standard deviation of the population. As already stated, when we wish to fit a normal curve to a sample distribution, the equation is written

$$Y_c = \frac{Ni}{2.5066s}\, 2.71828^{\frac{-x^2}{2s^2}}.$$

Applications. The normal curve is sometimes used to describe the errors made in repeated measurements of the same object or

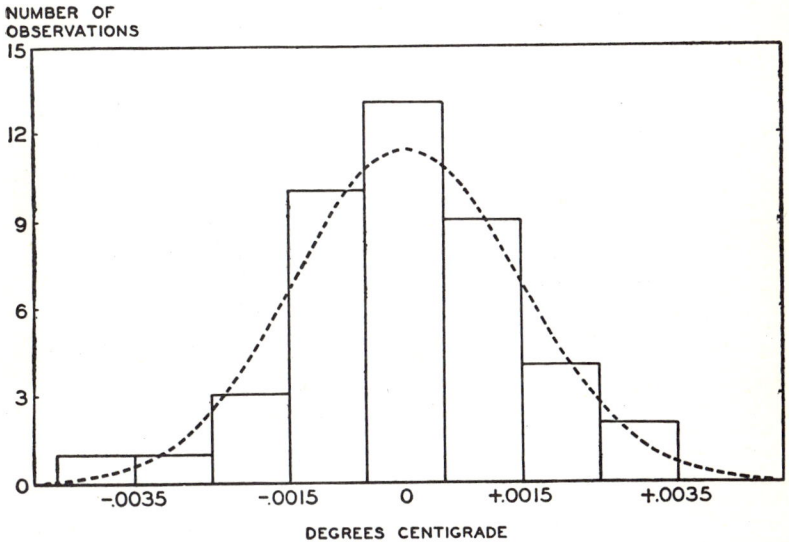

Chart 8.6. Normal Curve Fitted to 43 Observations of the Freezing Point of Water. The 43 observations are from T. B. Crumpler and J. H. Yoe, *Chemical Computations and Errors*, John Wiley and Sons, New York, 1940, p. 142.

phenomenon. Its early application by Gauss to errors made in astronomical measurements resulted in its also being known as the Gaussian Curve and the "normal curve of error." Chart 8.6 shows a normal curve fitted to a series of measurements of the freezing point of water. The observed data are represented by means of a column diagram; a curve is used to indicate the fitted normal curve. Not all distributions of repeated measurements will be of such a nature that a normal curve may appropriately be fitted, but, if a normal curve does fit the data, it may reasonably be assumed that the errors were random. This might also be a reasonable assumption if some other symmetrical, yet non-normal, curve were applicable, but not if a skewed curve were required to describe the data.

Chart 8.7 shows a normal curve fitted to a distribution of 1,000 arithmetic means, each of which was computed from a random sample of four items drawn from a normal population of 998 items.

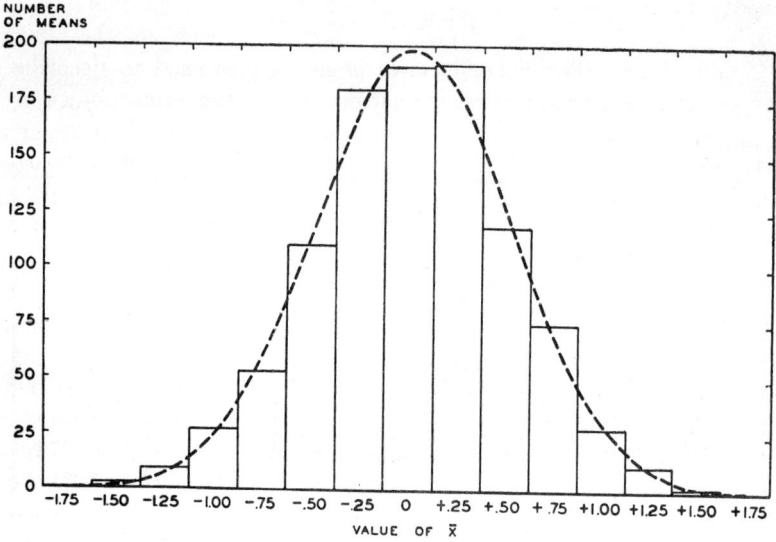

Chart 8.7. Normal Curve Fitted to Shewhart's 1,000 Sample Arithmetic Means. A chi-square test of "goodness of fit" (see pages 282, 283) shows that the fit is satisfactory. To avoid crowding, class mid-values rather than class limits are shown on the horizontal scale. Based on data from W. A. Shewhart, *Economic Control of Quality of Manufactured Product*, D. Van Nostrand Company, Inc., New York, 1931, pp 442–445, and 454–463.

This illustrates a point which will be more fully discussed in Chapter 9, that arithmetic means of random samples drawn from a normal population tend to form a normal curve around the arithmetic mean of the population from which they were drawn. While this is true for arithmetic means, it is not true that all statistical measures computed from samples will tend to form a normal curve; some follow other types of curves, as will be pointed out in Chapters 9, 10, 11, and 12. Applying to the data of Chart 8.7 methods to be described later in this chapter, we may determine: (1) the proportion of sample arithmetic means falling beyond an ordinate erected at any value greater (or less) than the arithmetic mean of the population, for example, an ordinate erected at $+1.10$; (2) the proportion of sample arithmetic means falling beyond ordinates erected one on one side and one on the other side of the arithmetic mean of the population, say, ordinates at ± 1.10 or one ordinate at $+1.10$ and the other at -1.00; (3) the proportion of sample arithmetic means falling between any two ordinates when one ordinate is on one side of the arithmetic mean of the population and the other is on the other side; and (4) the proportion of sample arithmetic means falling between any two ordinates when both ordinates are on the same side of the arithmetic mean of the population. Problems similar to these with applications to sample arithmetic means, proportions, standard deviations, and correlation coefficients will make up the subject matter of Chapters 9, 10, 11, and 12.

The data of Chart 8.6 were repeated measurements of the same phenomenon. Those of Chart 8.7 represented 1,000 attempts to measure, by means of samples, one aspect of the same population. To the extent that both were repeated attempts to measure, they are alike; but while the data of the freezing point of water reflect primarily errors of measurement, the data of the sample arithmetic means show fluctuations attributable to errors of sampling. Data of a different nature are used as the basis for Chart 8.8. Here a normal curve has been fitted to a distribution of the red blood cell counts of 137 healthy young men. These data are for a number of different but similar individuals. Using methods which will be described in later paragraphs, we can generalize for healthy young men by saying that, if these 137 measurements are representative, 32.6 per cent of such young men may be expected to have erythrocyte counts of 5.6 millions per cubic millimeter (M^2/mm^3) or higher; 12.7 per cent may be expected to have red blood cell counts of 4.9 M^2/mm^3 or lower; 82.6 per cent may be expected to be between 4.8 and 6.0 M^2/mm^3. Similar statements may be made for any other erythrocyte counts that may be of interest.

A final application of fitting the normal curve has to do with fitting to a given series in order to generalize concerning a closely associated series. For example, a normal curve may be fitted to the distribution of the neck circumferences of a homogeneous sample group of males. From the fitted curve, a manufacturing schedule of collars of various sizes may be made[2] which would be applicable to the larger group of men from which the sample was taken. In like fashion, a normal curve fitted to the head circumferences of boys may be used to determine the number of caps of the different

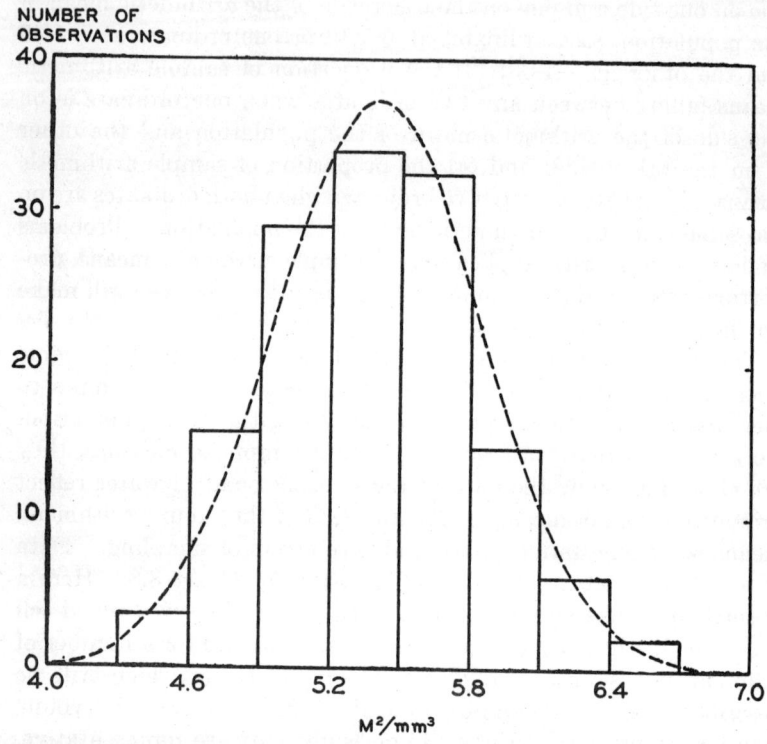

Chart 8.8. Normal Curve Fitted to Data of Red Blood Cell Count for 137 Healthy Young Men. Data of Tables 8.1 and 8.2.

sizes which might be required.[3] The reader will think of other similar applications, some calling for a normal curve, but others requiring a different sort of curve, symmetrical or skewed.[4]

One characteristic which all of the preceding illustrations have in

---

[2] See F. E. Croxton and D. J. Cowden, *Applied General Statistics*, Prentice-Hall, Inc., New York, 1939, pp. 281–283.

[3] See F. E. Croxton and D. J. Cowden, *Practical Business Statistics*, Prentice-Hall, Inc., New York, 1948, rev. ed., pp. 343–345.

[4] There are many types of skewed curves. The fitting of two is discussed in the reference in note 2, pp. 293–303.

common is that each set of data was a sample from a much larger group, called a *population*. Whenever a curve is fitted to a set of data, we are generalizing, from the limited information before us, in an attempt to say what the underlying distribution may be. In the case of the measurements of the freezing point of water, we have a few readings which are a sample from a much larger (infinite) number that might be made. The 1,000 arithmetic means, each computed from a sample of 4 items, shown in Chart 8.7, constitute only a relatively small group, since 992,023,968,016 samples of four items each may be drawn from a population of 998 items.[5] The 137 red blood cell counts of Chart 8.8 likewise represent only an extremely small portion of the counts which might be had. When we generalize by fitting a normal, or other, curve to a sample distribution, we cannot be sure that the curve we have used is appropriate. In Chapter 11 we shall consider a method of assaying the "goodness of fit" of a curve.

The fitting process. Fitting a normal curve to a set of observed data involves two steps: first, the computation of the ordinates and the drawing of the fitted curve, and, second, the determination of the proportionate areas in whatever part or parts of the curve may concern us. When ascertaining areas under the fitted curve, we shall make use of the classes as set up in the observed distribution. This would always be done if a test of "goodness of fit" (described in Chapter 11) is to be made. Sometimes classes quite different from those of the original data are employed. This might be the case if we were to ascertain men's collar sizes from data of neck circumferences. The class intervals and the class limits might both be different for the two distributions. At times we may not be interested in the areas for all parts of a distribution but may wish to know only the area or areas associated with one or more sections on the X-axis of the curve. Examples of this have already been given on pages 184 and 185. In Chapters 9–12 we shall have numerous occasions to ascertain the proportionate areas occurring in one or both tails of a curve.

---

[5] This is obtained from the expression $\mathcal{P}^N = 998^4 = 992,023,968,016$ and represents the number of combinations and permutations if each item is replaced after being drawn. $\mathcal{P}$ is the number of items in the population.

188   THE NORMAL CURVE   [Chap. 8

The data of the red blood cell counts for 137 young men, shown in Table 8.1, will be used to illustrate the procedure for fitting a normal curve. As explained in Chapter 3, the fractional frequencies are the result of splitting cases which had values falling on class limits. The figures in the first two columns of Table 8.1 have been plotted as the column diagram of Chart 8.8.

TABLE 8.1

Computation of $\bar{X}$ and s for Data of Red Blood Cell Count for 137 Healthy Young Men

(Cell counts are millions per cubic millimeter.)

Cell count X	Number of men f	d'	fd'	$f(d')^2$
4.3–4.6	3.5	−3	−10.5	31.5
4.6–4.9	15.5	−2	−31	62
4.9–5.2	29	−1	−29	29
5.2–5.5	34			
5.5–5.8	32.5	1	+32.5	32.5
5.8–6.1	14.5	2	+29	58
6.1–6.4	6	3	+18	54
6.4–6.7	2	4	+ 8	32
Total	137	...	+17	299

Data from *Archives of Internal Medicine*, Vol. 37, pp. 685–706, "Hemoglobin, Color Index, Saturated Index, and Volume Index Standards—Determinations Based on the Findings in One Hundred and Thirty-Seven Healthy Young Men," by Edwin E. Osgood. The men were medical students 19–30 years of age. Osgood's data, which were given to two decimal places, were rounded to one before grouping.

$$\bar{X} = 5.35 + \left(\frac{17}{137}\right)0.3 = 5.4 \text{ M}^2/\text{mm}^3.$$

$$s = 0.3\sqrt{\frac{299}{137} - \left(\frac{17}{137}\right)^2} = 0.44 \text{ M}^2/\text{mm}^3.$$

Computing the ordinates. The sole purpose of this step is to furnish us with a picture of the fitted curve such as has already been given in Charts 8.6, 8.7, and 8.8. It will be remembered that the equation is

$$Y_c = \frac{Ni}{2.5066s} 2.71828^{\frac{-x^2}{2s^2}}.$$

The values of $\bar{X}$ and s have been computed in Table 8.1, where it is seen that $\bar{X} = 5.4$ and $s = 0.44$ M^2/mm^3 (millions per cubic millimeter).

We first compute the value of the maximum ordinate, which is at $\bar{X}$. At $\bar{X}$, the value of $x = 0$. Rewriting the equation with $x = 0$ and using Y_0 to indicate the maximum ordinate, erected at $\bar{X}$, we have

$$Y_0 = \frac{Ni}{2.5066s} \, 2.71828^{\frac{-0^2}{2s^2}},$$

$$= \frac{Ni}{2.5066s} \, 2.71828^0,$$

$$= \frac{Ni}{2.5066s}.$$

Substituting the values for N, i and s gives

$$Y_0 = \frac{(137)(0.3)}{(2.5066)(0.44)} = 37.3.$$

The location of the first point for the fitted curve is therefore given by $X = \bar{X} = 5.4$ M^2/mm^3 and $Y_c = Y_0 = 37.3$.

Having determined the value of $\frac{Ni}{2.5066s}$, we may now get other ordinates by solving $2.71828^{\frac{-x^2}{2s^2}}$ for each of the various X values at which we wish to erect ordinates, and multiplying the two parts of the equation. However, before we can proceed, we must decide where we are going to erect the additional ordinates. Since the curve is symmetrical, an ordinate erected at a given distance on one side of the mean will have the same height as one erected at the same distance on the other side of the mean. We need, therefore, to consider how many ordinates we want to erect on one side of the arithmetic mean. We already know that, in theory, the normal curve extends indefinitely on either side of the arithmetic mean. However, the height of an ordinate at $\pm 3s$ from the mean is only about $\frac{1}{100}$ of the height of the ordinate at $\bar{X}$, so, unless a very large chart is being drawn, it is nearly impossible to plot ordinates beyond $\pm 3s$, since they will virtually coincide with the X-axis. If six ordinates were to be erected (at $+0.5s$, $+1.0s$, $+1.5s$, $+2.0s$, $+2.5s$, and $+3.0s$ and similarly on the other side of the arithmetic mean), a very small amount of computing would be involved, but the resulting curve would not be very smooth. If 60 ordinates were to be erected on either side of the arithmetic mean, a very smooth curve would result, but an unnecessarily large amount of computing would be necessary. A reasonably smooth curve will be obtained if 12 ordinates are erected (at $+0.25s$, $+0.50s$, $+0.75s$, and so on, to $+3.0s$, and similarly on the other side of the arithmetic mean), and only a reasonable amount of computing will be called for.

Having already determined Y_0 to be 37.3, we shall ascertain the value of $2.71828^{\frac{-x^2}{2s^2}}$ for $\pm 0.25s$, which, since $s = 0.44$ M²/mm³, is, for $x = \pm 0.11$, M²/mm³. This is

$$2.71828^{\frac{-(0.11)^2}{2(0.44)^2}} = 0.96923,$$

and

$$Y_c = (37.3)(0.96923) = 36.2,$$

which is the height of the ordinates at $x = \pm 0.11$ M²/mm³, or $X = \bar{X} \pm 0.11 = 5.4 \pm 0.11 = 5.29$ and 5.51 M²/mm³.

It is not necessary to perform the calculations apparently needed to determine that

$$2.71828^{\frac{-(0.11)^2}{2(0.44)^2}} = 0.96923;$$

we merely need to note that $\dfrac{x}{s} = \dfrac{0.11}{0.44} = 0.25$ and look up the desired value of $2.71828^{\frac{-x^2}{2s^2}}$ in Appendix I.

The next step is to determine the height of the ordinate at $X = 5.18$ and 5.62 M²/mm³, which is $x = \pm 0.22$ M²/mm³, and $\dfrac{x}{s} = 0.50$. From the table of Appendix I we find that

$$2.71828^{\frac{-(0.22)^2}{2(0.44)^2}} = 0.88250,$$

and

$$Y_c = (37.3)(0.88250) = 32.9.$$

The remaining ordinates are computed in similar fashion, as shown in Table 8.2. It is preferable to perform the computations of this table vertically rather than horizontally. This enables one to look up all the values of $2.71828^{\frac{-x^2}{2s^2}}$ at one operation, and thus to save an appreciable amount of time. The 25 ordinates shown in column 5 of Table 8.2 enable us to plot the fitted normal curve which is shown in Chart 8.8.

TABLE 8.2

COMPUTATION OF ORDINATES FOR FIT OF NORMAL CURVE TO DATA OF RED BLOOD CELL COUNT FOR 137 HEALTHY YOUNG MEN

$\bar{X} = 5.4$ M^2/mm^3. $s = 0.44$ M^2/mm^3. $Y_0 = 37.3$.

X in millions per cubic millimeter, where ordinates are erected	$x = X - \bar{X}$	$\dfrac{x}{s}$	Proportionate height of ordinate $2.71828^{\dfrac{-x^2}{2s^2}}$ (From Appendix I)	Y_c height of ordinate $[Y_0 \times \text{Col }(4)]$
(1)	(2)	(3)	(4)	(5)
4.08	−1.32	−3.00	0.01111	0.4
4.19	−1.21	−2.75	0.02280	0.9
4.30	−1.10	−2.50	0.04394	1.6
4.41	−0.99	−2.25	0.07956	3.0
4.52	−0.88	−2.00	0.13534	5.0
4.63	−0.77	−1.75	0.21627	8.1
4.74	−0.66	−1.50	0.32465	12.1
4.85	−0.55	−1.25	0.45783	17.1
4.96	−0.44	−1.00	0.60653	22.6
5.07	−0.33	−0.75	0.75484	28.2
5.18	−0.22	−0.50	0.88250	32.9
5.29	−0.11	−0.25	0.96923	36.2
5.4	0	0	1.00000	37.3
5.51	+0.11	+0.25	0.96923	36.2
5.62	+0.22	+0.50	0.88250	32.9
5.73	+0.33	+0.75	0.75484	28.2
5.84	+0.44	+1.00	0.60653	22.6
5.95	+0.55	+1.25	0.45783	17.1
6.06	+0.66	+1.50	0.32465	12.1
6.17	+0.77	+1.75	0.21627	8.1
6.28	+0.88	+2.00	0.13534	5.0
6.39	+0.99	+2.25	0.07956	3.0
6.50	+1.10	+2.50	0.04394	1.6
6.61	+1.21	+2.75	0.02280	0.9
6.72	+1.32	+3.00	0.01111	0.4

Determining areas. To ascertain the area under any portion of a normal curve, it is necessary to integrate the curve. However, this has been reduced to a table, shown in Appendix II, so that no knowledge of the mathematics of integration is necessary. First, let it be recalled that half of the area of a normal curve is to the right of

$\bar{X}$ and half is to the left. The table of Appendix II shows the area enclosed between an ordinate erected at $\bar{X}$ and ordinates erected at various specified $\frac{x}{s}$ distances *in one direction* from $\bar{X}$, as shown in the small chart accompanying this appendix. Since the area under the entire curve is indicated by 1.0, the maximum proportionate area shown in Appendix II is 0.50.

Suppose that we wish to know the proportionate area under the normal curve of Chart 8.8 which is enclosed between a vertical line drawn at $\bar{X} = 5.4$ M^2/mm^3 and another at $X = 5.84$ M^2/mm^3. This value is 0.44 M^2/mm^3 from $\bar{X}$, so that $x = +0.44$ M^2/mm^3, and, since $s = 0.44$ M^2/mm^3, $X = 5.84$ M^2/mm^3 is exactly $+1s$ removed from the mean. Therefore, $\frac{x}{s} = 1.0$. From Appendix II it is seen that 0.3413 of the area under the curve is included between $\frac{x}{s} = 0$ and $\frac{x}{s} = 1.0$ in one direction.[6] Consequently, 0.3413 of the area is included between 5.4 and 5.84 M^2/mm^3. What has just been done is illustrated in part A of Chart 8.9. It will be noticed that, while $x = +0.44$ M^2/mm^3, we wrote $\frac{x}{s}$ as 1.0 without any sign. The sign merely tells us whether we are working to the right or left of $\bar{X}$. The tabled areas in Appendix II are for either $+$ or $-$ values of $\frac{x}{s}$.

If we desire the proportion of the normal curve to the right of $X = 5.84$ M^2/mm^3, we obtain the figure by subtracting 0.3413 from 0.5000, obtaining 0.1587. This, too, is shown in part A of Chart 8.9.

In the event that we wish to know the proportionate area between $X = 4.9$ M^2/mm^3 and $X = 5.3$ M^2/mm^3, we must determine first the proportionate area from $\bar{X}$ to $X = 4.9$ M^2/mm^3, then the proportionate area from $\bar{X}$ to $X = 5.3$ M^2/mm^3, and finally subtract the second figure from the first. This is necessary because integration proceeds from $\bar{X}$ as a point of reference. The value $X = 4.9$ M^2/mm^3 is 0.5 M^2/mm^3 less than $\bar{X}$, so that $x = -0.5$

---

[6] An ordinate drawn at exactly $\pm 1s$ from $\bar{X}$ meets the normal curve at the point of inflection. See Chart 8.9A.

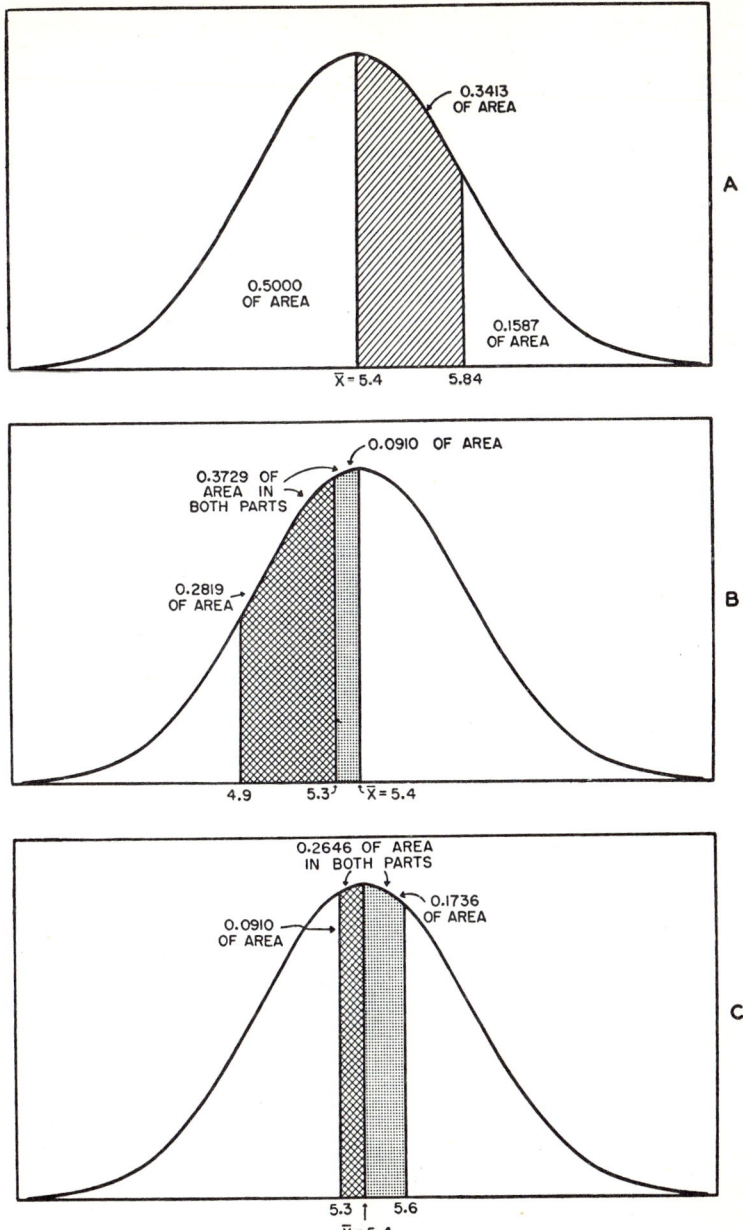

Chart 8.9. **Proportionate Areas Under the Normal Curve Between $\bar{X}$ and Selected Values.** The horizontal scale values are in terms of millions per cubic millimeter.

M²/mm³, $\dfrac{x}{s} = \dfrac{0.5}{0.44} = 1.14$, and the proportionate area from $\bar{X}$ to $X = 4.9$ M²/mm³ is 0.3729. When $X = 5.3$ M²/mm³, $x = -0.1$ M²/mm³, $\dfrac{x}{s} = \dfrac{0.1}{0.44} = 0.23$, and the proportionate area from $\bar{X}$ to $X = 5.3$ M²/mm³ is 0.0910. Subtracting these two decimal fractions gives

$$0.3729 - 0.0910 = 0.2819$$

as the proportionate area from $X = 4.9$ M²/mm³ to $X = 5.3$ M²/mm³. The foregoing is shown in part B of Chart 8.9.

Perhaps we want the proportion of the area under the curve between $X = 5.3$ M²/mm³ and $X = 5.6$ M²/mm³. This problem differs from any of the preceding, since one X value is smaller than $\bar{X}$ while the other is larger. The procedure consists merely of determining the two proportionate areas separately and adding. For the area from $\bar{X}$ to $X = 5.3$ M²/mm³: $x = -0.1$ M²/mm³, $\dfrac{x}{s} = \dfrac{0.1}{0.44} = 0.23$, and the proportionate area is 0.0910, as found in the preceding paragraph. For the area from $\bar{X}$ to $X = 5.6$ M²/mm³: $x = +0.2$ M²/mm³, $\dfrac{x}{s} = \dfrac{0.2}{0.44} = 0.45$, and the proportionate area is 0.1736. Adding these two results gives 0.2646, as shown in part C of Chart 8.9.

If we wish to determine the proportional frequencies under the normal curve corresponding to the classes shown in Table 8.1 and then to prorate those frequencies on a basis of $N = 137$, we proceed as in Table 8.3, which involves the procedure illustrated in part B of Chart 8.9 for all classes except the one which is split by $\bar{X}$, the class "5.2–5.5 million per cubic millimeter." The area for this class is computed by the procedure illustrated in part C of Chart 8.9. Since the normal curve is of unlimited range in both directions, there will ordinarily be proportionate and computed frequencies beyond the range of the observed data as shown in the first and last rows of figures in Table 8.3. This result is not unreasonable, since, if the sample of healthy young men were very large, it is conceivable that a few rare cases below 4.3 and above 6.7 M²/mm³ might be found. The column of computed frequencies with $N = 137$ compares well with the observed frequencies of Table 8.1. The two sets of frequencies will form the basis of a test of "goodness of fit"

TABLE 8.3

Determination of Computed Frequencies in Each Class for Data of Red Blood Cell Count for 137 Healthy Young Men

$\bar{X} = 5.4 \text{ M}^2/\text{mm}^3.$ $s = 0.44 \text{ M}^2/\text{mm}^3.$

Cell count	Limit of class		x Deviation from mean to limit	$\dfrac{x}{s}$	Cumulative proportion of area between mean and limit (From Appendix II)	Proportion of area in each class	Computed frequencies in each class $N = 137$
	Lower	Upper					
(1)	(2)	(3)	(4)	(5)	(6)	(7)	(8)
4.3 or fewer	...	...	...	...	0.5000	0.0062	0.8
4.3–4.6	4.3	...	1.1	2.50	0.4938	0.0282	3.9
4.6–4.9	4.6	...	0.8	1.82	0.4656	0.0927	12.7
4.9–5.2	4.9	...	0.5	1.14	0.3729	0.1993	27.3
5.2–5.5 {	5.2	...	0.2	0.45	0.1736	} 0.2646	36.3
{	...	5.5	0.1	0.23	0.0910		
5.5–5.8	...	5.8	0.4	0.91	0.3186	0.2276	31.2
5.8–6.1	...	6.1	0.7	1.59	0.4441	0.1255	17.2
6.1–6.4	...	6.4	1.0	2.27	0.4884	0.0443	6.1
6.4–6.7	...	6.7	1.3	2.95	0.4984	0.0100	1.4
6.7 or more	...	...	...	...	0.5000	0.0016	.2
Total	...	...	...	...	...	1.0000	137.1

in Chapter 11. As in the case of Table 8.2, the computations in Table 8.3 should be carried out vertically rather than horizontally.

When to fit the normal curve. Before fitting a normal curve to a sample distribution, some consideration should be given to the appropriateness of such a fit. The crudest check consists of merely looking at column diagrams (or curves) of the observed data such as those shown in Charts 8.6, 8.7, and 8.8. It is somewhat more satisfactory to compute cumulative frequencies and cumulative percentage frequencies, as shown in Table 8.4, and then to

TABLE 8.4

Cumulative Distribution of Red Blood Cell Count for 137 Healthy Young Men

(Cell counts are in millions per cubic millimeter.)

Cell count	Number of men	Per cent of men
4.6 or less	3.5	2.6
4.9 or less	19	13.9
5.2 or less	48	35.0
5.5 or less	82	59.9
5.8 or less	114.5	83.6
6.1 or less	129	94.2
6.4 or less	135	98.5
6.7 or less	137	100.0

Based on data of Table 8.1.

plot these cumulative percentage frequencies on a sheet of arithmetic probability paper, as shown in Chart 8.10. The vertical ruling of arithmetic probability paper is so designed that a normal curve will yield a straight line. Consequently, if a set of observed data are represented by a line which is approximately straight, one may proceed to fit a normal curve to the data. It is even better, but more time-consuming, to compute measures of skewness and kurtosis, as described in Chapter 5, and to test these measures to ascertain whether their values do or do not depart significantly from the values for a normal curve, as described in Chapter 12. If significant differences are not present, a normal curve may be fitted.

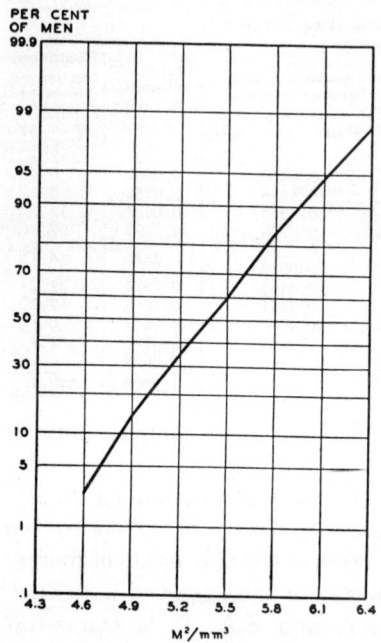

Chart 8.10. Cumulative Percentage Distribution of Red Blood Cell Counts, for 137 Healthy Young Men, Shown on Arithmetic Probability Paper. Data of Table 8.4.

Mention has already been made of a test of "goodness of fit" which is described in Chapter 11 and which tells us, after a normal curve has been fitted, whether the hypothesis that the sample was drawn at random from a normal population is or is not tenable.

The Binomial

We shall make use of the binomial, not only to describe a set of observed discrete data in this chapter, but also in Chapter 10 to test the reliability of a proportion computed from a small sample and to make an exact statement of the confidence limits (see page 259) of a population proportion (π) based upon a knowledge of the proportion (p) occurring in a sample and of the size of the sample.

The binomials shown in Charts 8.2, 8.3, 8.4, and 8.5 were all symmetrical, since π, the probability of occurrence of a head, was equal to τ, the probability of non-occurrence. If π and τ are not equal, the curve of the resulting binomial is skewed; and the greater the difference between π and τ, the greater the skewness. Since we write $(\tau + \pi)^N$, rather than $(\pi + \tau)^N$, and show increasing powers of π from left to right on the horizontal axis when plotting a binomial, the skewness is positive when $\pi < 0.5$ and negative when $\pi > 0.5$. This is clearly shown in Chart 10.4.

The data in Table 8.5 show the number of families of four living children which have 0, 1, 2, 3, or 4 males, as found in a survey in

TABLE 8.5

NUMBER OF MALE LIVE BIRTHS IN FAMILIES OF FOUR LIVE BIRTHS, INDIANAPOLIS SAMPLE, 1941

Number of male live births	Number of families
0	5
1	24
2	44
3	19
4	11
Total	103

Data are from the Milbank Memorial Fund, which obtained a sample, of families of various sizes, of relatively fecund couples in Indianapolis in 1941.

Indianapolis. We shall undertake to describe this series, which is shown by means of the separated bars of Chart 8.11, by use of a binomial. When fitting a binomial to a set of data, the proportion of occurrences and non-occurrences may be determined either from actual or hypothetical information concerning the population or from the sample data themselves. When population information is used, the proportion of occurrences is designated by π and the proportion of non-occurrences by τ. The binomial to be expanded would then be $(\tau + \pi)^N$, where N would be equal to one less than the number of categories in the data, since an expanded binomial has one more term than the power to which it is raised. N is also the number of items in a sample. In Table 8.5 there are 103 samples ($k = 103$), each consisting of four living children. If the sample data are used as the basis for determining the proportion of occurrences and non-occurrences, the proportion of occurrences is designated by p and the proportion of non-occurrences by q. The binomial to be expanded would then be $(q + p)^N$.

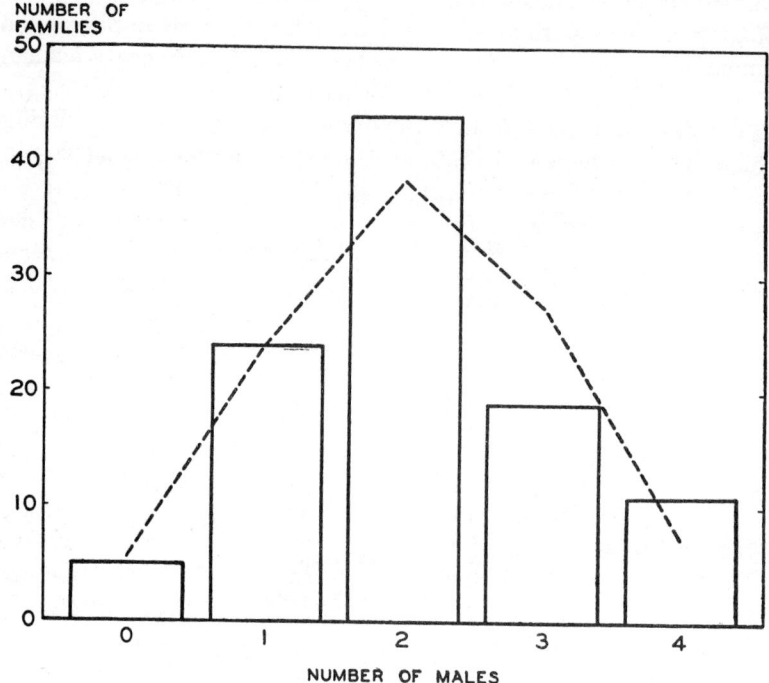

Chart 8.11. Binomial Fitted to Number of Male Live Births in Families of Four Live Births, Indianapolis Sample, 1941. Data of Tables 8.5 and 8.6.

For the present illustration, the value of p will be determined by computing the proportion of male live births in the 103 families.[7] Since there was a total of $4 \times 103 = 412$ live births, and since $(0 \times 5) + (1 \times 24) + (2 \times 44) + (3 \times 19) + (4 \times 11) = 213$ of them were male, we have

$$p = \frac{213}{412} = 0.5170,$$

---

[7] Alternatively, π could be computed by ascertaining the proportion of male live births in Indianapolis or in the United States for a selected period or π could be taken as 0.50 on the (incorrect) hypothesis that there are equal proportions of live births of the two sexes.

and $q = 1 - p = 0.4830$. Five terms will be needed (the samples are families of four), so the binomial will be raised to the fourth power, $N = 4$. We shall therefore fit a binomial by ascertaining the values of the five terms in the expression

$$(q + p)^4 = (0.4830 + 0.5170)^4.$$

These will yield the proportionate frequencies for the five classes, and the five terms will total 1.0. Each of the five terms will then be multiplied by 103 to give the computed frequencies for $k = 103$ to agree with the total of the observed data of Table 8.5. The computations are carried out by means of logarithms, as shown in Table 8.6, and the fitted binomial is shown by the broken curve of Chart 8.11. If a χ^2 test, described in Chapter 11, is made, the fit is found to be good.

The fitting of a binomial is often considered a test of randomness. We may therefore say that the satisfactory fit of the binomial to the data of Table 8.5 gives us no reason to conclude that other than chance factors are operating. However, it must be remembered that our sample dealt with but 103 families. The discrepancies between the observed and computed frequencies might be more pronounced if we had more extensive data. R. A. Fisher[8] has fitted a binomial to nineteenth-century data for 53,680 German families in the Kingdom of Saxony, each of eight children. He shows that his fit is not good and points out that there is an excess of very unequally divided families, owing in small part to multiple births, which show more instances of like sex than of unlike sex. An interesting feature of the basic data[9] (not commented on by Fisher) is that they were not a cross section but were based on registrations over the years 1876–1885. Extensive data of the sort shown in Table 8.5 for United States families are not available, but New Zealand data for 3,866 families of six children (having one or more members under 16 years of age present) are shown in Chart 8.12, together with a fitted binomial. In this instance $p = 0.5094$ and the binomial which was fitted was $(0.4906 + 0.5094)^6$.

---

[8] R. A. Fisher, *Statistical Methods for Research Workers*, Hafner Publishing Co., New York, 1946, 10th ed., pp. 66–68.

[9] The data are from *Zeitschrift des K. Sächsischen Statistischen Bureaus*, Vol. 35, 1889, "Beiträge zur Frage des Geschlechtsverhältnisses der Gebornen," by Arthur Geissler.

TABLE 8.6

Fitting of Binomial $(q + p)^N$ to Data of Male Live Births in Families of Four Live Births

$k = 103; q = 0.4830; p = 0.5170; N = 4;$
$\text{Log } q = 9.683947 - 10; \log p = 9.713491 - 10.$
$\text{Log } q = 9.683947 - 10.$

Number of males (power of p) (1)	Expression* (2)	Log C (3)	Log of indicated power of q (4)	Log of indicated power of p (5)	Sum of logs in Cols. (3), (4), and (5) (6)	Proportionate frequencies [antilog of Col. (6)] (7)	Computed frequencies $k = 103$ (8)
0	$C_0 \cdot q^4 \cdot p^0 = 1(0.4830)^4(0.5170)^0$	...	8.735788 − 10	...	8.735788 − 10	0.0544	5.6
1	$C_1 \cdot q^3 \cdot p^1 = 4(0.4830)^3(0.5170)^1$	0.602060	9.051841 − 10	9.713491 − 10	9.367392 − 10	0.2330	24.0
2	$C_2 \cdot q^2 \cdot p^2 = 6(0.4830)^2(0.5170)^2$	0.778151	9.367894 − 10	9.426982 − 10	9.573027 − 10	0.3741	38.5
3	$C_3 \cdot q^1 \cdot p^3 = 4(0.4830)^1(0.5170)^3$	0.602060	9.683947 − 10	9.140473 − 10	9.426480 − 10	0.2670	27.5
4	$C_4 \cdot q^0 \cdot p^4 = 1(0.4830)^0(0.5170)^4$	...	...	8.853964 − 10	8.853964 − 10	0.0714	7.4
Total						1.0000	103.0

* C_0, C_1, C_2, etc. are the binomial coefficients, obtained as follows:

$$C_0 = 1;\ C_1 = N;\ C_2 = \frac{N(N-1)}{2!};\ C_3 = \frac{N(N-1)(N-2)}{3!};\ \text{etc.}$$

Although there is an excess of families with no males and with 6 males, a χ^2 test shows that the over-all fit is satisfactory.

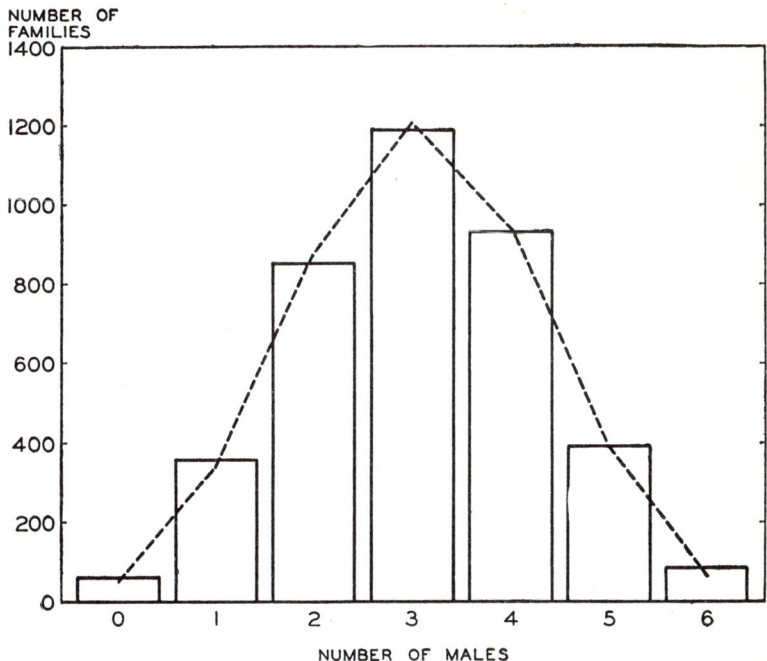

Chart 8.12. Binomial Fitted to Number of Males in Families of Six Children, New Zealand, 1926. The data are for members present under 16 years of age. Some families included stepchildren and adopted children. Data from Dominion of New Zealand, *Population Census*, 1926, *Vol. XII, Families and Households*, Table 15, p. 37, Wellington, 1931.

The Poisson Distribution

It was pointed out earlier in this chapter that the normal curve is the limit of the binomial $(\frac{1}{2} + \frac{1}{2})^N$ as N approaches infinity. The Poisson distribution is the limit of the binomial under different conditions. If, in the binomial $(\tau + \pi)^N$ the value of π (or τ) is allowed to become very small while N approaches infinity, it can be shown[10] that the binomial approaches the Poisson distribution

---

[10] See S. S. Wilks, *Elementary Statistical Analysis*, Princeton University Press, Princeton, 1948, p. 133f.

as a limit, the various terms of which are given by the expression

$$\frac{1}{e^{\bar{X}}} \cdot \frac{\bar{X}^0}{0!}, \quad \frac{1}{e^{\bar{X}}} \cdot \frac{\bar{X}^1}{1!}, \quad \frac{1}{e^{\bar{X}}} \cdot \frac{\bar{X}^2}{2!}, \quad \frac{1}{e^{\bar{X}}} \cdot \frac{\bar{X}^3}{3!}, \text{ etc.}$$

and the probability of exactly a occurrences is given by

$$\frac{\bar{X}^a}{a! e^{\bar{X}}}.$$

The Poisson distribution may be used to describe a distribution when the value of π is small (say, less than 0.10) and when the value of N is large enough so that the product πN is finite but not large. It should be clearly understood that, under these conditions, the Poisson is an approximation to the binomial $(\tau + \pi)^N$ but is easier to fit. Like the binomial, it is used to describe discrete variables. Unlike the binomial, which can be fitted only if the value of π (or p computed from the sample) is known, the Poisson may be fitted without reference to the actual value of π or p. In fact, the value of π or p is sometimes not ascertainable; we merely need to be sure that it is small.

There is still another point of contrast between the binomial and the Poisson distribution. We cannot fit a binomial unless our data consist of a specific number of categories, since a binomial has $N + 1$ terms. It will be recalled that the data of Table 8.5 formed 5 categories, and that the exponent of the binomial fitted to those data was 4. However, if our observed data should fall into a number of categories (say, 10), but if an indefinite number of additional categories are possible, though not observed, it is impossible to fit a binomial, since N is not known, but a Poisson distribution may be employed.

As is apparent, from the expressions already given for the Poisson, the fitting is accomplished from a knowledge of only the value of the arithmetic mean of the sample. For a given set of data

$$\bar{X} = pN;$$

but, since p and N are often not known, we compute $\bar{X}$ from the data.

As an illustration, we shall fit a Poisson distribution to data (from a single blood specimen) of the number of erythrocytes which were found in each of 400 squares (that is, 400 samples, $k = 400$) in a graduated counting chamber. The data are shown in Table 8.7.

THE POISSON DISTRIBUTION

To make the count in each square, the field under the microscope was enlarged 220 times and photographed, after which each cell (which was then about 1.5 mm in diameter) was pierced with a pointed stylus and the count made electrically. There was therefore no error in the count.

TABLE 8.7

NUMBER OF ERYTHROCYTES PER SQUARE, FROM A SINGLE BLOOD SPECIMEN, IN EACH OF 400 SQUARES IN A GRADUATED COUNTING CHAMBER

Number of erythrocytes a	Number of squares
0	2
1	10
2	21
3	52
4	63
5	77
6	62
7	46
8	41
9	11
10	8
11	5
12 or more*	2
Total	400

* Considered to have been counts of 12, which results in a value of $\bar{X}$ in agreement with that given in the reference below.

Data from J. Berkson, T. B. Magath, and M. Hurn, "Laboratory Standards in Relation to Chance Fluctuations of the Erythrocyte Count as Estimated with the Hemocytometer," *Journal of the American Statistical Association*, Vol. 30, No. 190, pp. 414–426.

To fit a Poisson distribution to the data of Table 8.7, we first compute $\bar{X}$, the mean number of erythrocytes per sample, which is $[(2 \times 0) + (10 \times 1) + (21 \times 2) + \cdots + (2 \times 12)] \div 400 = 5.31$, and then proceed to ascertain the proportional frequencies by evaluating the terms

$$\frac{1}{e^{\bar{X}}} \cdot \frac{\bar{X}^0}{0!}, \quad \frac{1}{e^{\bar{X}}} \cdot \frac{\bar{X}^1}{1!}, \quad \frac{1}{e^{\bar{X}}} \cdot \frac{\bar{X}^2}{2!}, \quad \frac{1}{e^{\bar{X}}} \cdot \frac{\bar{X}^3}{3!}, \text{ etc.}$$

Consideration of these expressions reveals that each term may be computed from the preceding one by multiplying the preceding term by $\dfrac{\bar{X}}{a}$; thus,

1st term $(a = 0)$.........$\dfrac{1}{e^{\bar{X}}}$,

2nd term $(a = 1)$.........(1st term) $\times \dfrac{\bar{X}}{1}$,

3rd term $(a = 2)$.........(2nd term) $\times \dfrac{\bar{X}}{2}$,

4th term $(a = 3)$.........(3rd term) $\times \dfrac{\bar{X}}{3}$,

etc.   etc.

TABLE 8.8

FITTING OF POISSON DISTRIBUTION TO DATA OF ERYTHROCYTES PER SQUARE

Number of erythrocytes a (1)	$\dfrac{\bar{X}}{a}$ for all terms except first (2)	Proportionate frequency, preceding term $\times \dfrac{\bar{X}}{a}$ except for first entry (3)	Computed frequency $k = 400$ (4)
0	$\dfrac{1}{e^{\bar{X}}} =$	0.004942	2.0
1	5.31	0.02624	10.5
2	2.655	0.06967	27.9
3	1.77	0.1233	49.3
4	1.3275	0.1637	65.5
5	1.062	0.1738	69.5
6	0.885	0.1538	61.5
7	0.7586	0.1167	46.7
8	0.6638	0.07747	31.0
9	0.59	0.04571	18.3
10	0.531	0.02427	9.7
11	0.4827	0.01172	4.7
12 or more	...	0.00868*	3.5
Total	...	1.00000	400.1

* This figure computed as a residual.

The computations in the above table could be further simplified by using $k \div e^{\bar{X}}$ for the first term. This would eliminate one column of figures.

Approximate values for column (3) may be read directly from Table LI on pages 113–121 of Karl Pearson, *Tables for Statisticians and Biometricians*, Cambridge University Press, 1914. In this table proportionate frequencies are given corresponding to values of $\bar{X}$ ranging from 0.1 to 15.0 by steps of 0.1.

Table 8.8 shows the fit of a Poisson distribution by this procedure, the proportional frequencies being given in column (3) and the computed frequencies, for $k = 400$, appearing in column (4).

The observed frequencies of Table 8.7 and the computed frequencies of Table 8.8 are shown in Chart 8.13; the agreement appears to be good. If a test of goodness of fit is made, as described in

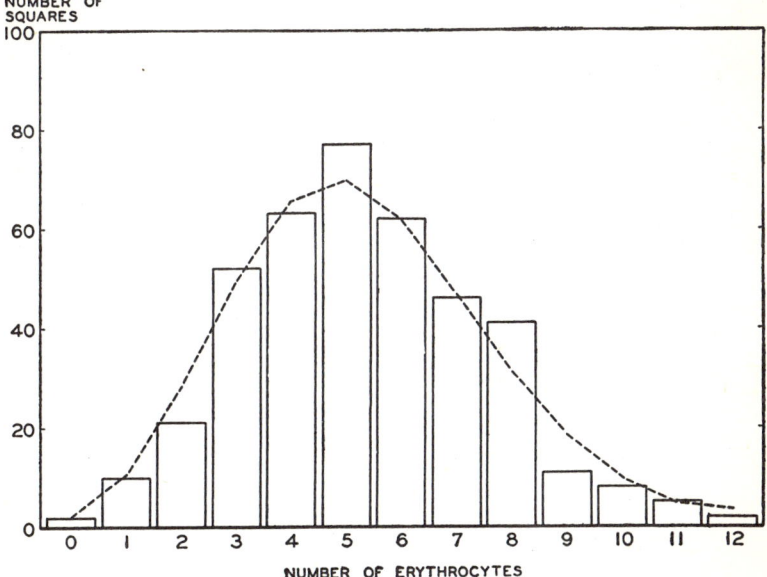

Chart 8.13. Poisson Distribution Fitted to Data of Erythrocytes per Square. Data of Tables 8.7 and 8.8.

Chapter 11, the fit is found to be satisfactory. This result is often interpreted to mean that the distribution is a random one.

Although we do not need the value of p or N to accomplish the fit of a Poisson, it is possible to approximate them for the particular set of illustrative data which we used. Berkson, Magath, and Hurn point out, in the reference from which the data of Table 8.7 were taken, that a droplet of diluted blood will cover about 100,000 squares in a counting chamber, and that the probability of a cell entering a square is therefore approximately .000 01 ($\pi \approx 0.000\ 01$). They also state that the number of cells in a droplet would be in the neighborhood of 500,000. It follows, then, that $\pi N \approx 5$, which agrees approximately with the value of 5.31 for $\bar{X}$ as determined from the data. The binomial which was approximated by use of the fit of the Poisson distribution in Table 8.8 is

$$(\tau + \pi)^N = (0.999\ 99 + 0.000\ 01)^{500,000}.$$

However, Berkson, Magath, and Hurn call attention to the fact that only about 50 cells can possibly be in a square, and that the actual situation therefore departs from the theory on which the Poisson series is based and which assumes that π is constant, irrespective of the number of cells already in a square. Actually, the more cells in a square, the smaller the probability that another cell will fall in that square. This discrepancy does not appreciably affect the goodness of fit of the Poisson to the observed data, but it does result in a figure of $s = 2.18$ cells per square, *computed from the data* of Table 8.7. This is smaller than the theoretical value of s for a Poisson, which is $\sqrt{\overline{X}}$, and which would therefore be 2.30 cells per square. Now, it is not surprising that these two values should differ, but Berkson, Magath, and Hurn found that the standard deviation computed from the data was smaller than $\sqrt{\overline{X}}$ for every one of ten series similar to the one used for our illustration.

Symbols Used in

CHAPTER 9

$\beta_{1\wp}$: lower-case Greek beta, skewness in a population.
$\beta_{1\bar{x}}$: skewness of the distribution of sample $\bar{X}$ values.
$\beta_{2\wp}$: kurtosis in a population.
$\beta_{2\bar{x}}$: kurtosis of the distribution of sample $\bar{X}$ values.
D: a difference between paired values.
$F: \dfrac{\hat{\sigma}_1^2}{\hat{\sigma}_2^2}$, see Chapter 12.
K: the number of different possible samples of N items from a population of $\wp$ items.
n: degrees of freedom in a sample. When two samples are under consideration, $n = n_1 + n_2$.
N: the number of items in a sample. When two samples are under consideration, we use N_1 and N_2.
P: probability, varies from 0 to 1.
$\wp$: the number of items in a population. As a subscript, $\wp$ means "population"; thus, $\bar{X}_\wp$ is the arithmetic mean of a population.
r: the correlation coefficient.
s: the standard deviation of a sample.
σ: lower-case Greek sigma, the standard deviation of a population.
$\hat{\sigma}$: the estimated standard deviation of a population, computed from a single sample. Referred to as "sigma caret" or "sigma hat."
  $\hat{\sigma}_1$ is an estimate based on sample 1.
  $\hat{\sigma}_2$ is an estimate based on sample 2.
  $\hat{\sigma}_{1+2}$ is an estimate computed by pooling x^2 values and degrees of freedom from two samples.
$\hat{\sigma}_D$: the estimated population standard error for a series of D values.
$\sigma_{\bar{x}}$: the standard error of $\bar{X}$. When two samples are under consideration, we use $\sigma_{\bar{x}_1}$ and $\sigma_{\bar{x}_2}$.
$\hat{\sigma}_{\bar{x}}$: the estimated standard error of $\bar{X}$.
$\hat{\sigma}_{\bar{x}_1 - \bar{x}_2}$: the estimated standard error of the difference between two sample arithmetic means.
$\hat{\sigma}_{\bar{x}_D}$: the estimated standard error of $\bar{X}_D$.

SYMBOLS USED IN CHAPTER 9

Σ: upper-case Greek sigma, meaning "take the sum of."

$t: \dfrac{\bar{X} - \bar{X}_\mathcal{P}}{\hat{\sigma}_{\bar{X}}}, \dfrac{\bar{X}_1 - \bar{X}_2}{\hat{\sigma}_{\bar{X}_1 - \bar{X}_2}}, \text{ or } \dfrac{\bar{X}_D}{\hat{\sigma}_{\bar{X}_D}}.$

$x: X - \bar{X}.$
$x_1: X_1 - \bar{X}_1.$
$x_2: X_2 - \bar{X}_2.$
X: an observed value in a sample.
X_1: an observed value in sample 1.
X_2: an observed value in sample 2.
$\bar{X}$: the arithmetic mean of a sample.
$\bar{X}_1$: the arithmetic mean of sample 1.
$\bar{X}_2$: the arithmetic mean of sample 2.
$\bar{X}_D$: the arithmetic mean of a series of D values.
$\bar{X}_\mathcal{P}$: the arithmetic mean of a population.
$\bar{X}_{\mathcal{P}_1}$: the lower confidence limit of $\bar{X}_\mathcal{P}$.
$\bar{X}_{\mathcal{P}_2}$: the upper confidence limit of $\bar{X}_\mathcal{P}$.
$\dfrac{x}{\sigma}$: a deviation divided by its standard error, for example, $\dfrac{\bar{X} - \bar{X}_\mathcal{P}}{\sigma_{\bar{X}}}$.

Chapter 9
RELIABILITY AND SIGNIFICANCE OF ARITHMETIC MEANS

The evidence obtained by a research worker will almost always be based upon sample data. There are several reasons why this is true. In the first place, it is often not possible to take into consideration all the items in a population. If a study is to be made of the reaction of male hamsters to a particular drug, it is obvious that it would not be possible to include all male hamsters in the investigation. In the second place, it is more economical of time and money to analyze a representative sample than to attempt to include all existing cases. Finally, it is not necessary to study an entire population to arrive at a reliable conclusion; information covering a suitable sample will ordinarily be satisfactory.

In this chapter we shall deal with arithmetic means computed from random samples. Other statistical measures will be considered in Chapters 10, 11, and 12, but in every instance we shall be concerned only with random samples. *A random sample may be defined as one which is obtained in such a manner that at each selection of an item from the population, each item is drawn independently of each other item in the population and each item in the population has the same probability of being selected.* When a sample is drawn in this way, each possible sample of N items will have an equal chance of being selected. When heterogeneity is present in a population, and when that heterogeneity is believed to have a bearing upon the problem under investigation, the data may be divided into strata and a random sample selected from each stratum. This volume will not consider the reliability of measures computed from stratified samples.

From this point on, we shall usually refer to arithmetic means computed from random samples merely as *sample means*, since we are dealing only with random samples and only with arithmetic (not geometric, harmonic, or other) means.

Behavior of Arithmetic Means of Random Samples

Walter A. Shewhart[1] has provided useful experimental data to illustrate the behavior of arithmetic means of random samples drawn from a normal population. He set up a population of 998 items consisting of circular chips bearing the values -3.0, -2.9, -2.8, $\cdots$, -0.2, -0.1, 0, 0.1, 0.2, $\cdots$, 2.8, 2.9, 3.0. The number of chips bearing each of the 61 values was so designed that the population was as nearly normal as possible for a population of 998 items. The distribution had

$$\overline{X}_\mathcal{P} = 0, \qquad \sigma = 1.0070,$$

$$\beta_{1\mathcal{P}} = 0, \qquad \beta_{2\mathcal{P}} = 2.9302.$$

Individual chips were drawn at random from the population. After a chip was drawn, and the value upon it recorded, the chip was replaced before another draw was made.

Sample means vary on either side of the population mean. Shewhart was interested in studying the behavior of the means of samples of four items each ($N = 4$). In the preceding chapter (page 187) it was noted that 992,023,968,016 samples of four might have been drawn from the population of 998 items ($\mathcal{P} = 998$). Shewhart drew 1,000 samples each consisting of four items, and for each of the 1,000 samples he computed the arithmetic mean. For the first sample he obtained $\overline{X}_1 = 0.950$, for the second sample $\overline{X}_2 = 0.350$. Neither of these agrees with the arithmetic mean of the population, $\overline{X}_\mathcal{P} = 0$, but that is not surprising. The sample means will vary above (positive) and below (negative) the value for the mean of the population. If we consider the first ten samples, we find:

$$\overline{X}_1 = 0.950,$$
$$\overline{X}_2 = 0.350,$$
$$\overline{X}_3 = 0.325,$$
$$\overline{X}_4 = -0.400,$$

---

[1] Walter A. Shewhart, *Economic Control of Quality of Manufactured Product*, D. Van Nostrand Co., New York, 1931, pp. 167, 442–445, and 454–462.

$$\overline{X}_5 = 0.400,$$
$$\overline{X}_6 = -0.150,$$
$$\overline{X}_7 = -0.275,$$
$$\overline{X}_8 = -0.075,$$
$$\overline{X}_9 = -0.075,$$
$$\overline{X}_{10} = -0.400.$$

The arithmetic mean of a series of sample means. It will be seen that four of the sample means are positive while six are negative. If the ten values are totaled, we get 0.650, and the mean of the ten sample arithmetic means is therefore 0.065. For the 1,000 sample means obtained by Shewhart, the arithmetic mean was found to be 0.014. If all of the possible 992,023,968,016 samples of $N = 4$ were to be considered, the value of the arithmetic mean of all these sample arithmetic means would equal 0, which is $\overline{X}_\varphi$.

Dispersion of sample means. As a measure of the dispersion of a series of means of random samples, we may compute their standard deviation in the same fashion that we computed the standard deviation of a series of values in Chapter 5, the deviations being the difference between each sample mean and $\overline{X}_\varphi$. For the first 10 sample means, this would be[2]

$$\sqrt{\frac{(0.950 - 0)^2 + (0.350 - 0)^2 + \cdots + (-0.400 - 0)^2}{10}} = 0.415.$$

If the standard deviation is computed for all of the 1,000 sample means obtained by Shewhart, it would be ascertained by taking

$$\sqrt{\frac{(\overline{X}_1 - \overline{X}_\varphi)^2 + (\overline{X}_2 - \overline{X}_\varphi)^2 + \cdots + (\overline{X}_{1,000} - \overline{X}_\varphi)^2}{1,000}},$$

and its value is found to be 0.503.

Suppose, now, that, instead of employing merely the 1,000 sample means obtained by Shewhart, we were to consider all the 992,023,968,016 possible different samples of four items, indicated by K.

---

[2] If the deviations are taken from the mean of the sample means instead of from $\overline{X}_\varphi$, we get 0.410 for the 10 sample means and 0.502 for the 1,000 sample means.

This is

$$\sigma_{\bar{x}} = \sqrt{\frac{(\bar{X}_1 - \bar{X}_\mathcal{P})^2 + (\bar{X}_2 - \bar{X}_\mathcal{P})^2 + \cdots + (\bar{X}_K - \bar{X}_\mathcal{P})^2}{K}},$$

which reduces to[3]

$$\sigma_{\bar{x}} = \frac{\sigma}{\sqrt{N}}.$$

$\sigma_{\bar{x}}$ is termed *the standard error of sample means*, or, more briefly, *the standard error of the mean*. For the samples of four, we have

$$\sigma_{\bar{x}} = \frac{1.0070}{\sqrt{4}} = 0.5035.$$

Notice the close agreement between the figure 0.503, obtained from the data for 1,000 sample means, and this figure. Of course, it is most unusual to have a large number of sample means, so that $\sigma_{\bar{x}}$ is ordinarily computed by using

$$\sigma_{\bar{x}} = \frac{\sigma}{\sqrt{N}}.$$

Skewness and kurtosis of sample means. Another important observation concerning the behavior of means of random samples must be made before we are in a position to consider the significance of the difference between a sample mean and a population mean. It is that means of random samples, drawn from a normal population, may be expected to describe a normal curve. This has already been clearly shown in Chart 8.7, which is repeated here as Chart 9.1 and which portrays a normal curve fitted to Shewhart's 1,000 sample means. Chart 9.2 shows the distribution of the 1,000 sample means compared with the distribution of the population of 998 items.

---

[3] For a demonstration, see F. E. Croxton and D. J. Cowden, *Applied General Statistics*, Prentice-Hall, Inc., New York, 1939, pp. 834–837. If $\mathcal{P}$ is finite and the individual items are replaced only after each sample has been drawn, use

$$\sigma_{\bar{x}} = \frac{\sigma}{\sqrt{N}} \sqrt{\frac{\mathcal{P} - N}{\mathcal{P} - 1}}.$$

The expression under the second radical may be dropped if $\mathcal{P}$ is large in relation to N.

Even if the population is not normal, the distribution of random sample arithmetic means will tend toward normality according to the relationships

$$\beta_{1\bar{x}} = \frac{\beta_{1\wp}}{N} \text{ and}$$

$$\beta_{2\bar{x}} - 3 = \frac{\beta_{2\wp} - 3}{N},$$

where $\beta_{1\bar{x}}$ and $\beta_{2\bar{x}}$ indicate, respectively, the skewness and kurtosis of sample means, and $\beta_{1\wp}$ and $\beta_{2\wp}$ refer to the skewness and kurtosis

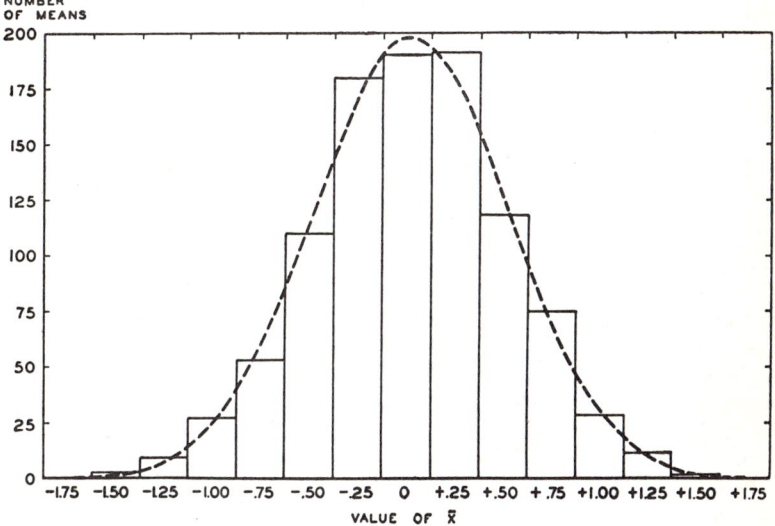

Chart 9.1. Normal Curve Fitted to Shewhart's 1,000 Sample Arithmetic Means. A chi-square test of "goodness of fit" (see pages 282–283) shows that the fit is satisfactory. To avoid crowding, class mid-values rather than class limits are shown on the horizontal scale. Based on data from W. A. Shewhart, *Economic Control of Quality of Manufactured Product*, D. Van Nostrand Company, Inc., New York, 1931, pp. 442–445 and 454–463.

in the population. From these expressions it may be seen that, even though a population departs from normal, the random sample arithmetic means drawn from it will tend to depart even less from normal[4] and, the larger the size of the sample, the more marked

---

[4] A chart showing the distribution of a series of sample means drawn from a skewed population is given in F. E. Croxton and D. J. Cowden, *Applied General Statistics*, Prentice-Hall, Inc., New York, 1939, p. 306.

this tendency will be. Consequently, we usually consider that random sample arithmetic means are distributed normally unless the population from which they are taken is known to depart markedly from normal.

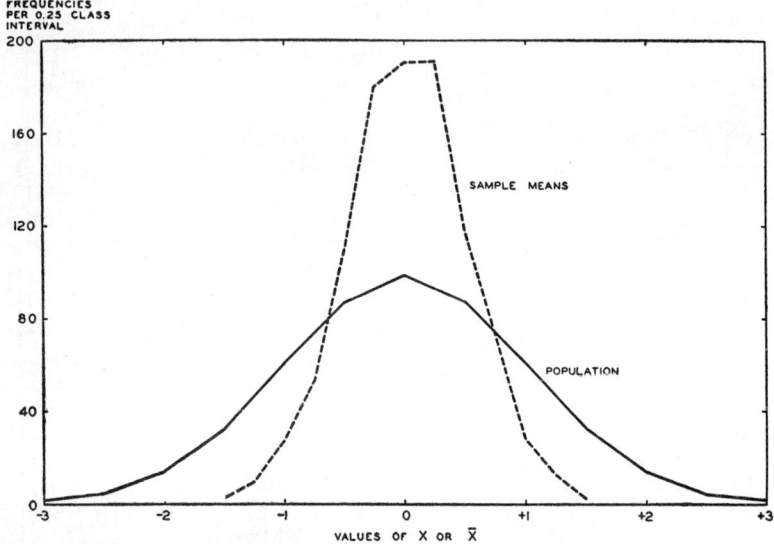

Chart 9.2. Distribution of Shewhart's Normal Population of 998 Items and of 1,000 Sample Arithmetic Means. The class intervals are 0.50 for the population, 0.25 for the sample means. Based on data from W. A. Shewhart, *Economic Control of Quality of Manufactured Product*, D. Van Nostrand Co., Inc., New York, 1931, pp. 167, 442–445, and 454–463.

Illustrative distributions of sample means. It is clear from the expression

$$\sigma_{\bar{X}} = \frac{\sigma}{\sqrt{N}}$$

that the dispersion of sample means varies directly with the dispersion of the population and inversely as the square root of the size of the sample. A few simple illustrations will help to fix this in the reader's mind.

If we have a normally distributed population of infinite size having $\bar{X}_\varphi = 80$ grams and $\sigma = 12$ grams, and we propose to draw samples of $N = 25$, we find that

$$\sigma_{\bar{X}} = \frac{12}{\sqrt{25}} = 2.4 \text{ grams,}$$

and the distribution of the sample means is shown by the solid curve of Chart 9.3. If we draw samples of the same size from a normally

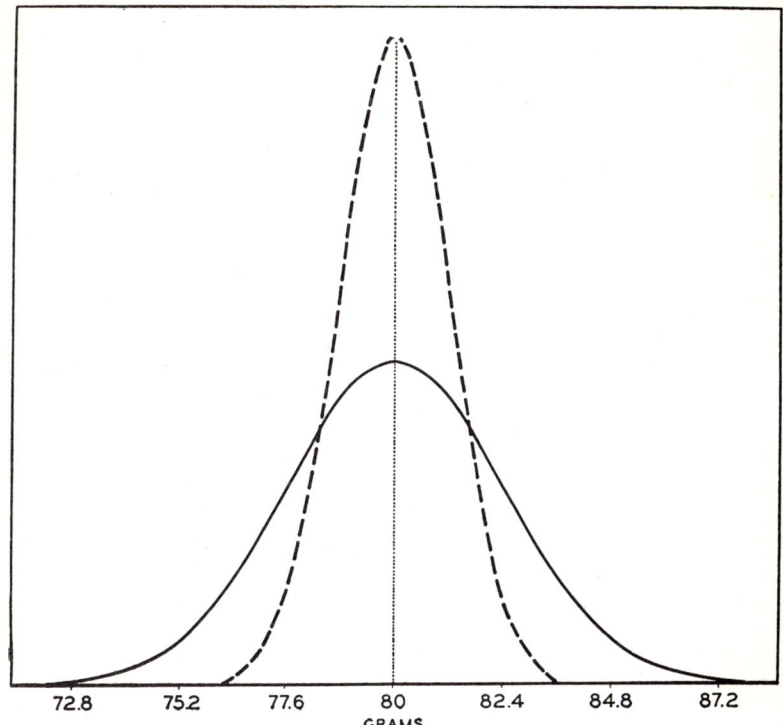

Chart 9.3. Distribution of Sample Arithmetic Means for $N = 25$ When $\bar{X}_{\wp} = 80$ Grams and $\sigma = 12$ Grams (Solid Curve) and When $\bar{X}_{\wp} = 80$ Grams and $\sigma = 6$ Grams (Broken Curve).

distributed population of infinite size having $\bar{X}_{\wp} = 80$ grams and $\sigma = 6$ grams, we have

$$\sigma_{\bar{x}} = \frac{6}{\sqrt{25}} = 1.2 \text{ grams.}$$

The distribution of sample means from this population is indicated by the broken curve of Chart 9.3. It is apparent that the smaller the value of σ, the less the dispersion of sample means.

Suppose that random samples of $N = 16$ are to be drawn from a normally distributed population of infinite size having $\bar{X}_{\wp} = 50$

mm and $\sigma = 8$ mm. Then

$$\sigma_{\bar{x}} = \frac{8}{\sqrt{16}} = 2 \text{ mm},$$

and the distribution of the sample means is shown by the solid

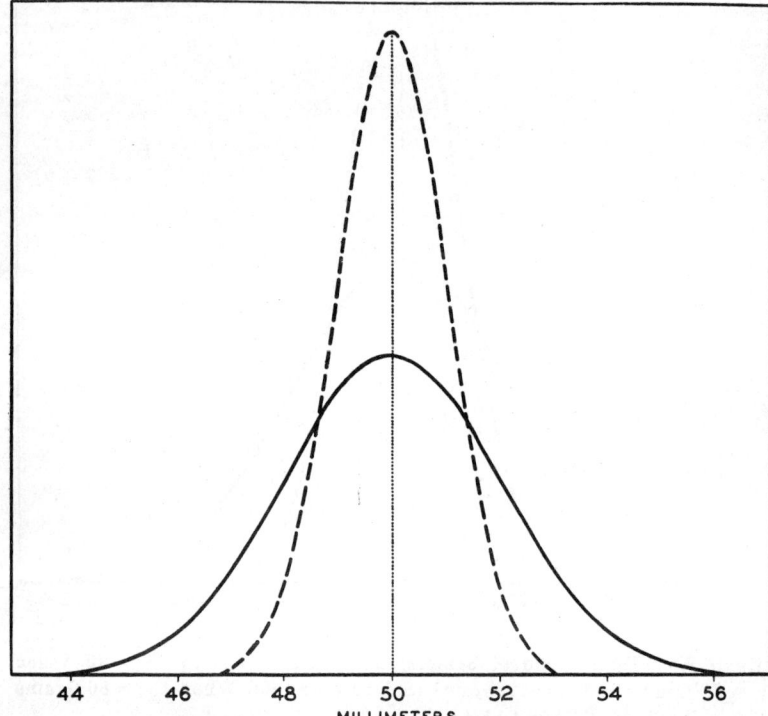

Chart 9.4. Distribution of Sample Arithmetic Means for $\bar{X}_{\varphi} = 50$ mm and $\sigma = 8$ mm, When $N = 16$ (Solid Curve) and When $N = 64$ (Broken Curve).

curve of Chart 9.4. If, now, we consider random samples of $N = 64$, we have

$$\sigma_{\bar{x}} = \frac{8}{\sqrt{64}} = 1 \text{ mm},$$

and the distribution of sample means from samples of 64 is shown by the broken curve of Chart 9.4. Increasing the size of the samples drawn results in decreasing the dispersion of sample means.

Consider the third of the four illustrations just mentioned, where $\overline{X}_\wp = 50$ mm, $\sigma = 8$ mm, $N = 16$, and $\sigma_{\bar{x}} = 2$ mm, and suppose that we wish to know the proportion of sample means that may be expected to equal or exceed 53 mm. This may be ascertained from the table of areas of the normal curve, given as Appendix II, but it is more easily determined from the table of areas in one tail of the normal curve, shown as Appendix III. We merely compute

$$\frac{x}{\sigma} = \frac{\overline{X} - \overline{X}_\wp}{\sigma_{\bar{x}}} = \frac{53 - 50}{2} = 1.5,$$

and, from the entries in Appendix III, learn that the proportion is 0.0668, or 6.68 per cent. This is shown as the cross-hatched area

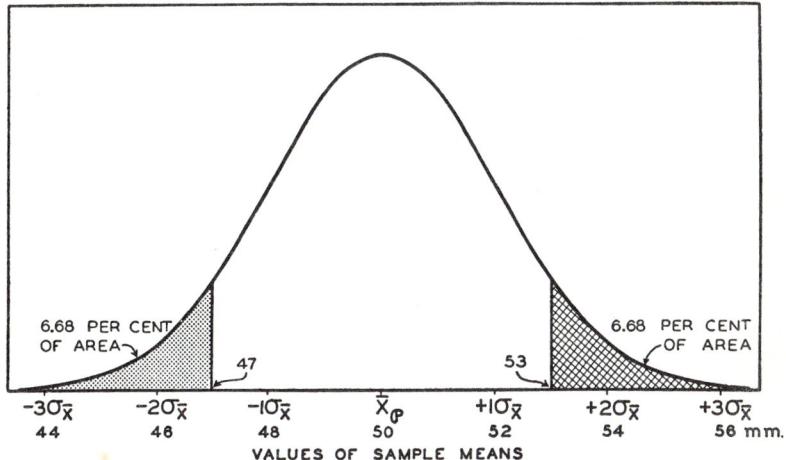

Chart 9.5. Expected Distribution of Sample Means and Chances of Obtaining Sample Means Differing from $\overline{X}_\wp$ by $\pm 1.5\sigma_{\bar{x}}$ or more.

of Chart 9.5. The proportion of sample means that may be expected to equal or fall below 47 mm is, similarly, 0.0668, or 6.68 per cent, and is represented graphically by the opposite tail of the curve, which is the stippled area of Chart 9.5. If we wish to know the proportion of sample means which differ from $\overline{X}_\wp$ by ± 3 mm or more, we may add the two percentages just obtained or we may make use of the table of areas in two tails of the normal curve, shown as Appendix IV. In either case, the proportion is 0.1336, or 13.36 per cent, which is indicated by the cross-hatched and stippled areas of Chart 9.5.

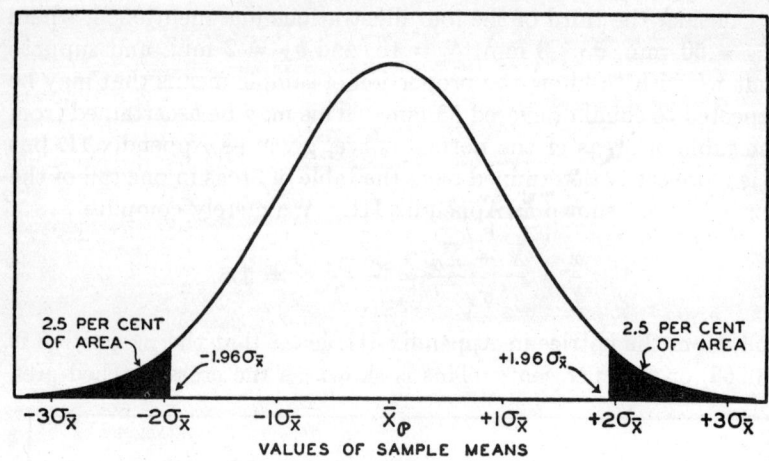

Chart 9.6. Expected Distribution of Sample Means Showing $\bar{X}_{\wp} \pm 1.96\sigma_{\bar{x}}$.

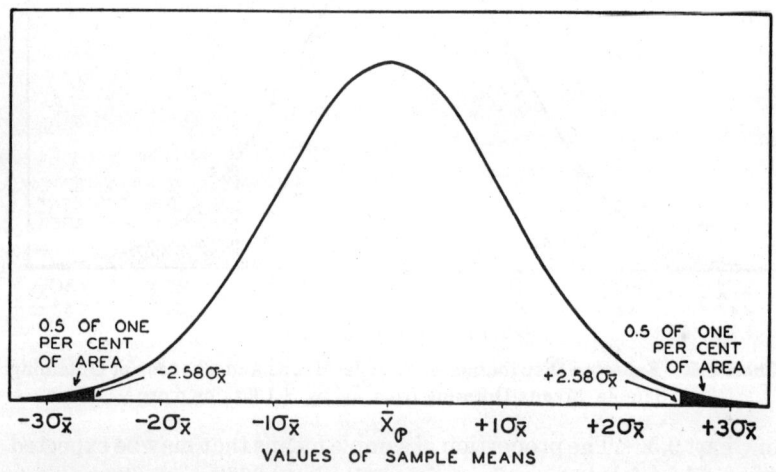

Chart 9.7. Expected Distribution of Sample Means Showing $\bar{X}_{\wp} \pm 2.58\sigma_{\bar{x}}$.

For use in later sections of this chapter, we shall be interested in the $\dfrac{x}{\sigma}$ value cutting off two tails of the curve which together include 5 per cent ($P = 0.05$) of the area of the curve and the $\dfrac{x}{\sigma}$ value which cuts off two tails including 1 per cent ($P = 0.01$) of the area.

CHAP. 9]   RELIABILITY AND SIGNIFICANCE   219

Referring to Appendix IV, it is seen that, for $P = 0.05$, the $\frac{x}{\sigma}$ value is 1.96 (see Chart 9.6), and that, for $P = 0.01$, the $\frac{x}{\sigma}$ value is 2.58 (see Chart 9.7), to the nearest tenth, or 2.576 if an additional decimal is desired.

Significance of Difference Between $\bar{X}$ and $\bar{X}_{(P)}$ When Population Values Are Known

Presence of a non-significant difference. It will be recalled that the population from which Shewhart selected his samples had $\bar{X}_{(P)} = 0$ and $\sigma = 1.0070$. Suppose that we are interested in the second

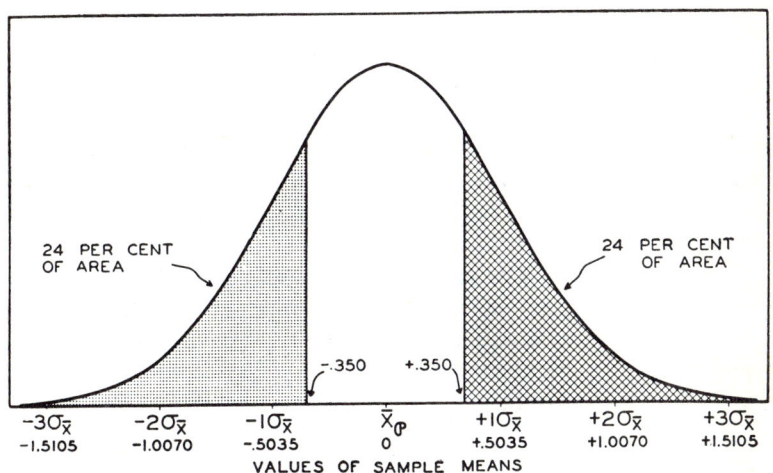

Chart 9.8. Expected Distribution of Sample Means and Chances of Obtaining Sample Means Differing from $\bar{X}_{(P)}$ by $\pm 0.70\sigma_{\bar{x}}$ or More.

sample of four items which he drew. This sample yielded $\bar{X} = 0.350$. Is it reasonable to believe that $\bar{X} = 0.350$ differs more than a mean of a sample of four items might be expected to differ from the mean of this population? In other words, is there a significant difference between $\bar{X}$ and $\bar{X}_{(P)}$? Since sample means are distributed normally around $\bar{X}_{(P)}$, we can draw a diagram such as Chart 9.8, having

$$\sigma_{\bar{x}} = \frac{\sigma}{\sqrt{N}} = \frac{1.0070}{\sqrt{4}} = 0.5035.$$

Then we can indicate the value of $\overline{X} = 0.350$ on Chart 9.8. Now, sample means vary on either side of $\overline{X}_\varphi$ and there is no reason for believing that sample means will always *exceed* $\overline{X}_\varphi$. Since we are interested in knowing whether the observed *difference* between $\overline{X}$ and $\overline{X}_\varphi$ is significant, we consider not only $\overline{X} = 0.350$ but also the equally probable $\overline{X} = -0.350$, which is also noted on Chart 9.8. From the chart it is clear that a divergence equal to ± 0.350 or greater may be expected to occur rather often.

To be more specific,

$$\frac{x}{\sigma} = \frac{\overline{X} - \overline{X}_\varphi}{\sigma_{\overline{x}}} = \frac{0.350 - 0}{0.5035} = 0.70.$$

and, looking up $\frac{x}{\sigma} = 0.70$ in Appendix IV, we find that $P = 0.4839$, indicating that a difference equal to or greater than that observed might be expected to occur in about 48 out of 100 random samples. Since the observed difference may occur this often as a result of the operation of chance factors, it can hardly be thought of as attributable to a real difference between $\overline{X}$ and $\overline{X}_\varphi$. The difference is not significant.

What we have just done was first to set up the hypothesis that the observed sample mean was the mean of a random sample from the population having $\overline{X}_\varphi = 0$ and $\sigma = 1.0070$. This is called a "null hypothesis," meaning that it is a hypothesis of no difference between $\overline{X}$ and $\overline{X}_\varphi$. We then proceeded to test the hypothesis by computing a significance ratio $\frac{x}{\sigma}$ and ascertaining the probability of obtaining, through the operation of random sampling, a difference equal to or greater than that observed. In essence, our test consists of casting doubt upon the hypothesis. Had P been small (just how small will be considered later), much doubt would have been cast upon the hypothesis, and we would have considered it discredited or impugned. However, P was found to be 0.4839, meaning that a difference such as the one under consideration or larger would be expected to occur rather often merely because of the variations attributable to random sampling. We have therefore cast little doubt on the hypothesis and consider it not to be discredited. Notice that, statistically, we cannot prove or disprove a hypothesis: we merely cast much or little doubt upon it. Experimentally, a hypothesis might be considered proved or disproved after many consistent repetitions, but a statistical test of a null hypothesis merely discredits or fails to discredit it.

Presence of a significant difference. Suppose that we are presented with the results of one sample of four items having[5] $\bar{X} = 1.72$. Is there a significant difference between $\bar{X}$ and $\bar{X}_\varphi$? Our null hypothesis is that $\bar{X} = 1.72$ is the mean of a random sample

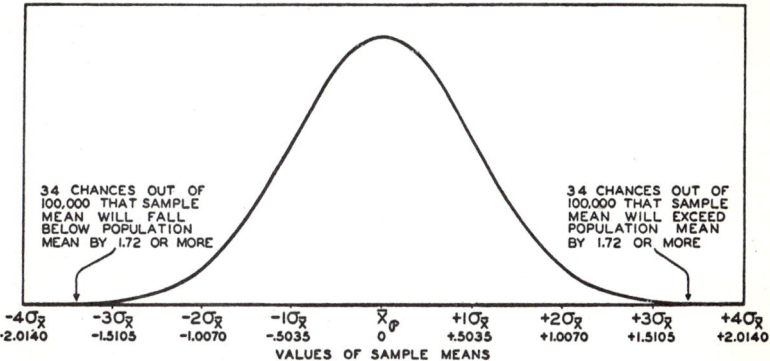

Chart 9.9. Expected Distribution of Sample Means and Chances of Obtaining Sample Means Differing from $\bar{X}_\varphi$ by $\pm 3.4\sigma_{\bar{x}}$ or More.

from the population having $\bar{X}_\varphi = 0$ and $\sigma = 1.0070$. We compute

$$\sigma_{\bar{x}} = \frac{\sigma}{\sqrt{N}} = \frac{1.0070}{\sqrt{4}} = 0.5035 \text{ and}$$

$$\frac{x}{\sigma} = \frac{\bar{X} - \bar{X}_\varphi}{\sigma_{\bar{x}}} = \frac{1.72 - 0}{0.5035} = 3.4.$$

Chart 9.9 shows the expected distribution of sample means with the values of $\bar{X} = 1.72$ and $\bar{X} = -1.72$ shown by means of arrows. It is obvious from the chart that a chance difference of ± 1.72 or more would occur but rarely. The probability is obtained from Appendix IV; $P = 0.000674$. Only about 7 times in 10,000 would a difference equal to or greater than that observed be expected to occur as the result of random sampling. We have discredited the null hypothesis. There is a significant difference between $\bar{X}$ and $\bar{X}_\varphi$.

---

[5] None of Shewhart's samples showed so great a departure from $\bar{X}_\varphi$.

Our declaration of the existence of a significant difference means that we believe that the sample was either not a random sample or not from the population under consideration or both. In the present instance, if the population of 998 chips was the only one available, and if there was no other population in existence from which a sample might erroneously have been drawn, it would appear that the sample mean under consideration was not from a sample drawn at random.

The judgments, based upon probabilities, which were just made may seem to the reader to embody a new and unusual principle, but just the opposite is true. Nearly all of our everyday activities involve decisions based upon probabilities. Consider, for example, the matter of crossing a busy road. One looks to the left, then to the right, judges the distance and speed of approaching traffic, and decides, upon the basis of subjective probability (not numerically stated), that he can or cannot safely reach the other side. Occasionally one decides that he can make it across and finds he is wrong. Sometimes one decides to wait and finds that waiting was not necessary. A young man, courting a young lady, may unconsciously make a judgment based on probability when he decides whether tonight, tomorrow night, or indeed any night, is the time to propose, and she, in turn, in making up her mind whether or not to accept him may very likely base her decision upon probability. The football player who decides what plays his team will use when on the offense must make a quick decision each time concerning the probable success of the various plays used by his team. When his team is on the defensive, he or another player must estimate the best probable deployment of his team against each play which he thinks his opponents will use.

What probability constitutes a suitable criterion of significance? The two tests of significance which were used as illustrations embodied clear-cut situations. The first one was manifestly not significant; the second was obviously significant. No question was raised concerning how small P should be in order for a difference to be declared significant. It is also worth while to point out that, even though P was only 0.000674 in the second illustration, and we had no hesitation in declaring the presence of a significant difference, our conclusion nevertheless may have been wrong, because truly random samples *would* show a deviation equal to or greater than that observed 674 times in 1,000,000. However, our chance of being wrong is exactly that small. This leads to a consideration of the ways in which we may be wrong (and right) when making a statistical inference and to a choice of a probability level for declaring significance or the lack of it.[6]

Two types of errors. Suppose that we set up a null hypothesis that a sample mean is the mean of a random sample drawn from a particular population, and that *the hypothesis is actually true.* If we test an observed difference and conclude that it is not significant, we are right. On the other hand, if we test an observed difference and declare it to be significant, we are wrong. This is referred to as a "Type I error," and if we have used $P = 0.05$ (often referred to as "the 0.05 level") as a criterion of significance, we shall make exactly 1 out of 20 such Type I errors in the long run. Using $P = 0.05$ as a criterion of significance means that we shall declare significant all differences having $P \leq 0.05$. Similarly, if we use $P = 0.01$ (the 0.01 level) as a criterion, declaring significant all differences having $P \leq 0.01$, we shall make 1 out of 100 Type I errors in the long run.

Consider, now, that we set up a null hypothesis that a sample mean is the mean of a random sample drawn from a particular population, and that *the hypothesis is actually false.* If we test an observed difference and conclude that it is significant, we are right. However, if we test an observed difference and declare it to be not significant, we are wrong, and this is referred to as a "Type II error." If we use $P = 0.05$ as the criterion, it is not possible to say how often Type II errors will occur. This is so because we have no way of knowing how false the hypothesis is, since the sample may be (1) a non-random sample from the population under consideration or (2) a random or non-random sample from some other population. About all that can be said[7] is that we shall make fewer Type II errors when we use $P = 0.05$ as a criterion than when we use $P = 0.01$.

The choice of a criterion of significance depends largely upon the relative seriousness of Type I and Type II errors. If it is very important to avoid Type I errors, we may employ $P = 0.01$ or $P = 0.001$. If Type II errors are more important to avoid, we

---

[6] For a more complete discussion, see Paul G. Hoel, *Introduction to Mathematical Statistics*, John Wiley and Sons, New York, 1947, Ch. XI.

[7] But see the reference given in note 6.

would be likely to employ $P = 0.05$ or possibly $P = 0.10$, although this would be unusual. Three illustrations will serve to clarify this point.

An institution using a number of short-lived pieces of laboratory equipment considers replacing them with a new, improved model. The new apparatus, although alleged to have a longer life than that formerly used, can be installed only at considerable expense. If, in the comparison of the life of the new and the old device, a Type I error is made, the new device would be installed and a large amount. of money wasted, when actually the new device is no better than the old. The consequence of this error is a sizable financial loss. However, if a Type II error is made in comparing the two devices in respect to length of life, the new device would not be installed, although actually having a longer life. The institution fails to get the advantages accruing from the use of apparatus having a longer life, but no positive loss has occurred. It would seem more important to avoid a Type I error than a Type II error, and therefore the value of P might be 0.01, or even 0.001, for the declaration of a significant difference. Whenever it is particularly important to have a high degree of assurance that the declaration of the presence of a significant difference is correct, one should use a small value of P as the criterion.

As a second illustration, consider the problem of manufacturing a powerful drug which must be of exactly the right potency, neither too weak nor too strong. If a batch is manufactured and, upon being compared with the standard (population), a Type I error is made, the batch will be rejected although it was really satisfactory. The consequence of this error is destruction or remanufacture of the batch. On the other hand, if a batch is compared with the standard and a Type II error is made, a quantity of the drug which is actually not standard may be released for use. The consequence of an error of this type may be the death of a number of persons. In such a situation, it is more important to avoid Type II errors than Type I errors, and P may well be taken as 0.05, or possibly 0.10 or larger.

Sometimes it is not easy to say whether Type I or Type II errors are more important to avoid. If a new treatment (which is expensive, painful, or dangerous) has been developed for a disease, it would, of course, be compared with the conventional method. If a Type I error is made, concluding that the new treatment is better when it actually is not, patients would experience no more beneficial

RELIABILITY AND SIGNIFICANCE

results than before but would be put to additional expense, endure more pain, or be subject to more danger. If a Type II error is made, concluding that the new treatment is no better than the former one when actually it is superior, patients would fail to reap the advantage of the superior treatment. Under these conditions, one would be likely to use $P = 0.05$ or possibly 0.02.

In any situation, the investigator should consider the probability which he will use as a criterion in the light of the problem on which he is working. It is not satisfactory to use one level of probability and apply it indiscriminately to all problems.

When making a test of significance, one should select, *before* the computations are made, the probability level which he will use. This precaution, obviously, is taken to avoid any possibility of wishful thinking after the calculations have been completed. If the investigator, instead of merely concluding "significant" or "not significant," indicates what level of significance he is using as a criterion and then states the value of P which is obtained, he is not only being frank with his readers in revealing the basis of his conclusion, but he is also indicating the probability of the occurrence of Type I errors.

The reader may have wondered why our initial test of the difference between a sample mean and a population mean dealt with Shewhart's second sample rather than with his first one. The reason is that it was desired to present an example that would clearly show non-significance, without the necessity of entering into a discussion of what level of significance to employ. Using the 0.05 level of significance as our criterion, let us now consider Shewhart's first sample. The data are: $\overline{X}_{\wp} = 0$, $\sigma = 1.0070$, $\overline{X} = 0.950$, and $N = 4$. As before, $\sigma_{\overline{X}} = 0.5035$, and we have

$$\frac{x}{\sigma} = \frac{\overline{X} - \overline{X}_{\wp}}{\sigma_{\overline{X}}} = \frac{0.950 - 0}{0.5035} = 1.89.$$

Referring to Appendix IV, we find that $P = 0.0588$, and the difference is not significant.

Throughout the preceding part of this chapter we have been concerned with only those situations in which $\overline{X}_{\wp}$ and σ were known. It was necessary to know σ in order to obtain $\sigma_{\overline{X}}$. Suppose that σ was known but $\overline{X}_{\wp}$ was not. First let us recognize that such a condition could hardly obtain, since σ is computed around $\overline{X}_{\wp}$ and, therefore, if σ is known, $\overline{X}_{\wp}$ would almost certainly be known.

In the unlikely event that only σ were known, it would still be possible (1) to test the significance of the difference between $\bar{X}$ and one or more hypothetical values of $\bar{X}_{\wp}$ or (2) to compute confidence limits of $\bar{X}_{\wp}$ as described on pages 231–235 but referring to the normal curve rather than to the t distribution.

Significance of Difference Between $\bar{X}$ and $\bar{X}_{\wp}$ When σ Is Unknown

Although, in the illustrations dealt with in the preceding sections of this chapter, σ and $\bar{X}_{\wp}$ were known, this is not often the case. There are relatively few situations under which population values are known. Sometimes they are known because a complete census has been taken. From the 1950 United States Census of Population it would be possible to ascertain $\bar{X}_{\wp}$ and σ for the ages of all the inhabitants of the United States.[8]

Occasionally population values are known, or approximately known, because of extensive experience. Although no complete enumeration has been made, enough information may be available so that $\bar{X}_{\wp}$ and σ may be computed and treated as if they were actually population values. Such a condition would occur if one had data of the weights of hundreds, or thousands, of healthy male mice of the same age and breed. A somewhat similar situation arises in quality-control work, when a manufacturer sets up a control population. A large amount of product is turned out under carefully controlled conditions which involve too great expense for day-to-day production. Values computed from the control population are considered as population values, and sample values obtained from day-to-day production are compared to them.

Finally, population values may be known on the basis of hypothesis or theory. Cases of this sort occur most often when proportions, rather than means, are being considered.[9] Thus, we might compare the observed proportions of the sexes among a group of laboratory animals to ascertain whether they differ from hypothetical population proportions of 0.50 male and 0.50 female. Or we might compare an inherited characteristic with an expected Mendelian ratio of 3:1.

---

[8] Even in the population census there are some inhabitants with "age unknown" and many others for whom ages are inaccurately reported.

[9] See Chapter 10.

A research worker studying the shape of cells in living matter[10] made three experiments employing lead shot in a compression cylinder. One experiment used small shot, 1.27 millimeters in diameter, which were shaken down before the application of pressure; another made use of small shot which were not shaken down before pressure was applied; while a third used large shot, 2.54 millimeters in diameter, not shaken down. After pressure had been applied to the shot in a cylinder until all the interstices were eliminated, the pressure was removed and the number of faces on each shot was counted for a sample drawn from the outer layer and for a sample drawn from each of three inner layers. Thus a total of 12 samples were drawn. Data are shown in Table 9.1 of the

TABLE 9.1

DISTRIBUTION OF NUMBER OF FACES ON LEAD SHOT* IN AN OUTER LAYER OF A COMPRESSION CYLINDER

Number of faces	Number of shot f	d'	fd'	$f(d')^2$
8	1	−3	− 3	9
9	2	−2	− 4	8
10	11	−1	−11	11
11	15	0	0	0
12	9	1	+ 9	9
13	1	2	+ 2	4
Total	39	...	− 7	41

* Small shot not shaken down before application of pressure.
Data from James Marvin, "The Shape of Compressed Lead Shot and Its Relation to Cell Shape," *American Journal of Botany*, May 1939, pp. 280–288.

$$\bar{X} = \bar{X}_d + \frac{\Sigma fd'}{N} i = 11 - \frac{7}{39} 1 = 11 - 0.18 = 10.82 \text{ faces.}$$

$$\hat{\sigma} = i \sqrt{\frac{\Sigma f(d')^2}{N-1} - \frac{(\Sigma fd')^2}{N(N-1)}} = 1 \sqrt{\frac{41}{38} - \frac{(7)^2}{39(38)}} = 1.023 \text{ faces.}$$

number of faces per shot for the sample of 39 small shot selected from the outer layer of a compression cylinder and which had not been shaken down before pressure was applied. From these data the value of $\bar{X} = 10.82$ faces is computed. Another investigator has indicated that epidermal cells in living matter can be expected to average 11 faces, $\bar{X}_\mathcal{P} = 11$. Does $\bar{X} = 10.82$ represent a sig-

---

[10] James Marvin, "The Shape of Compressed Lead Shot and Its Relation to Cell Shape," *American Journal of Botany*, May 1939, pp. 280–288.

nificant deviation from $\bar{X}_{\varphi} = 11$? Now we have a (hypothetical) value for $\bar{X}_{\varphi}$ but we do not know σ, and therefore we are unable to compute $\sigma_{\bar{x}}$. What we shall do is to *make an estimate of σ from the sample*, and we shall identify this estimate by the symbol $\hat{\sigma}$. It is computed from the expression

$$\hat{\sigma} = \sqrt{\frac{\Sigma x^2}{N-1}},$$

$$= \sqrt{\frac{\Sigma X^2}{N-1} - \frac{(\Sigma X)^2}{N(N-1)}} \text{ for ungrouped data,}$$

$$= i\sqrt{\frac{\Sigma f(d')^2}{N-1} - \frac{(\Sigma f d')^2}{N(N-1)}} \text{ for grouped data.}$$

$\hat{\sigma}^2$ is known as an "unbiased" estimate of σ^2, since it can be shown[11] that

$$\frac{\hat{\sigma}_1^2 + \hat{\sigma}_2^2 + \cdots + \hat{\sigma}_K^2}{K} = \sigma^2.$$

We are now in a position to ascertain the standard error of $\bar{X}$, but we shall use the symbol $\hat{\sigma}_{\bar{x}}$ to indicate that we have employed $\hat{\sigma}$ instead of σ, and we write[12]

$$\hat{\sigma}_{\bar{x}} = \frac{\hat{\sigma}}{\sqrt{N}}.$$

The computation of $\hat{\sigma}$ is shown below Table 9.1, and we get

$$\hat{\sigma}_{\bar{x}} = \frac{1.023}{\sqrt{39}} = 0.16 \text{ faces.}$$

Using this value, we now compute the significance ratio, which is

---

[11] s^2 is a biased estimate of σ^2, since

$$\frac{s_1^2 + s_2^2 + \cdots + s_K^2}{K} < \sigma^2.$$

For a proof that $\hat{\sigma}^2$ is an unbiased estimate of σ^2, see F. E. Croxton and D. J. Cowden, *Applied General Statistics*, Prentice-Hall, Inc. New York, 1939, pp. 837–840.

[12] If s is given for a set of data, we can obtain $\hat{\sigma}$ from the expression $\hat{\sigma} = \sqrt{\frac{N}{N-1}}\, s$. Alternatively, we can compute $\hat{\sigma}_{\bar{x}} = \frac{s}{\sqrt{N-1}}$.

designated t rather than $\dfrac{x}{\sigma}$, because we are using $\hat{\sigma}$.

$$t = \frac{\overline{X} - \overline{X}_{\wp}}{\hat{\sigma}_{\overline{X}}} = \frac{10.82 - 11.00}{0.16} = \frac{0.18}{0.16} = 1.125.$$

Because we have made use of $\hat{\sigma}$ instead of σ, we cannot employ normal curve areas to ascertain whether the observed difference is

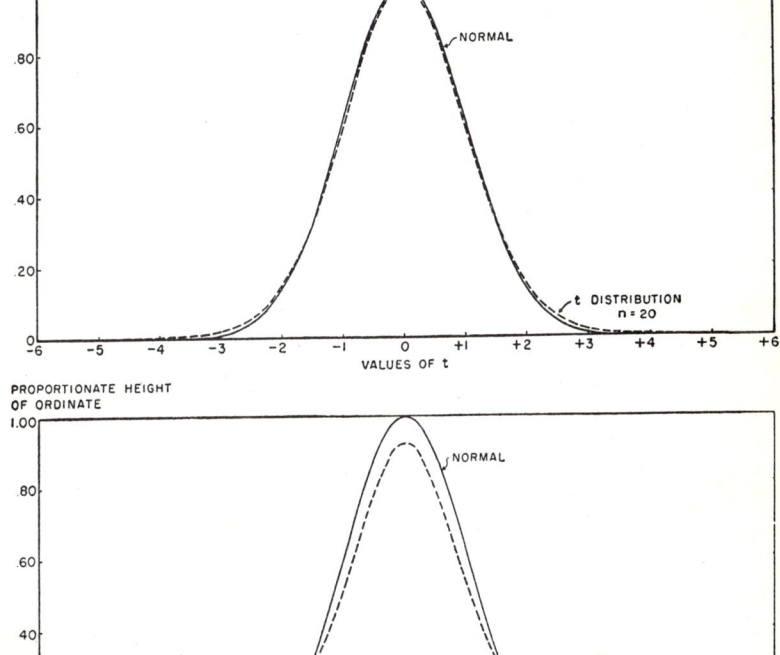

Chart 9.10. The t-Distribution for $n = 20$ and $n = 3$ Compared with the Normal Distribution. The expression used for computing the ordinates of the t-distribution is $Y_c = \sqrt{\dfrac{2}{n}} \dfrac{\left(\dfrac{n-1}{2}\right)!}{\left(\dfrac{n-2}{2}\right)!\left(1 + \dfrac{t^2}{n}\right)^{\frac{n+1}{2}}}$.

significant. While $\dfrac{\bar{X} - \bar{X}_\mathcal{P}}{\sigma_{\bar{x}}}$ is distributed normally, $\dfrac{\bar{X} - \bar{X}_\mathcal{P}}{\hat{\sigma}_{\bar{x}}}$ follows the t distribution. The t distribution is symmetrical, but it is more widely dispersed than the normal curve, as may be seen in Chart 9.10. The exact shape of the t distribution depends upon the number of "degrees of freedom" (n) present, the dispersion being greatest for one degree of freedom and becoming less as n increases, with the t distribution approaching the normal distribution as n approaches infinity. For the type of problem under consideration, $n = N - 1$, because, in computing $\hat{\sigma}$, we have employed the devia-

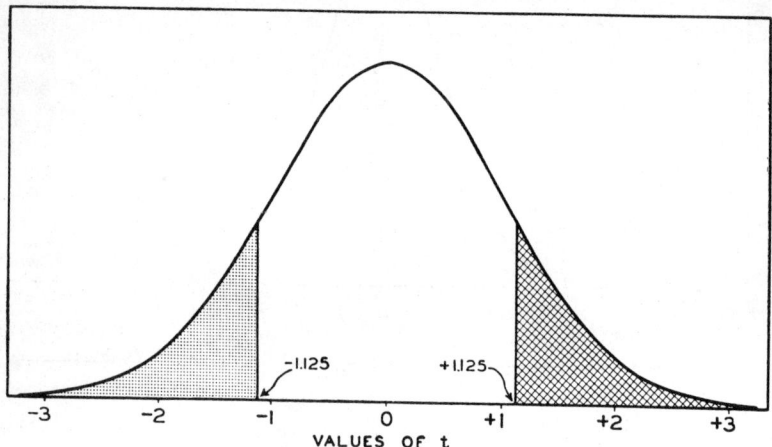

Chart 9.11. The t-Distribution for $n = 38$ Showing Probability of Obtaining $t = \pm 1.125$ or More.

tions of a series of N values around their own arithmetic mean, leaving us with $N - 1$ independent deviations. For the lead shot, we have $t = 1.125$ and $n = 39 - 1 = 38$. Referring to the t table of Appendix V, we find no entries for $n = 38$, but we do have $n = 30$ and $n = 40$. It is not necessary to interpolate, since P is greater than 0.25 but less than 0.30 ($0.25 < P < 0.30$), for $t = 1.125$ when n is either 30 or 40. The hypothesis that $\bar{X} = 10.82$ is the mean of a random sample from a population having $\bar{X}_\mathcal{P} = 11$ is not discredited. The difference is not significant. Chart 9.11, which shows a t distribution for $n = 38$, illustrates what has just been done.

If our conclusion had been based on the normal curve (Appendix IV or the bottom row of Appendix V), the result would have been the same: "not significant." Actually, the t distribution begins to resemble the normal curve rather closely in the neighborhood of $n = 20$, as may be seen from Chart 9.10 and Appendix V. Some investigators are in the habit of using the normal table for testing means when $n \geq 30$, but it is better to make a habit of using the t table in all cases where $\hat{\sigma}$ is employed in place of σ.

When making inferences concerning a sample mean which are based upon the use of $\hat{\sigma}$ rather than σ, it should be understood that the value of t is affected by sampling variations of $\hat{\sigma}$ as well as by sampling variations of $\bar{X}$. A large value of t and a corresponding small value of P may arise because $\bar{X}$ differs greatly from $\bar{X}_\wp$, or because $\hat{\sigma}$ is smaller than σ, or because of both conditions. Similarly, a small value of t and a corresponding large value of P may occur because $\bar{X}$ is very nearly the same as $\bar{X}_\wp$, or because $\hat{\sigma}$ is larger than σ, or both.

Confidence Limits of $\bar{X}_\wp$

A team of investigators studying wound healing[13] ascertained the pressure required to cause disruption of the abdomens of 20 unoperated rats, as shown in Table 9.2. Their purpose was to establish a control group (not a population) with which to compare the strength of healing wounds after various numbers of days following an operation and with the use of a number of different suture materials. From the data of Table 9.2 we obtain $\bar{X} = 97.7$ mm and $\hat{\sigma} = 7.81$ mm. We have no information concerning $\bar{X}_\wp$ or σ, but we may ascertain whether $\bar{X}$ departs from various selected values of $\bar{X}_\wp$.

Using the 0.02 level as a criterion, is it reasonable to believe that $\bar{X} = 97.7$ mm is the mean of a random sample from a population having $\bar{X}_\wp = 99.4$ mm? We compute

$$\hat{\sigma}_{\bar{X}} = \frac{\hat{\sigma}}{\sqrt{N}} = \frac{7.81}{\sqrt{20}} = \frac{7.81}{4.47} = 1.75 \text{ mm, and}$$

$$t = \frac{\bar{X} - \bar{X}_\wp}{\hat{\sigma}_{\bar{X}}} = \frac{97.7 - 99.4}{1.75} = \frac{1.7}{1.75} = 0.97.$$

---

[13] S. A. Localio, W. Casale, and J. W. Hinton, "Wound Healing—Experimental and Statistical Study: IV. Results," *Surgery, Gynecology, and Osbtetrics*, October 1943, pp. 376–388.

TABLE 9.2

Pressure, in Millimeters of Mercury Necessary to Cause Disruption of Abdomens of 20 Unoperated Rats

X	X^2	X	X^2
93	8,649	95	9,025
98	9,604	96	9,216
93	8,649	115	13,225
87	7,569	95	9,025
101	10,201	90	8,100
87	7,569	104	10,816
93	8,649	108	11,664
96	9,216	111	12,321
93	8,649	1,954	192,064
98	9,604		
93	8,649		
108	11,664		

Data from source given in footnote 13.

$$\bar{X} = \frac{\Sigma X}{N} = \frac{1,954}{20} = 97.7 \text{ mm.}$$

$$\hat{\sigma} = \sqrt{\frac{\Sigma X^2}{N-1} - \frac{(\Sigma X)^2}{N(N-1)}} = \sqrt{\frac{192,064}{19} - \frac{(1,954)^2}{20(19)}},$$
$$= 7.808 \text{ mm.}$$

$$\hat{\sigma}_{\bar{X}} = \frac{\hat{\sigma}}{\sqrt{N}} = \frac{7.808}{\sqrt{20}} = 1.75 \text{ mm.}$$

To ascertain the significance of the observed t, we refer to Appendix V for $n = 20 - 1 = 19$ and $t = 0.97$, and find $0.30 < P < 0.40$. The difference is not significant. Since the hypothesis that $\bar{X} = 97.7$ is the mean of a random sample drawn from a population having $\bar{X}_\mathcal{P} = 99.4$ is not discredited, the answer to our question is "Yes."

Now let us try another hypothetical value for $\bar{X}_\mathcal{P}$. Again using the 0.02 level is it reasonable to believe that $\bar{X} = 97.7$ mm is the mean of a random sample from a population having $\bar{X}_\mathcal{P} = 92.0$ mm? As before, $\hat{\sigma}_{\bar{X}} = 1.75$ mm

$$t = \frac{\bar{X} - \bar{X}_\mathcal{P}}{\hat{\sigma}_{\bar{X}}} = \frac{97.7 - 92.0}{1.75} = \frac{5.7}{1.75} = 3.26.$$

Referring once more to the t table of Appendix, V we find that, when $n = 19$ and $t = 3.26$, the value of P is less than 0.01 but more than 0.001. The difference is significant and the answer to our question is "No."

RELIABILITY AND SIGNIFICANCE

It must be obvious that we might have selected many other $\bar{X}_{\mathcal{P}}$ values which would qualify as perhaps having been the mean of the population from which the sample mean of $\bar{X} = 97.7$ mm may have come. Also, many $\bar{X}_{\mathcal{P}}$ values would fail to qualify. Is it possible to select two values, one smaller than $\bar{X}$ and the other greater than $\bar{X}$, which will give us limits within which the population mean can be expected to fall? We can do this, and we shall call these two values the "confidence limits" of $\bar{X}_{\mathcal{P}}$. First, however, we must decide how frequently we can afford to be wrong in the statement of confidence limits. For purposes of illustration, let us say that we can afford to be wrong not more than 2 times in 100. We will therefore compute the 98 per cent confidence limits of $\bar{X}_{\mathcal{P}}$ and this will be accomplished by (1) ascertaining a value $\bar{X}_{\mathcal{P}_1}$, *smaller* than $\bar{X}$, such that the value of $\bar{X}$ cuts off the *upper* 1 per cent tail of the distribution of sample means around $\bar{X}_{\mathcal{P}_1}$, and (2) determining a value of $\bar{X}_{\mathcal{P}_2}$, *larger* than $\bar{X}$, such that the value of $\bar{X}$ cuts off the *lower* 1 per cent tail of the distribution of sample means around $\bar{X}_{\mathcal{P}_2}$. We shall obtain these values by using the expression

$$\bar{X} = \bar{X}_{\mathcal{P}} \pm t\hat{\sigma}_{\bar{X}},$$

in which we shall substitute the already computed values $\bar{X} = 97.7$ mm and $\hat{\sigma}_{\bar{X}} = 1.75$ mm and the value of t for $P = 0.02$ when $n = 19$. From Appendix V we get $t = 2.539$, and

$$97.7 = \bar{X}_{\mathcal{P}} \pm (2.539)(1.75).$$
$$\bar{X}_{\mathcal{P}} = 97.7 \pm 4.4 = 93.3 \text{ and } 102.1 \text{ mm.}$$
$$\bar{X}_{\mathcal{P}_1} = 93.3 \text{ mm}; \; \bar{X}_{\mathcal{P}_2} = 102.1 \text{ mm.}$$

Chart 9.12 shows what has just been done.

The 98 per cent confidence limits, $\bar{X}_{\mathcal{P}_1} = 93.3$ mm and $\bar{X}_{\mathcal{P}_2} = 102.1$ mm, do not necessarily include the unknown population mean, but it is quite likely that the population mean is between 93.3 and 102.1 mm. To be more specific, if many determinations of 98 per cent confidence limits are made, one can expect to be right 98 times in 100 and wrong 2 times in 100. This may be demonstrated experimentally, and Roger P. Doyle[14] computed the 95 per cent confidence limits of $\bar{X}_{\mathcal{P}}$ for each of the 1,000 samples drawn by Shewhart. In each case he used only $\bar{X}$ and $\hat{\sigma}$, and then

---

[14] From unpublished material.

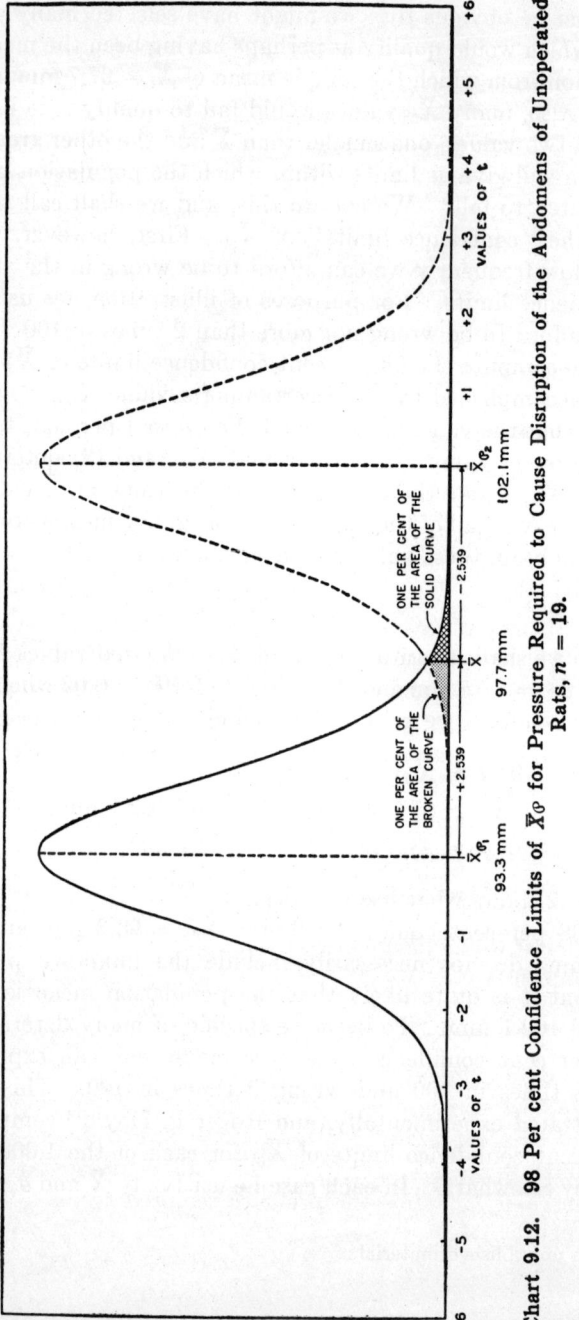

Chart 9.12. 98 Per cent Confidence Limits of $\bar{X}_\sigma$ for Pressure Required to Cause Disruption of the Abdomens of Unoperated Rats, $n = 19$.

referred to $\bar{X}_\mathcal{P}$ to ascertain whether $\bar{X}_\mathcal{P}$ did or did not fall within the limits of $\bar{X}_{\mathcal{P}_1}$ and $\bar{X}_{\mathcal{P}_2}$ computed as above, but for $n = 3$. He found that his statements of confidence limits were correct in 951 and wrong in 49 of the instances.

If we desire the 99.9 per cent confidence limits for the population mean of pressure required to disrupt the abdomens of unoperated rats, the procedure is the same, except that we use $t = 3.883$ and

$$\bar{X} = \bar{X}_\mathcal{P} \pm t\hat{\sigma}_{\bar{x}} \text{ becomes}$$
$$97.7 = \bar{X}_\mathcal{P} \pm (3.883)(1.75).$$
$$\bar{X}_\mathcal{P} = 97.7 \pm 6.8 = 90.9 \text{ and } 104.5 \text{ mm}.$$
$$\bar{X}_{\mathcal{P}_1} = 90.9 \text{ mm}; \bar{X}_{\mathcal{P}_2} = 104.5 \text{ mm}.$$

If we make a great number of statements of 99.9 per cent confidence limits, we can expect to be right 999 times out of 1,000 and wrong once in a thousand.

The reader may have wondered why $\bar{X}_\mathcal{P}$ was not placed initially on the left side of the equations just used for computing $\bar{X}_{\mathcal{P}_1}$ and $\bar{X}_{\mathcal{P}_2}$. The reason is that putting $\bar{X}$ on the left stresses the fact that sample means vary around $\bar{X}_\mathcal{P}$, not vice versa. The design of Chart 9.12 is also intended to emphasize this point.

Any appropriate confidence limits may be computed, but it is unusual to determine limits representing less than 90 per cent confidence, since, if one were to compute, say, 80 per cent confidence limits, he would not be expressing a very high degree of confidence.

A warning concerning the use of confidence limits of $\bar{X}_\mathcal{P}$ (or of any statistical value) is in order. The investigator should consider, at the outset, the maximum and minimum values of $\bar{X}_\mathcal{P}$ which could occur. The nature of the phenomenon being measured might be such that it would be impossible for $\bar{X}_\mathcal{P}$ to fall below, or to exceed, certain values.

Significance of Difference Between Two Sample Means

Independent samples. The three doctors studying wound healing[15] gave data of the pressure in millimeters of mercury required to disrupt healing wounds sutured with five different materials and for 1, 2, 3, 4, and subsequent days after the operation. The figures in Table 9.3 show the pressure required to disrupt wounds

---

[15] See note 13.

sutured with silk and with wire four days after the operation. As indicated below the table, the mean strength of the wounds sutured with silk was 81.8 mm ($\bar{X}_1 = 81.8$ mm), while the mean strength of the wounds sutured with wire was 74.6 mm ($\bar{X}_2 = 74.6$ mm). Is there a significant difference at the 0.01 level (the criterion used by Localio, Casale, and Hinton) between $\bar{X}_1$ and $\bar{X}_2$? The null hypothesis which we shall test is that $\bar{X}_1$ and $\bar{X}_2$ are means of random samples from the same population in regard to $\bar{X}_\varphi$. To test this hypothesis, we need the standard error of the difference between two sample means, which is[16]

$$\sigma_{\bar{X}_1-\bar{X}_2} = \sqrt{\sigma_{\bar{X}_1}^2 + \sigma_{\bar{X}_2}^2},$$

$$= \sqrt{\frac{\sigma^2}{N_1} + \frac{\sigma^2}{N_2}},$$

$$= \sigma \sqrt{\frac{1}{N_1} + \frac{1}{N_2}}.$$

TABLE 9.3

MILLIMETERS OF MERCURY REQUIRED TO DISRUPT HEALING WOUNDS SUTURED WITH SILK (FOUR RATS) AND WIRE (FIVE RATS), FOUR DAYS AFTER OPERATION

Silk		Wire	
X_1	X_1^2	X_2	X_2^2
76	5,776	71	5,041
84	7,056	70	4,900
83	6,889	77	5,929
84	7,056	76	5,776
		79	6,241
327	26,777	373	27,887

Data from source given in footnote 13.

$$\bar{X}_1 = \frac{\Sigma X_1}{N_1} = \frac{327}{4},$$
$$= 81.8 \text{ mm.}$$

$$\Sigma x_1^2 = \Sigma X_1^2 - \frac{(\Sigma X_1)^2}{N_1},$$
$$= 26{,}777 - \frac{(327)^2}{4},$$
$$= 44.75.$$

$$\bar{X}_2 = \frac{\Sigma X_2}{N_2} = \frac{373}{5},$$
$$= 74.6 \text{ mm.}$$

$$\Sigma x_2^2 = \Sigma X_2^2 - \frac{(\Sigma X_2)^2}{N_2},$$
$$= 27{,}887 - \frac{(373)^2}{5},$$
$$= 61.2.$$

---

[16] For a development, see F. E. Croxton and D. J. Cowden, *Applied General Statistics*, Prentice-Hall Inc., New York, 1939, pp. 841–842.

CHAP. 9] RELIABILITY AND SIGNIFICANCE   237

Two important observations must be made about this expression. First, it is applicable only if the two samples are independent. This is true of the present illustration, since the items of sample 1 are not inherently paired with the items of sample 2. The first item of sample 1 and the first item of sample 2 were not paired of necessity; they simply happened to be the first readings for each sample. The same may be said of the second, third, and following items of the two samples. Independence will be present in the vast majority of tests of significance of the difference between two sample means. However, occasional instances occur in which the samples are not independent. Such a situation would obtain if we were to test the significance of the difference between the mean weights of the first-born and second-born of a group of monozygotic male twins. An illustration involving non-independence because of inherent pairing is discussed on pages 240–242. Parenthetically, it may be noted that inherent pairing can hardly occur when $N_1 \neq N_2$. Second, the expression for $\sigma_{\bar{X}_1 - \bar{X}_2}$ calls for the value of σ, which is unknown. As a matter of fact, if we knew σ, we would almost certainly know $\bar{X}_\varphi$; and if we knew $\bar{X}_\varphi$, it would be much more meaningful to test the significance of the difference between $\bar{X}_1$ and $\bar{X}_\varphi$ and between $\bar{X}_2$ and $\bar{X}_\varphi$ than to test the significance of the difference between $\bar{X}_1$ and $\bar{X}_2$.

Inasmuch as σ is unknown, we substitute an estimate of σ based on the information available from both samples. This estimate may be denoted $\hat{\sigma}_{1+2}$ and is obtained from the expression

$$\hat{\sigma}_{1+2} = \sqrt{\frac{\Sigma x_1^2 + \Sigma x_2^2}{N_1 - 1 + N_2 - 1}},$$

where $\Sigma x^2 = \Sigma X^2 - \frac{(\Sigma X)^2}{N}$ for ungrouped data, and

$$\Sigma x^2 = i^2 \left[\Sigma f(d')^2 - \frac{(\Sigma fd')^2}{N} \right] \text{ for grouped data.}$$

The values of Σx_1^2 and Σx_2^2 are shown below Table 9.3 and

$$\hat{\sigma}_{1+2} = \sqrt{\frac{44.75 + 61.2}{3 + 4}} = 3.89 \text{ mm.}$$

We now compute the value of the estimated standard error of the difference between two sample means from the expression[17]

$$\hat{\sigma}_{\bar{X}_1-\bar{X}_2} = \hat{\sigma}_{1+2}\sqrt{\frac{1}{N_1} + \frac{1}{N_2}},$$
$$= 3.89\sqrt{\tfrac{1}{4} + \tfrac{1}{5}} = 3.89(0.67),$$
$$= 2.61 \text{ mm.}$$

Using this value and the observed difference between the two sample means, we get

$$t = \frac{\bar{X}_1 - \bar{X}_2}{\hat{\sigma}_{\bar{X}_1-\bar{X}_2}} = \frac{81.8 - 74.6}{2.61} = \frac{7.2}{2.61} = 2.76.$$

The degrees of freedom present are $n = N_1 - 1 + N_2 - 1 = 3 + 4 = 7$, since the deviations of the N_1 items of sample 1 were taken around $\bar{X}_1$ and the deviations of the N_2 items of sample 2 were taken around $\bar{X}_2$. Referring to the t table of Appendix V, we find that, when $n = 7$ and $t = 2.76$, $P \approx 0.03$. This is shown in Chart 9.13. Since a value of t this great or greater may be expected to occur about 3 times in 100, the difference is not significant at the 0.01 level. Had the investigators chosen to use the 0.05 level as a criterion of significance, the conclusion would have been "significant." In a situation such as this, the conclusion is sometimes stated: "Significant at the 0.05 level but not at the 0.01 level."

---

[17] Our procedure assumes that the two samples were drawn from the same population with respect to variance, σ^2. An F test of $\hat{\sigma}_1^2$ and $\hat{\sigma}_2^2$ (as described on pages 293–295) shows that the assumption is not unwarranted.

When the samples are believed to be from populations of unequal variance, and when $N_1 = N_2$, or $N_1 \approx N_2$, and are large, an approximate test may be made by using the expression

$$\hat{\sigma}_{\bar{X}_1-\bar{X}_2} = \sqrt{\frac{\hat{\sigma}_1^2}{N_1} + \frac{\hat{\sigma}_2^2}{N_2}}.$$

For a further treatment of the situation in which population variances are unequal, see Maurice G. Kendall, *The Advanced Theory of Statistics*, Charles Griffin and Co., Ltd., London, 1948, Vol. II, pp. 111–114.

When $N_1 = N_2$,

$$\hat{\sigma}_{1+2}\sqrt{\frac{1}{N_1} + \frac{1}{N_2}} = \sqrt{\frac{\hat{\sigma}_1^2}{N_1} + \frac{\hat{\sigma}_2^2}{N_2}}.$$

Confidence limits of $\bar{X}_{\mathcal{P}_1} - \bar{X}_{\mathcal{P}_2}$. The confidence limits of $\bar{X}_{\mathcal{P}_1} - \bar{X}_{\mathcal{P}_2}$ may be ascertained by a procedure paralleling that for the determination of the confidence limits of $\bar{X}_{\mathcal{P}}$, which was previously described. The expression to use is

$$\bar{X}_1 - \bar{X}_2 = (\bar{X}_{\mathcal{P}_1} - \bar{X}_{\mathcal{P}_2}) \pm t\hat{\sigma}_{\bar{x}_1 - \bar{x}_2}.$$

For the data of the preceding illustration, $n = 7$. Consequently, if we compute the 95 per cent confidence limits of $\bar{X}_{\mathcal{P}_1} - \bar{X}_{\mathcal{P}_2}$ for

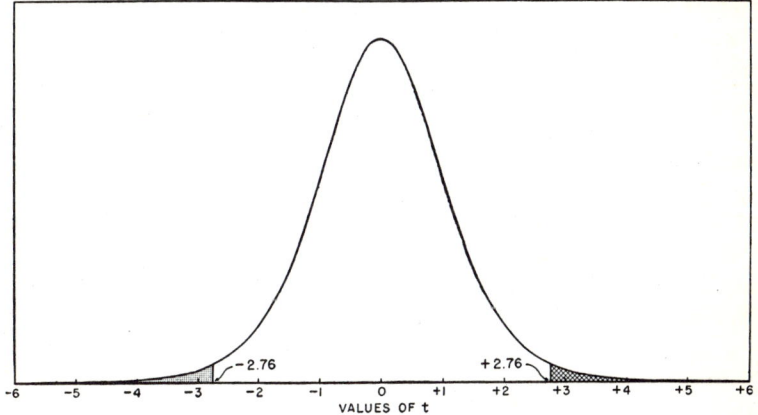

Chart 9.13. The t-Distribution for $n = 7$ Showing Probability of Obtaining $t = \pm 2.76$ or More. Approximately 0.03 of the area under the curve is in the two tails.

those data, we use $t = 2.365$. Substituting values already given, we have

$$81.8 - 74.6 = (\bar{X}_{\mathcal{P}_1} - \bar{X}_{\mathcal{P}_2}) \pm 2.365 \, (2.61).$$
$$\bar{X}_{\mathcal{P}_1} - \bar{X}_{\mathcal{P}_2} = 7.2 \pm 6.17,$$
$$= 1.0 \text{ mm and } 13.4 \text{ mm}.$$

These two results are perhaps too divergent to be useful; they would have been closer together if $\bar{X}_1 - \bar{X}_2 = 7.2$ mm had been significantly different at the 0.01 or 0.001 level, since that would have necessitated a smaller value for $\hat{\sigma}_{\bar{x}_1 - \bar{x}_2}$. While one can go through the arithmetic of computing the confidence limits of $\bar{X}_{\mathcal{P}_1} - \bar{X}_{\mathcal{P}_2}$, whether $\bar{X}_1 - \bar{X}_2$ is or is not significantly different, it is meaningful to determine the confidence limits only when a significant difference between $\bar{X}_1$ and $\bar{X}_2$ is present.

Non-independent samples. The data of Table 9.4 show the percentage of solids in the shaded and exposed havles of 25 grapefruit. We want to know if there is a significant difference between the means of these two sets of data. Here, it is obvious that the data are not independent: they are inherently paired. The shaded side of grapefruit #1 had 8.59 per cent solids, while the exposed side of the same grapefruit had 8.49 per cent solids. These two figures are inherently paired with each other because they refer to the same individual fruit. The same is true of the figures for the other 24 grapefruit.

In order to make the desired significance test, we shall obtain the difference D between each pair of values, determine the value of $\bar{X}_D$, and ascertain whether $\bar{X}_D$ differs significantly from 0. The null hypothesis is that $\bar{X}_D$ is the mean of a random sample from a population of differences having a mean of zero. Below Table 9.4 the computations are shown which give

$$\bar{X}_D = 0.194 \text{ per cent},$$
$$\hat{\sigma}_D = 0.307 \text{ per cent, and}$$
$$\hat{\sigma}_{\bar{X}_D} = 0.061 \text{ per cent}.$$

We then determine the value of t,

$$t = \frac{\bar{X}_D - 0}{\hat{\sigma}_{\bar{X}_D}} = \frac{0.194 - 0}{0.061} = 3.18.$$

Since there are 24 independent D values, $n = 24$, and reference to Appendix V shows that P is between 0.005 and 0.001. It is clear that the difference is significant.

It is very important that the lack of independence between the two samples be recognized in such a problem as this. Had we followed the usual procedure, which assumes the samples to be independent, computing $\bar{X}_1 = 8.22$ per cent, $\bar{X}_2 = 8.03$ per cent, and $\hat{\sigma}_{\bar{X}_1 - \bar{X}_2} = 0.092$ per cent, we would have obtained

$$t = \frac{8.22 - 8.03}{0.092} = \frac{0.19}{0.092} = 2.07,$$

which, for $n = 48$, has $0.025 < P < 0.05$. This probability differs greatly from that found first. In fact, if one were using the 0.02 or the 0.01 level as a criterion of significance, the method assum-

TABLE 9.4

Percentage of Solids in the Shaded and Exposed Halves of 25 Grapefruit

Fruit	Shaded X_1	Exposed X_2	$D = X_1 - X_2$	D^2
1	8.59	8.49	0.10	0.0100
2	8.59	8.59		
3	8.09	7.84	0.25	0.0625
4	8.54	7.89	0.65	0.4225
5	8.09	8.19	−0.10	0.0100
6	8.49	7.84	0.65	0.4225
7	7.89	7.89		
8	8.59	7.89	0.70	0.4900
9	8.54	7.79	0.75	0.5625
10	7.99	7.84	0.15	0.0225
11	7.89	7.79	0.10	0.0100
12	8.09	7.84	0.25	0.0625
13	7.89	7.89		
14	8.54	8.07	0.47	0.2209
15	7.84	7.97	−0.13	0.0169
16	7.49	7.57	−0.08	0.0064
17	7.89	7.92	−0.03	0.0009
18	7.79	7.97	−0.18	0.0324
19	7.84	8.17	−0.33	0.1089
20	8.89	8.67	0.22	0.0484
21	8.54	8.07	0.47	0.2209
22	8.04	7.97	0.07	0.0049
23	8.59	8.62	−0.03	0.0009
24	8.19	7.92	0.27	0.0729
25	8.59	7.97	0.62	0.3844
Total	205.50	200.66	4.84	3.1938

Data from Paul L. Harding, Plant Physiologist, Division of Fruit and Vegetable Crops and Diseases, Bureau of Plant Industry, Soils and Agricultural Engineering, Agricultural Research Administration, United States Department of Agriculture.

$$\bar{X}_D = \frac{\Sigma D}{N} = \frac{4.84}{25} = 0.194 \text{ per cent.}$$

$$\hat{\sigma}_D = \sqrt{\frac{\Sigma D^2}{N-1} - \frac{(\Sigma D)^2}{N(N-1)}} = \sqrt{\frac{3.1938}{24} - \frac{(4.84)^2}{25(24)}},$$

$$= \sqrt{0.133075 - 0.039043} = \sqrt{0.094032},$$

$$= 0.307 \text{ per cent.}$$

$$\hat{\sigma}_{\bar{X}_D} = \frac{\hat{\sigma}_D}{\sqrt{N}} = \frac{0.307}{\sqrt{25}} = 0.061 \text{ per cent.}$$

ing independence of the two samples would have led one erroneously to conclude "not significant."

The possible consequences of using the method which assumes independence of the two samples when they are not, in fact, independent may be clarified by writing $\hat{\sigma}_{\bar{X}_D}$ in its alternative form[18]

$$\hat{\sigma}_{\bar{X}_1 - \bar{X}_2} = \sqrt{\hat{\sigma}_{\bar{X}_1}^2 + \hat{\sigma}_{\bar{X}_2}^2 - 2r\hat{\sigma}_{\bar{X}_1}\hat{\sigma}_{\bar{X}_2}},$$

where r is the correlation between the two samples. If the shorter form

$$\hat{\sigma}_{\bar{X}_1 - \bar{X}_2} = \sqrt{\hat{\sigma}_{\bar{X}_1}^2 + \hat{\sigma}_{\bar{X}_2}^2},$$

which assumes independence, is used, the value of $\hat{\sigma}_{\bar{X}_1 - \bar{X}_2}$ will be too large when there is positive correlation between the two sets of data and too small when there is negative correlation present. Ignoring the lack of independence may cause us to fail to declare a significant difference when r is positive and erroneously to declare a difference to be significant when r is negative. In most problems involving inherent pairing, the correlation will be positive, but occasional cases occur in which the correlation is negative. In any event, when inherent pairing is present, correlation between the two series is also almost certain to be present. The chance correlation that may be present between two series having $N_1 = N_2$ and known to be independent is of no concern to us.

Conclusion

The reader may have observed that this chapter has not stressed "large-number methods" versus "small-number methods." The reason is that, when σ is known, the normal curve is appropriate for samples of any size, large or small. When σ is not known, but $\hat{\sigma}$ is used in its stead, the t distribution (a "small-number method") is always the proper distribution to use. As n increases in size, the t distribution approaches the normal curve, so that for large samples the normal distribution is sometimes employed. However, even when n is large, and σ is not known, the normal curve is an approximation. Sometimes, when a sample is large, $s = \sqrt{\dfrac{\Sigma x^2}{N}}$

---

[18] The two forms are exact equivalents, but the expression involving r requires much more computation. For the grapefruit data, using $r = +0.577$, $\hat{\sigma}_{\bar{X}_1 - \bar{X}_2} = 0.061$, which agrees with the value for $\hat{\sigma}_{\bar{X}_D}$.

rather than $\hat{\sigma} = \sqrt{\dfrac{\Sigma x^2}{N-1}}$ is used as an estimate of σ. The numerical difference is slight for large samples, but the use of s as an estimate of σ should be avoided.

Since the methods discussed in this chapter are just as applicable to small samples as to large samples, the question may arise: why bother to use large samples? The answer is that, when one makes use of large samples, a smaller observed difference $\bar{X} - \bar{X}_\varphi$ or $\bar{X}_1 - \bar{X}_2$ is necessary to obtain significance at a specified probability level. This is true (1) because $\hat{\sigma}_{\bar{x}}$ (or $\sigma_{\bar{x}}$) and $\hat{\sigma}_{\bar{x}_1 - \bar{x}_2}$ tend to decrease with an increase in sample size, while $\bar{X} - \bar{X}_\varphi$ and $\bar{X}_1 - \bar{X}_2$ do not have a corresponding tendency to decrease; also (2) because the t value required for the specified probability level decreases as n increases. Occasionally, as a result of using small samples, one may come to the conclusion that an observed difference is not significant when, if larger samples had been used, the difference (which itself would probably change) would likely have been significant. The illustration of lower fatalities from Rocky Mountain spotted fever through the use of para-aminobenzoic acid, described in Chapter 10, is a case of this sort.

Raymond Pearl[19] contrasts statistical significance and biological or medical significance. To be even more general than was Pearl, one might contrast a statistically significant difference on the one hand with a generic difference on the other, meaning by "generic difference" an actual difference in kind, whether that difference be in regard to two groups of adult males with different racial backgrounds, two batches of bolts of different kinds of metal, or two groups of plants which may be of different strains although not different as to genus or species. Generic difference may be present, but there may not be a statistically significant difference. For example, a group of men and a group of women are generically—in this case biologically—different, but there may not be a statistically significant difference in their reaction times, hair pigmentation, skin pigmentation, and various other measurements. Conversely, Pearl indicates that a statistically significant difference may be present but a biological difference may be absent. He indicates that such a situation may occur when one is unable to measure the

---

[19] Raymond Pearl, *Introduction to Medical Biometry and Statistics*, W. B. Saunders Co., Philadelphia, 1940, pp. 293–294.

individual observations accurately and when one has very large samples. For example, the measurement of oral temperature may be possible only to tenths of a degree, and the mean temperatures for two identical groups of men may be only very slightly different; yet for two very large samples, the value of $\hat{\sigma}_{\bar{x}_1-\bar{x}_2}$ might be extremely small, and a statistically significant difference might be present in spite of the absence of a generic difference. To the writer this seems to be more a matter of having employed more digits than are significant, and it is believed that the occurrence of a statistically significant difference when no generic difference is present would be unusual. However, such a situation could occur as a result of making a Type I error.

Symbols Used in
CHAPTER 10

a: number of occurrences in a sample.
α: lower-case Greek alpha, number of occurrences in a population.
A: indicating an occurrence, A has no numerical value.
b: number of non-occurrences in a sample.
β: lower-case Greek beta, number of non-occurrences in a population.
B: indicating a non-occurrence, B has no numerical value.
k: number of samples.
N: the number of items in a sample. When two samples are under consideration, we use N_1 and N_2.
p: proportion of occurrences in a sample.
p_1: proportion of occurrences in sample 1.
p_2: proportion of occurrences in sample 2.
$\bar{p}$: an estimate of π based on two samples; a weighted average of p_1 and p_2.
P: probability; varies from 0 to 1.
π: lower-case Greek pi, proportion of occurrences in a population.
π_1: the lower confidence limit of π.
π_2: the upper confidence limit of π.
q: proportion of non-occurrences in a sample. $q = 1 - p$.
q_1: proportion of non-occurrences in sample 1.
q_2: proportion of non-occurrences in sample 2.
$\bar{q}$: $1 - \bar{p}$.
σ_a: the standard error of a.
σ_p: the standard error of p.
$\hat{\sigma}_{p_1-p_2}$: estimated standard error of the difference between p_1 and p_2.
τ: lower-case Greek tau; proportion of non-occurrences in a population. $\tau = 1 - \pi$.
$\dfrac{x}{\sigma}$: a deviation divided by its standard error; for example, $\dfrac{p - \pi}{\sigma_p}$ and $\dfrac{a - \pi N}{\sigma_a}$.
$\approx$: means "is approximately equal to."

Chapter 10
RELIABILITY AND SIGNIFICANCE OF PROPORTIONS

In its general approach, this chapter will parallel the preceding one. We shall first consider the reliability of a proportion obtained from a random sample (p) when the proportion in the population (π) is known; then we shall attack the problem of determining the confidence limits of π when only p and the size of the random sample are known; finally, we shall test the significance of the difference between the proportions (p_1 and p_2) observed in two random samples.

The *number* of individuals in a population having a particular characteristic (generally: an "occurrence") may be designated by α; the *number* of individuals in a population not having the particular characteristic (generally: a "non-occurrence") may be designated by β. Provisional final figures for the census of 1950 showed 74,833,239 males and 75,864,122 females in the United States. Considering males as "occurrences" and females as "non-occurrences" (that is, non-occurrences of males), we have $\alpha = $ 74,833,239 and $\beta = $ 75,864,122. The *proportion* of occurrences in a population may be indicated by π and the *proportion* of non-occurrences by τ. The value of π is obtained from $\pi = \dfrac{\alpha}{\alpha + \beta}$ and $\tau = \dfrac{\beta}{\alpha + \beta}$. For the preceding data,

$$\pi = \frac{74{,}833{,}239}{74{,}833{,}239 + 75{,}864{,}122} = 0.497 \text{ and}$$

$$\tau = \frac{75{,}864{,}122}{74{,}833{,}239 + 75{,}864{,}122} = 0.503.$$

Note that $\pi + \tau = 0.497 + 0.503 = 1.0$. It must be obvious that $\pi + \tau$ will always equal 1.0 and that $\tau = 1 - \pi$.

Behavior of Proportions from Random Samples

Standard error of a proportion. For a sample we use the symbols: a, number of occurrences; b, number of non-occurrences; p, proportion of occurrences; and q, proportion of non-occurrences. The size of a sample is $a + b = N$. We may obtain p from $p = \dfrac{a}{a+b} = \dfrac{a}{N}$ and $q = \dfrac{b}{a+b} = \dfrac{b}{N}$. It is apparent that $p + q = 1.0$ and that $q = 1 - p$.

If many random samples of the same size were to be drawn from a population, we could compute the value of p for each of these samples. These proportions may be identified as $p_1, p_2, p_3, \cdots, p_k$, and we could ascertain the standard deviation of these proportions from the expression

$$\sqrt{\frac{(p_1 - \pi)^2 + (p_2 - \pi)^2 + (p_3 - \pi)^2 + \cdots + (p_k - \pi)^2}{k}},$$

where k is the number of samples. It would be very unusual to have many random samples from the same population. It can be shown, however, that if we have all possible random samples of the given size from a population, the standard error of p is

$$\sigma_p = \sqrt{\frac{\pi \tau}{N}}.$$

Since $\tau = 1 - \pi$, we have the following alternative forms of the expression for the standard error of p, which are sometimes useful:

$$\sigma_p = \sqrt{\frac{\pi(1 - \pi)}{N}},$$

$$= \sqrt{\frac{\pi - \pi^2}{N}}.$$

There are occasions when we shall wish to use σ_a instead of σ_p. The standard error of a is given by

$$\sigma_a = \sqrt{N \pi \tau}.$$

Distribution of p when $\pi = 0.50$. The values of p computed from random samples are distributed symmetrically around π, if $\pi = 0.50$. This will be clear when it is realized that values of p

may range from 0.50 *up to* 1.0 and from 0.50 *down to* 0. Chart 10.1 illustrates this for samples of 10, showing the values of a and of p which can occur as the result of expanding $(0.50B + 0.50A)^{10}$. In this expression A indicates an occurrence of the characteristic under

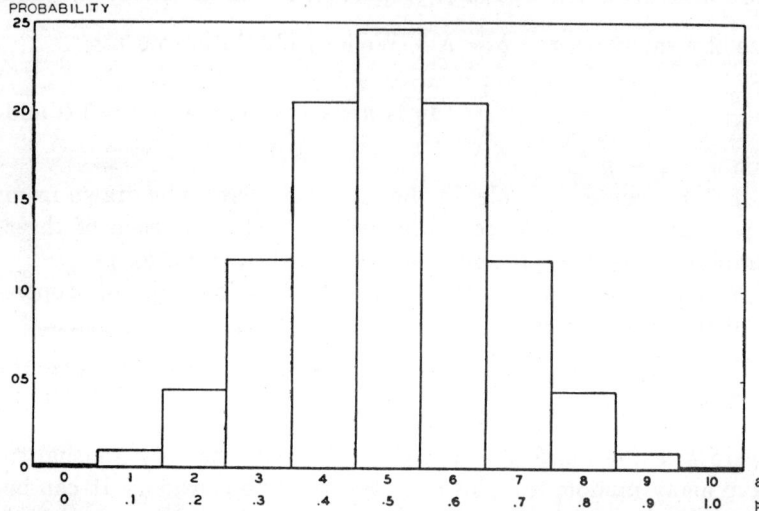

Chart 10.1. Probability of Occurrence of Values of a and p in Samples of 10 When $\pi = 0.50$. Obtained from the expansion of $(0.50B + 0.50A)^{10} = 0.0010B^{10} + 0.0098B^9A + 0.0439B^8A^2 + 0.1172B^7A^3 + 0.2051B^6A^4 + 0.2461 B^5A^5 + 0.2051B^4A^6 + 0.1172B^3A^7 + 0.0439B^2A^8 + 0.0098BA^9 + 0.0010A^{10}$.

consideration and B indicates a non-occurrence. Expansion of the binomial yields the eleven terms shown below Chart 10.1. These terms have values of a (the exponents of A) of 0, 1, 2, 3, $\cdots$, 10, which correspond to values of p of 0, 0.1, 0.2, 0.3, $\cdots$, 1.0, since $N = 10$. The terms may be summarized:

Number of occurrences a	Proportion of occurrences p	Probability
0	0	0.0010
1	0.1	0.0098
2	0.2	0.0439
3	0.3	0.1172
4	0.4	0.2051
5	0.5	0.2461
6	0.6	0.2051
7	0.7	0.1172
8	0.8	0.0439
9	0.9	0.0098
10	1.0	0.0010
		1.0000

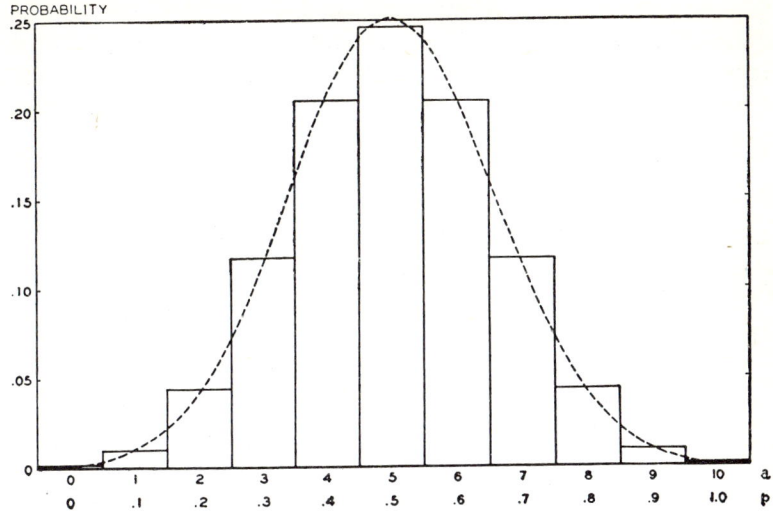

Chart 10.2. Normal Curve Fitted to $(0.50B + 0.50A)^{10}$.

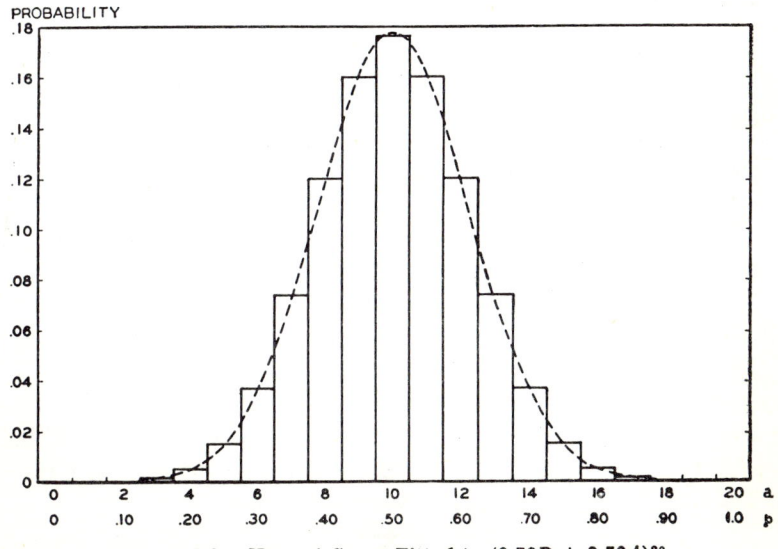

Chart 10.3. Normal Curve Fitted to $(0.50B + 0.50A)^{20}$.

As pointed out before, the column diagram of Chart 10.1 is symmetrical. It is not normal, however, since a normal curve is continuous and of unlimited range in each direction. Chart 10.2 shows a normal curve fitted to the column diagram of Chart 10.1.

If samples of larger size are drawn from a population having $\pi = 0.50$, the correspondence between the binomial, which expresses the exact distribution of sample p's, and the normal curve becomes even closer. Chart 10.3 shows a normal curve fitted to the expected

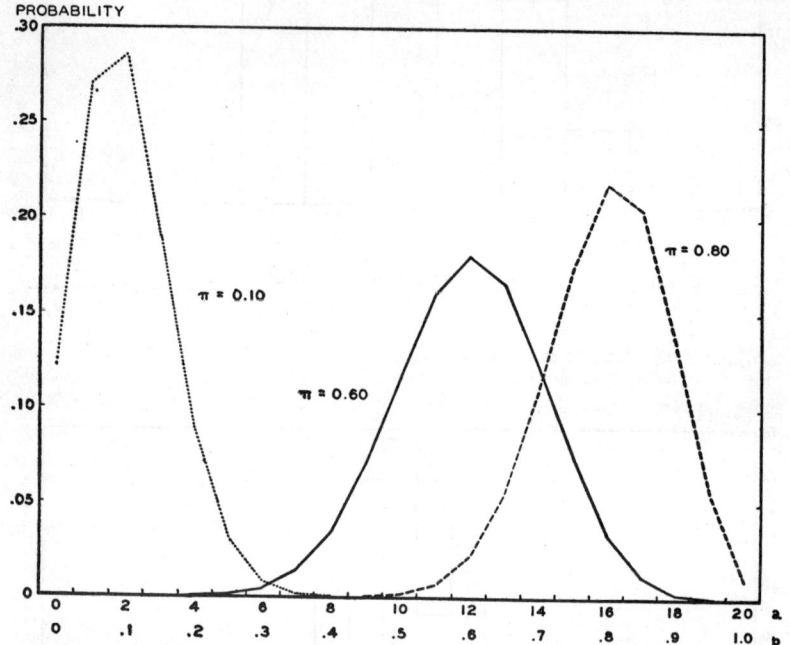

Chart 10.4. Distribution of Sample Values of a and p When $N = 20$, for $\pi = 0.10$, $\pi = 0.60$, and $\pi = 0.80$.

distribution of p's from samples of 20, that is, to the binomial $(0.50B + 0.50A)^{20}$.

Distribution of p when $\pi \neq 0.50$. When sample p's are drawn from a population having a value of π greater or less than 0.50, the distribution of sample p's is skewed: skewed to the right if π is less than 0.50; skewed to the left if π is greater than 0.50.

For a given sample size, the greater the departure of π from 0.50, the greater the skewness. Chart 10.4 shows the distribution of values of a and p from samples of 20 when $\pi = 0.10$, 0.60, and 0.80.

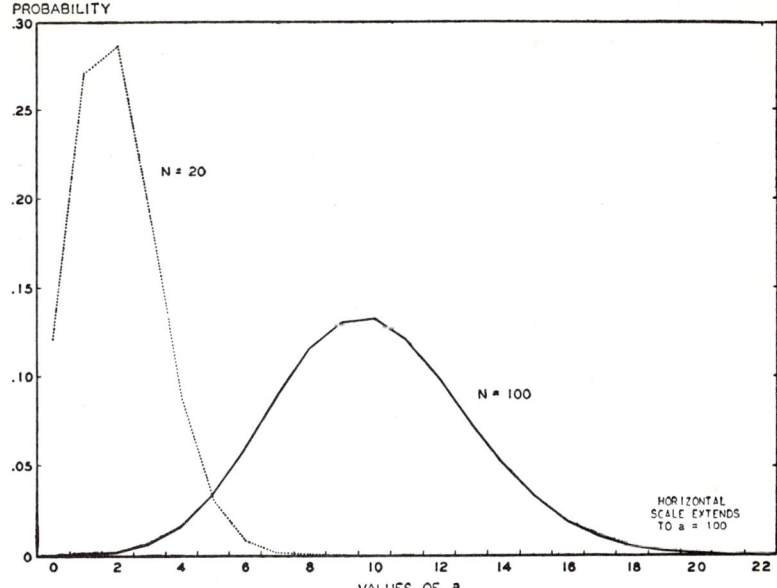

Chart 10.5. Distribution of Sample Values of a, When $\pi = 0.10$, for $N = 20$ and $N = 100$. Values of p cannot be shown on the horizontal scale, as they differ for the two curves. For example, when $N = 20$ and $a = 2$, $p = 0.10$; when $N = 100$ and $a = 2$, $p = 0.02$.

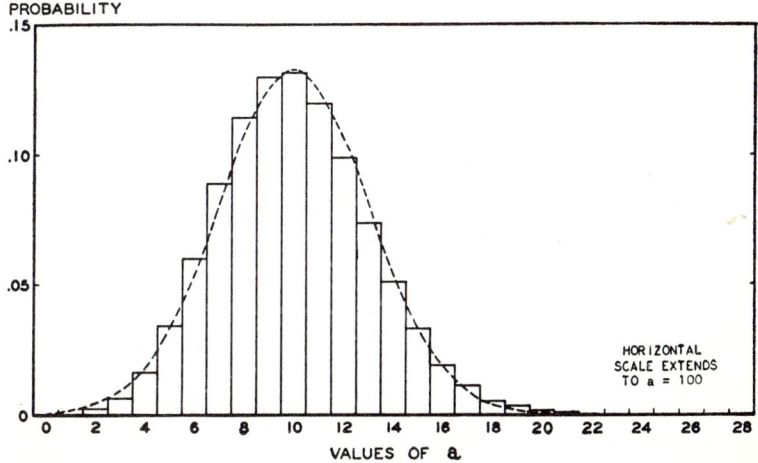

Chart 10.6. Normal Curve Fitted to $(0.90B + 0.10A)^{100}$. Values of p are not shown on the horizontal scale. They would be $\frac{1}{100}$ of the corresponding a values.

The skewness of the distribution of sample p's depends not only on π but upon the size of the sample. For a given value of π, the larger the size of the sample, the less the skewness. Chart 10.5 shows the distribution of values of a from a population having $\pi = 0.10$ for $N = 20$ and $N = 100$. The two curves are, respectively, the expansion of $(0.90B + 0.10A)^{20}$ and $(0.90B + 0.10A)^{100}$. It is evident that the skewness is much less for samples of 100 than for samples of 20. Chart 10.6 shows a normal curve fitted to the binomial $(0.90B + 0.10A)^{100}$.

The Reliability of p When π Is Known

Approximate method. From the preceding paragraphs it is apparent that the normal curve may be used to describe, at least approximately, the sampling distribution of p: (1) when $\pi = 0.50$ or thereabouts and N is moderate or large, and (2) when $\pi \neq 0.50$ and N is large.

A sample of 100 persons shows 54 males ($a = 54$, $p = 0.54$) and 46 females ($b = 46$, $q = 0.46$). Does this represent a significant departure from the value $\pi = 0.497$ as determined from the United States Census data? We first compute

$$\sigma_p = \sqrt{\frac{\pi\tau}{N}} = \sqrt{\frac{(0.497)(0.503)}{100}},$$

$$= \sqrt{\frac{0.249991}{100}} = \sqrt{0.00249991},$$

$$= 0.05,$$

and then

$$\frac{p - \pi}{\sigma_p} = \frac{0.54 - 0.497}{0.05} = \frac{0.043}{0.05},$$

$$= 0.9.$$

Referring to the table of areas in one tail of the normal curve shown in Appendix III, it appears that the probability of a divergence this great or greater and in this direction (that is, an excess of males) is 0.18. The tabled value is 0.1841. The probability of a divergence equal to or greater than that observed, but in either direction (Appendix IV) is 0.37. It is apparent that the observed p does not differ significantly from π.

In the preceding illustration, $\pi \approx 0.50$ and $N = 100$, so that there was little loss of accuracy through the use of the normal curve. An exact test would have employed the binomial $(0.503B + 0.497A)^{100}$, but its expansion entails much more labor than is warranted for this problem.

Exact method. Consider, now, a problem having $\pi = 0.50$ but N small. Each member of a group of eight male students was asked to fold his hands and then to note whether his left or right thumb was on top. Seven of the students had the right thumb on top ($a = 7$, $p = 0.875$); one had the left thumb on top ($b = 1$, $q = 0.125$). So far as is known, 0.50 persons place the right thumb on top ($\pi = 0.50$) and 0.50 place the left thumb[1] on top ($\tau = 0.50$).

Using the procedure of the previous illustration, we compute

$$\sigma_p = \sqrt{\frac{(0.50)(0.50)}{8}} = \sqrt{\frac{0.25}{8}},$$

$$= \sqrt{0.03125} = 0.1768, \text{ and}$$

$$\frac{p - \pi}{\sigma_p} = \frac{0.875 - 0.50}{0.1768} = \frac{0.375}{0.1768} = 2.12.$$

Alternatively, using a and σ_a (where πN is the number of right thumbs on top, if the sample agreed exactly with the population):

$$\sigma_a = \sqrt{8(0.50)(0.50)},$$

$$= \sqrt{2} = 1.414, \text{ and}$$

$$\frac{a - \pi N}{\sigma_a} = \frac{7 - 4}{1.414} = \frac{3}{1.414} = 2.12.$$

Observe that the two $\frac{x}{\sigma}$ ratios, $\frac{p - \pi}{\sigma_p}$ and $\frac{a - \pi N}{\sigma_a}$, yield the same result, 2.12. From the table of areas in one tail of the normal curve (Appendix III), it appears that 17 out of a thousand (0.017) random samples of eight might be expected to show this much or greater departure *in this direction*. For departures in either direction, that is, excesses of left thumbs on top as well as right thumbs on top, the above probability must be doubled, giving 0.034.

---

[1] There seems to be no inherited tendency concerning this. Interesting data for one-egg and two-egg twins are presented, but not tested, by Dahlberg. (Gunnar Dahlberg, *Statistical Methods for Medical and Biological Students*, George Allen and Unwin, Ltd., London, 1940, p. 28.) Some of Dahlberg's figures are tested in the following chapter.

Using the 0.05 level as a criterion, the conclusion to be drawn from the foregoing is that there is a significant difference between p and π. However, the use of the normal curve introduces an error. Owing to the fact that the normal curve is continuous while the actual distribution is discontinuous, *the probabilities are understated.* This will be clear from Chart 10.7, which shows, by means of bars, the expansion of the binomial $(0.50B + 0.50A)^8$, where an

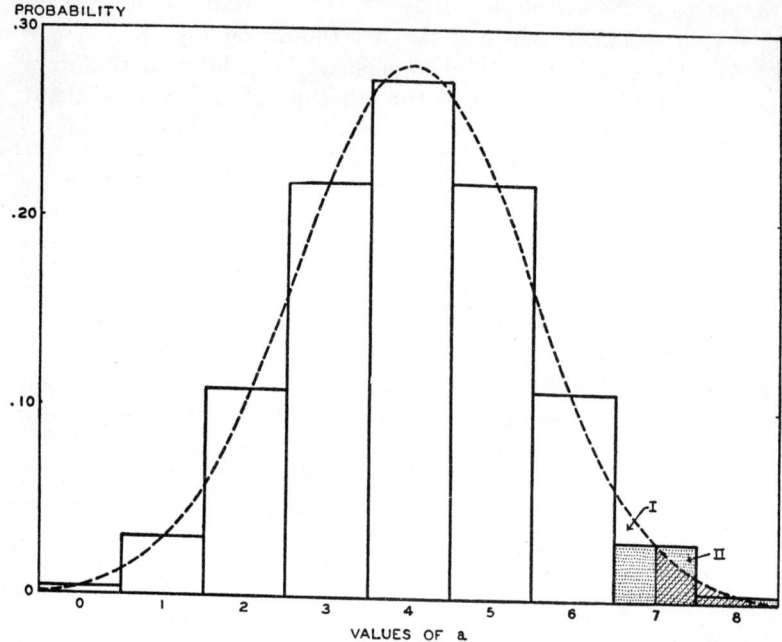

Chart 10.7. Explanation of Yates' Correction by Means of a Normal Curve Fitted to $(0.50B + 0.50A)^8$. The values of a indicate the number of right thumbs on top.

occurrence, A, is a right thumb on top and a non-occurrence, B, is a left thumb on top, and which shows, also, the normal curve. The diagonally hatched area shows the probability of 0.017 just ascertained. The *exact* probability of obtaining 7 or 8 right thumbs on top is shown by the two bars at the right and is represented by the stippled area. It is apparent that the normal curve must always understate the probabilities, when we are evaluating a tail of a curve, and that the understatement is serious when N is small. The numerical value of the two bars is obtained by evaluating the last two terms in the expression

CHAP. 10] RELIABILITY AND SIGNIFICANCE 255

$(0.50B + 0.50A)^8 = (0.50B)^8 + 8(0.50B)^7(0.50A)$
$\qquad + 28(0.50B)^6(0.50A)^2 + 56(0.50B)^5(0.50A)^3$
$\qquad + 70(0.50B)^4(0.50A)^4 + 56(0.50B)^3(0.50A)^5$
$\qquad + 28(0.50B)^2(0.50A)^6 + 8(0.50B)(0.50A)^7$
$\qquad + (0.50A)^8.$

The sum of these two terms is $0.03125 + 0.00391 = 0.03516$, and it is clear that 35 out of a thousand random samples of eight might be expected to show the observed divergence, or greater, in this direction. Also, 70 out of a thousand could be expected to show the observed divergence, or greater, in either direction. Using the 0.05 level as a criterion, we would conclude that there is not a significant difference between p and π. Note that the normal curve not only understated the probabilities but, in this instance, led us to an erroneous conclusion. To avoid possible confusion, it may be well to point out that, while the diagonally hatched area under the curve happens to be roughly one-half of the area of the stippled bars, this would not be likely to be true in another situation.

Yates' correction. A great deal of labor may be saved by employing Yates' correction for the continuity of the normal curve instead of solving the binomial. The correction yields results that are roughly in agreement with the exact method. Looking at Chart 10.7, it will be apparent that, if we were to consider not only the tail of the normal curve which is diagonally hatched, but *also* the portion of it extending from the hatched area one-half of a bar to the left (including the triangle I, which approximates in area the excluded triangle II), the area under the tail of the curve would be very nearly the same as the area of the two bars. We can accomplish this by making our test in terms of $\dfrac{a - \pi N}{\sigma_a}$ and *decreasing the absolute value* of $a - \pi N$ in the numerator by $\frac{1}{2}$. This gives

$$\frac{|a - \pi N| - \frac{1}{2}}{\sigma_a} = \frac{|7 - 4| - \frac{1}{2}}{\sqrt{8(0.50)(0.50)}} = \frac{2.5}{\sqrt{2}}$$

$$= \frac{2.5}{1.414} = 1.77.$$

Referring to the tables of areas of the normal curve in Appendices III and IV, we find that the probability is 0.0384 for a one-tail test or 0.0767 for a two-tail test. While this probability agrees roughly with that given by the exact test, Yates' correction has overcorrected.

Although Yates' correction is usually employed only when N is small, it may also be used when N is large. However when N is large, the normal curve and the binomial give so nearly the same results that the correction is unnecessary. It should be clearly understood that Yates' correction corrects for continuity only and gives a rough approximation of the exact probability only when π is equal to, or approximately equal to, 0.50. When π departs appreciably from 0.50 and N is small, the exact method should be used, as in the following illustration.

Exact method, $\pi \neq 0.50$. A medical research organization announced a new drug for the treatment of Rocky Mountain spotted fever and stated that, although the usual mortality was $\frac{1}{3}$, it had found that, of eight patients suffering from this disease and given the new drug, only one had died.[2] From the foregoing we have: $\pi = 0.33$; $a = 1$; $p = 0.125$; and $N = 8$. Does the observed value of $p = 0.125$ differ significantly from $\pi = 0.33$? To answer this question, we shall ascertain the probability of obtaining $p = 0.125$ or less (or $a = 1$ or fewer) from the expression $(0.67B + 0.33A)^8$. That is to say, we shall evaluate the first two terms of

$$(0.67B + 0.33A)^8 = (0.67B)^8 + 8(0.67B)^7(0.33A)$$
$$+ 28(0.67B)^6(0.33A)^2 + 56(0.67B)^5(0.33A)^3$$
$$+ 70(0.67B)^4(0.33A)^4 + 56(0.67B)^3(0.33A)^5$$
$$+ 28(0.67B)^2(0.33A)^6 + 8(0.67B)(0.33A)^7$$
$$+ (0.33A)^8,$$

where A is, as before, an occurrence (specifically, a death) and B a non-occurrence (that is, a recovery). These terms, in order, and their probabilities are

Number dying a	Proportion dying p	Probability
0	0	0.0406
1	0.125	0.1600
2	0.250	0.2758
3	0.375	0.2717
4	0.500	0.1673
5	0.625	0.0659
6	0.750	0.0162
7	0.875	0.0023
8	1.000	0.0001

---

[2] The exact source of the data is purposely not stated. The announcement was in the press in the summer of 1948.

The sum of the first two terms is 0.2006. This is the probability of one death or no deaths and leads to the conclusion that there is not a significant difference between $p = 0.125$ and $\pi = 0.33$ in this case. It does not necessarily follow that the new drug is not superior. It may, in fact, be a better medicine, but not enough cases were included in the sample to demonstrate its superiority. Note that the test made here was a one-tail test, since we wished to know if there were significantly fewer deaths as a result of using the new drug. For that reason we considered only the two terms having *negative* $p - \pi$ values of 0.205 or more. If the other tail of the distribution were to be evaluated, it would consist of those terms for which $p - \pi$ has *positive* values equal to or exceeding 0.205. They are the last four terms of the binomial.

Confidence Limits of π

The problem here is basically the same as for the arithmetic mean, which was considered in Chapter 9. For the 95 per cent confidence limits of π, we need to ascertain (1) a value of π (smaller than p) such that the observed p cuts off the upper $2\frac{1}{2}$ per cent tail of the distribution of sample p's around π_1, and (2) a value of π_2 (larger than p) such that the observed p cuts off the lower $2\frac{1}{2}$ per cent tail of the distribution of sample p's around π_2. Two methods of arriving at the confidence limits will be considered: an approximate method and the exact method.

As mentioned in the preceding chapter, before proceeding to compute confidence limits for any statistical value, the investigator should consider the range over which it is *possible* for a value to vary. For example, a sample might yield a value of $p = 0.40$, and the 90 per cent confidence limits of π might be computed as 0.30 and 0.52, yet the nature of the phenomenon might be such that π could not possibly be lower than 0.33.

Approximate method. In a group of 20 laboratory animals, four showed a particular characteristic. On the basis of these figures, $N = 20$, $a = 4$, and $p = 0.20$. What are the 95 per cent confidence limits of π? The approximate method consists of determining the values of π_1 and π_2 from the expression $\dfrac{p - \pi}{\sigma_p}$, the numerical value of this fraction being taken as 1.96, since we desire the 95 per cent confidence limits and are assuming a normal distribution of p's around π_1 and π_2. We have, then,

$$1.96 = \frac{0.20 - \pi}{\sqrt{\dfrac{\pi\tau}{20}}},$$

$$= \frac{0.20 - \pi}{\sqrt{\dfrac{\pi - \pi^2}{20}}}.$$

Squaring gives

$$3.8416 = \frac{0.04 - 0.40\pi + \pi^2}{\dfrac{\pi - \pi^2}{20}},$$

$$\frac{3.8416\pi - 3.8416\pi^2}{20} = 0.04 - 0.40\pi + \pi^2,$$

$$0.19208\pi - 0.19208\pi^2 = 0.04 - 0.40\pi + \pi^2,$$

$$0.04 - 0.59208\pi + 1.19208\pi^2 = 0.$$

This quadratic, $0 = a + b\pi + c\pi^2$, may be solved for π by using the expression

$$\pi = \frac{-b \pm \sqrt{b^2 - 4ac}}{2c},$$

$$= \frac{0.59208 \pm \sqrt{(0.59208)^2 - 4(0.04)(1.19208)}}{2(1.19208)},$$

$$= \frac{0.59208 \pm \sqrt{0.1598259}}{2.38416} = \frac{0.59208 \pm 0.39978}{2.38416},$$

$$= \frac{0.19230}{2.38416} \text{ and } \frac{0.99186}{2.38416}, \text{ giving}$$

$$\pi_1 = 0.081 \text{ and } \pi_2 = 0.416.$$

These are the 95 per cent confidence limits of π. Note that p is closer to π_1 than to π_2.

If a normal curve having $\sigma_p = \sqrt{\dfrac{(0.081)(0.919)}{20}} = 0.061$ is drawn around $\pi_1 = 0.081$ (the lower confidence limit), the observed value $p = 0.20$ will cut off the upper $2\frac{1}{2}$ per cent tail of this curve. If a normal curve having $\sigma_p = \sqrt{\dfrac{(0.416)(0.584)}{20}} = 0.110$ is drawn around $\pi_2 = 0.416$ (the upper confidence limit), the observed value $p = 0.20$ will cut off the lower $2\frac{1}{2}$ per cent tail of this curve. Both of these statements are illustrated in Chart 10.8. It is clear that the normal curve drawn around $\pi_2 = 0.416$, while not strictly accurate, is not unreasonable. However, the normal curve drawn around $\pi_1 = 0.081$ is obviously faulty, because a large portion of it extends below zero, which is impossible; a skewed distribution is clearly called for here.

The approximate method just described may be used when N is large and p is not too far removed from 0.50. These two restric-

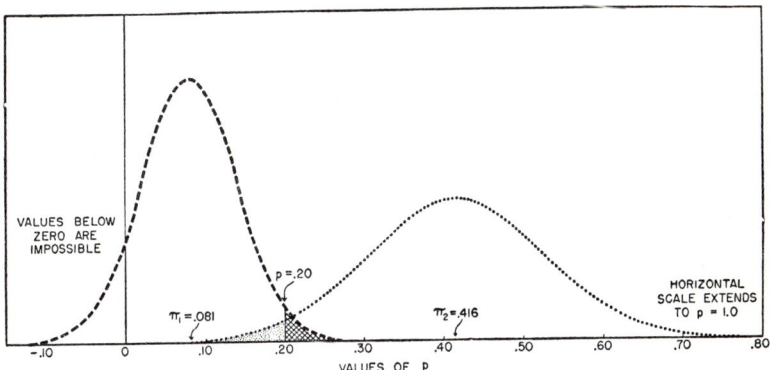

Chart 10.8. 95 Per cent Confidence Limits of π When $p = 0.20$ and $N = 20$, Computed by Use of $\dfrac{p - \pi}{\sqrt{\dfrac{\pi\tau}{N}}}$. The hatched area is $2\frac{1}{2}$ per cent of the left curve. The stippled area is $2\frac{1}{2}$ per cent of the right curve.

tions are complementary: if N is very large, p need not be as close to 0.50; if p is close to 0.50, N may be smaller. Let us see how much the approximate method errs by ascertaining π_1 and π_2 by a more exact procedure.

Exact method. The description of this method will be easier if we ascertain the value of π_2 first and then compute the value of π_1.

To determine the upper 95 per cent confidence limit, π_2, we need to know the value of π in the expression $(\tau + \pi)^{20}$ which will result in $a = 4$ ($p = 0.20$), cutting off the lower $2\frac{1}{2}$ per cent tail of the binomial. To say the same thing in other words: what value of π inserted in $(\tau + \pi)^{20}$ will yield a binomial, the first five terms ($a = 0, 1, 2, 3, 4$) of which will total 0.025? This question is easy to ask, but it is troublesome to answer, since successive approximations of π are required. The preceding computations gave $\pi_2 = 0.416$, but a normal curve centered around 0.416 was used. The curve should have been skewed, and, assuming that π_2 will turn out to be less than 0.50, skewed to the right. Since a curve having $\pi_2 = 0.416$ and skewed to the right would have more than 0.025 of the area in the left tail at and beyond $a = 4$, we must use a value for π_2 that is larger than 0.416. We shall first try $\pi_2 = 0.45$ and expand $(0.55B + 0.45A)^{20}$, with the results shown in columns 2 and 3 of Table 10.1. The sum of the first five terms is seen to be

TABLE 10.1

PROBABILITIES AND CUMULATIVE PROBABILITIES OF VALUES OF a IN $(\tau B + \pi A)^{20}$ WHEN $\pi = 0.45$, 0.44, AND 0.43

(Cumulations are from $a = 0$.)

a	$\pi = 0.45$		$\pi = 0.44$		$\pi = 0.43$	
	Probability	Cumulative* probability	Probability	Cumulative* probability	Probability	Cumulative* probability
(1)	(2)	(3)	(4)	(5)	(6)	(7)
0	0.0000	0.0000	0.0000	0.0000	0.0000	0.0000
1	0.0001	0.0001	0.0001	0.0002	0.0002	0.0002
2	0.0008	0.0009	0.0011	0.0012	0.0014	0.0016
3	0.0040	0.0049	0.0051	0.0063	0.0064	0.0080
4	0.0139	0.0189	0.0170	0.0233	0.0206	0.0286
5	0.0365	0.0553	0.0427	0.0660	0.0496	0.0783
6	0.0746					
7	0.1221	The terms for $a \geqq 6$ are not needed for this problem.				
8	0.1623					
9	0.1771					
10	0.1593					
11	0.1185					
12	0.0727					
13	0.0366					
14	0.0150					
15	0.0049					
16	0.0013	0.9997				
17	0.0002	>0.9999				
18	0.0000	>0.9999				
19	0.0000	>0.9999				
20	0.0000	1.0000				

* The cumulative figures were obtained from the non-cumulative figures before the non-cumulative figures were rounded to four decimals.

0.0189. This is shown in Chart 10.9. Since there is not enough area in the left tail of the binomial, a smaller value for π must be tried. Columns 4 and 5 of Table 10.1 show the results of expanding

$(0.56B + 0.44A)^{20}$, and it appears that the first five terms total 0.0233. One more expansion, using $\pi = 0.43$ is shown in columns 6 and 7 of Table 10.1; the first five terms of this series total 0.0286.

As a result of the three expansions, we conclude that $\pi_2 = 0.44$. If greater accuracy is required, we should try several values between 0.43 and 0.44, probably trying 0.435 first.

The determination of the value of π_1 will be similar to the foregoing, except that we wish to ascertain the value of π in the expression $(\tau B + \pi A)^{20}$ which will yield a total of 0.025 in the *last*

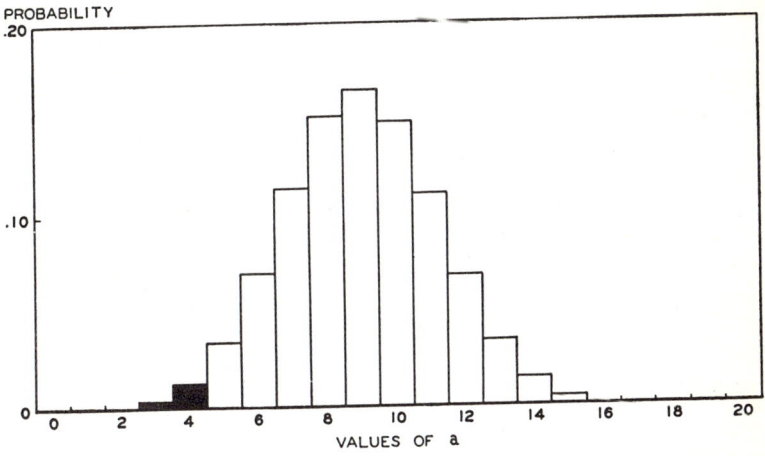

Chart 10.9. Expansion of $(0.55B + 0.45A)^{20}$. The first 5 bars, for $a = 0, 1, 2, 3,$ and 4, include 0.0189 of the area. The distribution is slightly skewed to the right. Values of p are not shown on the horizontal scale. They would be $\frac{1}{20}$ of the corresponding a values.

seventeen terms ($a = 4, 5, 6, \cdots, 20$). Referring to Chart 10.8 and realizing that the curve around π_1 will be markedly skewed, it appears that π_1 will be less than 0.081 as given by the approximate method. We shall therefore try $\pi = 0.05$, and the binomial $(0.95B + 0.05A)^{20}$ is seen, in columns 2 and 3 of Table 10.2, to have a total of 0.0159 in the last seventeen terms. This is shown in the sketch of Chart 10.10. Since there is less than 0.025 in the right tail of this binomial, we must try a larger value for π, and columns 4 and 5 of Table 10.2 show the result of using $\pi = 0.06$. The last seventeen terms of this binomial total 0.0290. Obviously, π_1 is between 0.05 and 0.06, but nearer to 0.06. For our purposes, we shall conclude that $\pi_1 = 0.06$ and note that, if greater accuracy

TABLE 10.2

Probabilities and Cumulative Probabilities of Values of a in $(\tau B + \pi A)^{20}$ when $\pi = 0.05$ and 0.06

(Cumulations are from $a = 20$.)

a	$\pi = 0.05$		$\pi = 0.06$	
	Probability*	Cumulative probability	Probability*	Cumulative probability
(1)	(2)	(3)	(4)	(5)
0	0.3585	1.0000	0.2901	1.0000
1	0.3773	0.6415	0.3703	0.7099
2	0.1887	0.2642	0.2246	0.3396
3	0.0596	0.0755	0.0860	0.1150
4	0.0133	0.0159	0.0233	0.0290
5	0.0022	0.0026	0.0048	0.0057
6	0.0003	0.0003		0.0009
7	0.0000	0.0000		
...	The balance of the terms for a are not needed for this			
...	problem.			
19				
20				

* Note that, instead of determining 17 values for $a = 4$ to $a = 20$ inclusive, the values were determined for $a = 0, 1, 2, 3$, and so forth, and subtracted from 1.0 to obtain the desired cumulative figures.

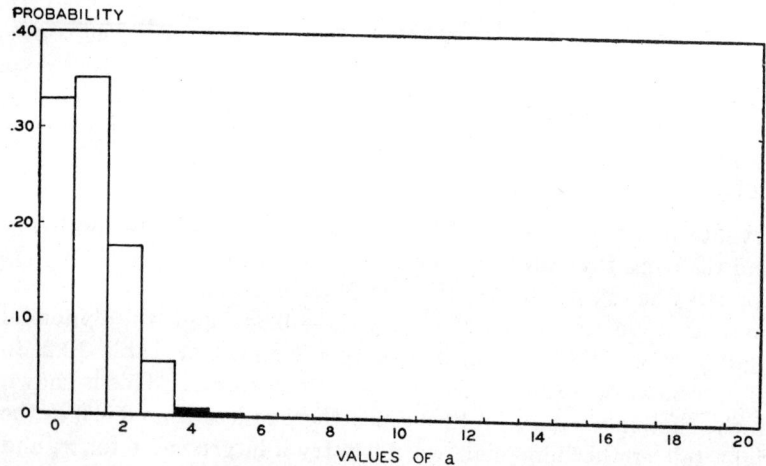

Chart 10.10. Expansion of $(0.95B + 0.05A)^{20}$. The last seventeen bars, for $a = 4, 5, 6, \ldots, 20$, include 0.0159 of the area. Values of p are not shown on the horizontal scale. They would be $\frac{1}{20}$ of the corresponding a values.

is required, additional values of π should be tried, probably using 0.059 first.

The approximate method gave $\pi_1 = 0.081$ and $\pi_2 = 0.416$. The exact method resulted in $\pi_1 = 0.06$ and $\pi_2 = 0.44$. The approximate method showed a greater relative discrepancy for π_1 than for π_2. A tremendous amount of labor is involved in expanding the binomials, and no general solution is possible. One could, of course, expand many binomials for various values of π and for (say) $N = 20$ and eventually arrive at a pair of curves giving the 0.95 (or other) confidence limits of π. Such a chart would appear thus:

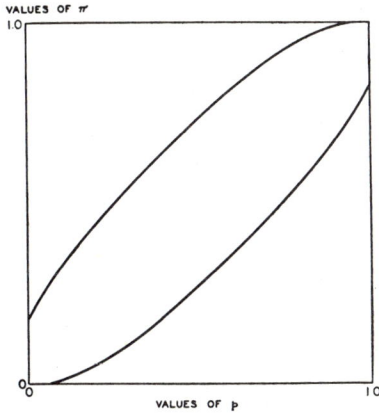

As a matter of fact, Clopper and Pearson, using certain approximations, have prepared charts of this type[3] for the 0.95 and 0.99 confidence limits of π and for selected values of N from 10 to 1000.

The Significance of the Difference between p_1 and p_2

A health study found that, among men 20–29 years old, 98 out of 359 $\left(p_1 = \dfrac{98}{359} = 0.273\right)$ in the chemical industry had hernia, while 58 out of 397 $\left(p_2 = \dfrac{58}{397} = 0.146\right)$ in the steel industry were

---

[3] See C. J. Clopper and E. S. Pearson, "The Use of Confidence or Fiducial Limits," *Biometrika*, Vol. 26, pp. 404–413. The charts are reproduced in F. E. Croxton and D. J. Cowden, *Practical Business Statistics*, Prentice-Hall, Inc., New York, 1949, 2nd ed., pp. 371 and 372.

similarly afflicted. Our null hypothesis is that these are random samples from the same population. The procedure is, in general, the same as that for testing the difference between two sample arithmetic means. We do not know π, and, as a matter of fact, if π were known, we should probably wish to test $p_1 - \pi$ and $p_2 - \pi$ rather than $p_1 - p_2$. An estimate of π, designated $\bar{p}$, is made from the two samples, using the expression[4]

$$\bar{p} = \frac{a_1 + a_2}{N_1 + N_2},$$
$$= \frac{98 + 58}{359 + 397} = \frac{156}{756} = 0.206.$$

The estimated standard error of the difference between two percentages is then computed from

$$\hat{\sigma}_{p_1-p_2} = \sqrt{\frac{\bar{p}\bar{q}}{N_1} + \frac{\bar{p}\bar{q}}{N_2}}$$
$$= \sqrt{\frac{(0.206)(0.794)}{397} + \frac{(0.206)(0.794)}{359}}$$
$$= \sqrt{0.000868} = 0.029.$$

We may now compare the observed difference between the two percentages with their estimated standard error:

$$\frac{p_1 - p_2}{\hat{\sigma}_{p_1-p_2}} = \frac{0.273 - 0.146}{0.029} = \frac{0.127}{0.029} = 4.4.$$

Because our samples are large, this ratio is evaluated by referring to the normal curve, and it appears that such a difference (in either direction) has a probability of less than 0.00001 for random samples from the same population. The difference is clearly significant. Possibly men with hernia can more readily do the work involved in the chemical industry than in the steel industry. Possibly some other explanation is in order.

---

[4] When p_1, N_1, p_2, and N_2 are given,

$$\bar{p} = \frac{N_1 p_1 + N_2 p_2}{N_1 + N_2}.$$

If N_1 and N_2 are small, Yates' correction should be used or an exact test should be made. We shall return to this problem in the following chapter in the section dealing with 2 x 2 tables.

SYMBOLS USED IN

CHAPTER 11

a_1: number of observed frequencies in the upper left cell of a 2 x 2 table.

a_2: number of observed frequencies in the lower left cell of a 2 x 2 table.

b_1: number of observed frequencies in the upper right cell of a 2 x 2 table.

b_2: number of observed frequencies in the lower right cell of a 2 x 2 table.

C: number of columns of observed frequencies (exclusive of totals) in a chi-square table which has its marginal totals set.

f: an observed frequency.

f_c: a computed frequency.

n: degrees of freedom.

N: number of items in a sample. For 2 x 2 and larger tables, where two or more samples are involved, N is the number of items in the entire table.

p: proportion of occurrences in a sample.

p_1: proportion of occurrences in sample 1.

p_2: proportion of occurrences in sample 2.

$\bar{p}$: an estimate of π based on two samples; a weighted average of p_1 and p_2.

P: probability, varies from 0 to 1.

π: lower-case Greek pi, proportion of occurrences in a population.

R: number of rows of observed frequencies (exclusive of totals) in a chi-square table which has its marginal totals set.

σ_p: the standard error of p.

$\hat{\sigma}_{p_1-p_2}$: estimated standard error of the difference between p_1 and p_2.

Σ: upper-case Greek sigma, meaning "take the sum of."

$\dfrac{x}{\sigma}$: a deviation divided by its standard error, for example, $\dfrac{p-\pi}{\sigma_p}$.

χ^2: chi-square. The symbol is a lower-case Greek chi.

χ_Y^2: chi-square with Yates' correction.

!: factorial. $4! = 1 \times 2 \times 3 \times 4$.

Chapter 11
THE χ^2 TEST

The two preceding chapters dealt with arithmetic means and proportions drawn from random samples. Before proceeding to discuss the reliability of standard deviations, in the following chapter, we shall digress for a consideration of some of the applications of the χ^2 test.

The first two sections of this chapter deal with the "1 x 2 table" and the "2 x 2 table," both situations in which one degree of freedom is present. For each of these we shall see that the χ^2 test gives results identical with those given by a previously considered procedure. Other aspects of the χ^2 test, discussed in the third and following sections of the chapter, are concerned with problems in which two or more degrees of freedom are present.

The 1 x 2 Table

Large numbers. In the *New York Times* for November 22, 1939, Dr. Richard E. Ching was quoted as having reported to the Southern Medical Association that, of 116 patients having pneumonia and treated with sulfapyridine, only 15 had died. Previously, when sulfapyridine had not been used, the ratio of those dying was twice as large. This information may be set up as follows:

Result	Observed (treated with sulfapyridine)	Expected* (not treated with sulfapyridine)
Recovered	101	86
Died	15	30
Total	116	116

* Based on extensive past experience and prorated to total 116.

This is referred to as a "1 x 2 table" because the observed data occupy one column and two rows.

We are interested in knowing whether Dr. Ching's sample figures for persons treated with sulfapyridine differ significantly from the population figures, which were determined from extensive experience over preceding years.

The chi-square test involves taking the difference between each observed frequency (f) and each corresponding expected, or computed, frequency (f_c), squaring this value, dividing by the expected frequency, and summing these quotients. Symbolically,[1] this is

$$\chi^2 = \Sigma \frac{(f - f_c)^2}{f_c}.$$

Having ascertained the numerical value of χ^2, the last step consists of determining the probability of its occurrence by chance.

For the data of pneumonia patients, χ^2 may be obtained as follows:

Result	Observed f	Expected f_e	$f - f_c$	$(f - f_c)^2$	$\frac{(f - f_c)^2}{f_c}$
Recovered	101	86	+15	225	2.62
Died	15	30	−15	225	7.50
Total	116	116	0	...	10.12

In a 1 x 2 table with the total given (116, in this case), it is possible to write any desired figure in one of the two cells. When this is done, the figure for the other cell is automatically determined. Therefore, we say that we have one degree of freedom ($n = 1$) in such a situation.

If a population is evenly divided into two categories, if samples are drawn from this population, and if χ^2 is computed for each sample, the various values of χ^2 will be distributed as shown in Chart 11.1 for one degree of freedom. The population values in our problem are not evenly divided; but, in view of the fact that $N = 116$, this is not important. From the table of χ^2 given in Appendix VI, we may determine the probability of the chance occurrence of $\chi^2 = 10.12$ or larger when $n = 1$. This is found to be slightly larger[2] than 0.001, and we conclude that, since a value of $\chi^2 = 10.12$ or larger may be expected to occur so infrequently by chance, the discrepancy between the observed and expected frequencies is real. If we are satisfied that the observed group and the

---

[1] An alternative expression is given below Table 11.5.

[2] The exact probability may be ascertained by use of the binomial $(0.259B + 0.741A)^{116}$, where A refers to a recovery and B to a death. This does not assume an even division between the two categories.

population differ in regard to no relevant characteristic, other than that the observed group was treated with sulfapyridine while the population was not, we may conclude that sulfapyridine appears to be efficacious.

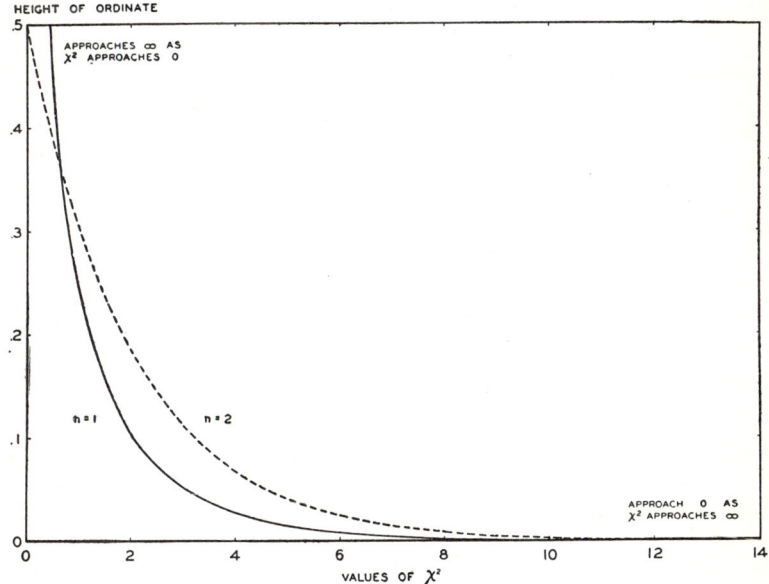

Chart 11.1. Distribution of χ^2 for One Degree of Freedom and for Two Degrees of Freedom. Horizontal and vertical scales extend to ∞. The ordinates of the distribution of χ^2 are obtained from the expression

$$Y_c = \frac{e^{\frac{-\chi^2}{2}} (\chi^2)^{\frac{n-2}{2}}}{2^{\frac{n}{2}} \left(\frac{n-2}{2}\right)!}.$$

It should be noted that the χ^2 test tells us the probability of getting a discrepancy equal to or greater than that observed *in either direction*. This is so because our $f - f_c$ values are squared. The χ^2 value of 10.12, which we found, might have arisen from the figures given by Dr. Ching or from figures of 71 recovered and 45 died. Although only one tail of the χ^2 distribution is involved, we have actually made a two-tail test, since the probability 0.001 refers to both of the divergences just mentioned.

Identity with $p - \pi$ test. The procedure which has just been described gives results which are identical with those of the $p - \pi$ test. The observed data showed $p = \dfrac{101}{116} = 0.871$, the proportion recovering when sulfapyridine was used, and $\pi = 0.741$, the proportion recovering during previous extensive experience when sulfapyridine was not used. The sample consisted of 116 cases. Proceeding as in the preceding chapter,

$$\sigma_p = \sqrt{\dfrac{(0.741)(0.259)}{116}} = 0.0407.$$

$$\dfrac{p - \pi}{\sigma_p} = \dfrac{0.871 - 0.741}{0.041} = \dfrac{0.130}{0.041},$$

$$= 3.17.$$

Looking up this value in the table of areas in two tails of the normal curve, Appendix IV, it is found that P is a little larger than 0.001. If we had more detailed normal and χ^2 tables, or could interpolate accurately into Appendices IV and VI, the probabilities obtained by the two procedures would be found to be identical, about 0.0015.

Notice that (within the permissible limits of errors due to rounding) the $\dfrac{p - \pi}{\sigma_p}$ value of 3.17 is the square root of the χ^2 value of 10.12. This relationship will always exist for this sort of problem. If the reader will look at the χ^2 table for $n = 1$ and at the normal-curve areas shown in the last row in Appendix V, he will find the following:

Probability	χ^2	$\dfrac{x}{\sigma}$
0.10	2.706	1.645
0.05	3.841	1.960
0.02	5.412	2.326
0.01	6.635	2.576
0.001	10.827	3.291

In every case, the χ^2 value is the square of the $\dfrac{x}{\sigma}$ value. It is interesting to note that, for $n = 1$, the values of χ (not χ^2) are distributed normally. Since the $p - \pi$ and the χ^2 procedures give exactly the same results, it does not matter which of the two is used.

Chap. 11]   THE χ² TEST   271

Small numbers. When N is small, the problem is exactly the same as in the case of the $p - \pi$ test. Either Yates' correction or the exact method, described in the preceding chapter, should be employed. If χ^2 is to be computed, Yates' correction may be applied by *decreasing* each $|f - f_c|$ by $\frac{1}{2}$. The expression then becomes

$$\chi_Y^2 = \Sigma \frac{(|f - f_c| - \frac{1}{2})^2}{f_c}.$$

The 2 x 2 Table

Large numbers. The seventeenth annual report of the medical department of the United States Fruit Company presented data referring to 5,501 persons classified according to whether or not their blood film showed malaria parasites and whether or not their spleens were enlarged. The figures are shown in Table 11.1, which is a 2 x 2 table, since the observed data occupy two columns and two rows.

TABLE 11.1

Presence of Malaria Parasites in Blood Film and Enlargement of Spleen for 5,501 Persons

Presence of malaria parasites in blood film	Enlarged spleen		Total
	Yes	No	
Yes................	740	743	1,483
No.................	1,287	2,731	4,018
Total............	2,027	3,474	5,501

The basic expression for χ^2 is the same as before:

$$\chi^2 = \Sigma \frac{(f - f_c)^2}{f_c}.$$

In this case, we have no population data from which to obtain the f_c values. They are obtained by making use of the marginal totals. If the groups with and without malaria parasites showed no difference in respect to the enlargement of the spleen, we would expect the first cell (row 1, column 1) to have $\frac{2,027}{5,501}$ of the 1,483 individuals with malaria parasites, and the second cell (row 1, column 2) to have $\frac{3,474}{5,501}$ of the 1,483 individuals with malaria parasites. Similarly, we would expect the third cell (row 2, column 1) to have $\dfrac{2,027}{5,501}$ of the 4,018 individuals without malaria parasites and the fourth cell (row 2, column 2) to have $\dfrac{3,474}{5,501}$ of the 4,018 individuals without malaria parasites. Table 11.2 is a worksheet for computing these

TABLE 11.2
COMPUTATION OF χ^2 FOR DATA OF MALARIA PARASITES IN BLOOD FILM AND ENLARGEMENT OF SPLEEN FOR 5,501 PERSONS

Cell	Computation of expected frequencies f_c		f	$f - f_c$	$(f - f_c)^2$	$\dfrac{(f - f_c)^2}{f_c}$
	Products of row and column totals	f_c Col. (2) ÷ 5,501				
(1)	(2)	(3)	(4)	(5)	(6)	(7)
Row 1, column 1...	1,483 × 2,027 = 3,006,041	546.5*	740	+193.5	37,442.25	68.5
Row 1, column 2...	1,483 × 3,474 = 5,151,942	936.5	743	−193.5	37,442.25	40.0
Row 2, column 1...	4,018 × 2,027 = 8,144,486	1,480.5	1,287	−193.5	37,442.25	25.3
Row 2, column 2...	4,018 × 3,474 = 13,958,532	2,537.5	2,731	+193.5	37,442.25	14.8
Total..........	...	5,501.0	5,501	0	...	148.6

* The f_c values are usually computed to tenths in order that Σf_c and Σf will not differ as much as 1. If f_c were computed to units, the two summations might differ by 1 or 2. The reader may wish to verify the fact that only one of the f_c values in column (3) need be computed, since the others may be obtained by subtraction from row and column totals.

four f_c values and also χ^2. Such a worksheet is not necessary for the determination of χ^2 for a 2 x 2 table, as an alternative procedure (described on page 273) is available. However, the worksheet of Table 11.2 helps explain the basic process. Furthermore, a computation form such as this is very useful for 3 x 3 and larger tables.

From Table 11.2 the value of χ^2 is seen to be 148.6. As will be explained in the following paragraph, a 2 x 2 table with marginal totals set has one degree of freedom, $n = 1$. Referring to the χ^2 table of Appendix VI, it is apparent that 148.6 is far beyond 0.001, and we conclude that there is a significant difference between the groups with and without parasites in regard to enlargement of the spleen. It should be noted that here, as in the case of χ^2 for the 1 x 2 table, we have a two-tail test. The four parts of the χ^2 value shown in Table 11.2 may arise from $f > f_c$ or $f < f_c$.

The reason why $n = 1$ for a 2 x 2 table with marginal totals set will be clear from the following illustration. Consider this 2 x 2 table with marginal totals but no entries in the cells:

		10
		18
15	13	28

If we now enter the figure 7 in the first cell, the figures are thereupon determined for the other three cells:

7	3	10
8	10	18
15	13	28

Since a figure may be entered freely in but one cell, we have one degree of freedom.

The same procedure may be followed in determining the number of degrees of freedom for tables having more than 2 columns and more than 2 rows and having the marginal totals set.[3] It is much simpler, however, to make use of the following relationships, where R is the number of rows and C is the number of columns:

Degrees of freedom lost because of presence of marginal totals............... $(R - 1) + (C - 1) + 1$
Degrees of freedom (remaining)......... $(R - 1)(C - 1)$
Total, i.e., number of cells............ RC

Simple computations will verify the statement above, that $[(R - 1) + (C - 1) + 1] + [(R - 1)(C - 1)] = RC$. For any problem of this type, the degrees of freedom may be readily ascertained from $n = (R - 1)(C - 1)$. This expression for n does not apply to single-column tables, such as the 1 x 2 table previously discussed or the 1 x 3 table to be discussed later. These and other one-column tables do not have the marginal totals fixed. If $n = (R - 1)(C - 1)$ were to be used for tables of this sort, $C - 1$ would equal zero, giving $n = 0$, which is incorrect.

An alternative procedure is available for computing χ^2 for a 2 x 2 table. If the cells of a 2 x 2 table are identified as in the accompanying table, we have

$$\chi^2 = \frac{(a_1 b_2 - b_1 a_2)^2 N}{(a_1+b_1)(a_2+b_2)(a_1+a_2)(b_1+b_2)}.$$

a_1	b_1	$a_1 + b_1$
a_2	b_2	$a_2 + b_2$
$a_1 + a_2$	$b_1 + b_2$	N

---

[3] A degree of freedom is not lost for every row total, column total, and the grand total. If any one row total and any one column total are deleted, they may be ascertained from the grand total and the other sub-totals.

Use will be made of this expression later, and the reader may wish to verify that it yields a value of 148.6 for the data of Table 11.1.

Identity with $p_1 - p_2$ test. The χ^2 test just described gives results which are exactly the same as those of the $p_1 - p_2$ test discussed in the preceding chapter. To apply the $p_1 - p_2$ test, we may consider our two samples as being the two rows or the two columns. The former seems more logical for this problem. Thus, we have:

With parasites:
$$p_1 = \frac{740}{1,483} = 0.4990. \quad N_1 = 1,483.$$

Without parasites:
$$p_2 = \frac{1,287}{4,018} = 0.3203. \quad N_2 = 4,018.$$

Estimate of π:
$$\bar{p} = \frac{2,027}{5,501} = 0.3685.$$

$$\hat{\sigma}_{p_1-p_2} = \sqrt{\frac{(0.3685)(0.6315)}{1,483} + \frac{(0.3685)(0.6315)}{4,018}},$$

$$= \sqrt{\frac{0.23270775}{1,483} + \frac{0.23270775}{4,018}} = \sqrt{0.00021484} = 0.01466.$$

$$\frac{p_1 - p_2}{\hat{\sigma}_{p_1-p_2}} = \frac{0.4990 - 0.3203}{0.01466} = \frac{0.1787}{0.01466} = 12.19.$$

Referring to the table of areas in two tails of the normal curve, Appendix IV, it is found that an $\frac{x}{\sigma}$ value of 12.19 is far beyond 0.001. Our χ^2 and normal tables do not extend far enough to enable us to verify the fact that $\chi^2 = 148.6$ for $n = 1$ and $\frac{x}{\sigma} = 12.19$ have the same probability of occurrence. However, the χ^2 value is seen to be the square of the $\frac{x}{\sigma}$ value.

Small numbers. Consider the illustrative data in Table 11.3:

TABLE 11.3

INCIDENCE OF DISEASE AMONG AN INOCULATED AND NOT INOCULATED GROUP

Inoculation status	Disease status		Total
	Not attacked	Attacked	
Inoculated............	10	3	13
Not inoculated.........	2	5	7
Total...............	12	8	20

The figures are those used by Rider in his discussion of the same topic and are apparently hypothetical. See Paul R. Rider, *An Introduction to Modern Statistical Methods*, John Wiley & Sons. New York, 1939, pp. 112–115.

If χ^2 is computed by means of either the expression

$$\chi^2 = \Sigma \frac{(f - f_c)^2}{f_c} \text{ or}$$

$$\chi^2 = \frac{(a_1 b_2 - b_1 a_2)^2 N}{(a_1 + b_1)(a_2 + b_2)(a_1 + a_2)(b_1 + b_2)},$$

it is found to be 4.43, and the associated probability ($n = 1$) is 0.036. In the absence of a detailed table for χ^2, we may obtain this value by using χ and referring to the table of areas of the normal curve, since, when $n = 1$, χ is distributed normally. If the 0.05 level is being used as a criterion, we would conclude from the foregoing that the inoculation is effective. We are, however, faced with exactly the same difficulty here as was described for the $p - \pi$ test in the preceding chapter. Either Yates' correction for continuity or, better, the exact method should be used.

Yates' correction. There are several ways in which Yates' correction may be applied. All of them yield the same result. As pointed out before, the correction consists basically of decreasing each $|f - f_c|$ by $\frac{1}{2}$, so that the expression for χ^2 with Yates' correction becomes

$$\chi_Y^2 = \Sigma \frac{(|f - f_c| - \frac{1}{2})^2}{f_c},$$

and this expression may be used in conjunction with a worksheet such as Table 11.2.

The value of χ_Y^2 may also be computed by applying a correction factor to the alternative formula for χ^2 mentioned before. Thus,

$$\chi_Y^2 = \frac{\left(|a_1 b_2 - b_1 a_2| - \frac{N}{2}\right)^2 N}{(a_1 + b_1)(a_2 + b_2)(a_1 + a_2)(b_1 + b_2)}.$$

This expression not only avoids the use of a worksheet but allows us to work entirely with integers when N is even. For our data,

$$\chi_Y^2 = \frac{[(10)(5) - (2)(3) - \frac{20}{2}]^2 20}{(13)(7)(12)(8)},$$

$$= \frac{23{,}120}{8{,}736} = 2.65.$$

Referring to the χ^2 table of Appendix VI for $n = 1$, we find that the probability is slightly larger than 0.10, and we conclude, *contrary to our previous statement*, that the inoculation does not appear to be effective. At least, further experimentation is in order.

Yates' correction may be applied to any 2 x 2 table. However, when N is very large, the difference between χ^2 and χ_Y^2 will be negligible. On the other hand, if N is small, the use of Yates' correction may overstate the probability.[4] As will be seen in the next section, that is exactly what has occurred in our present illustration.

Exact procedure. Although Yates' correction makes an adjustment for continuity of the χ^2 distribution, it does not allow for skewness. Both are taken care of by the exact method. The exact method consists of evaluating the probabilities of all the combinations of frequencies, in the 2 x 2 table, which show a divergence equal to or greater than that shown by the sample. If the cells of a 2 x 2 table are identified by a_1, b_1, a_2, b_2, as shown earlier in this chapter, the probability of any particular combination of frequencies is given by

$$\frac{(a_1 + b_1)!\,(a_2 + b_2)!\,(a_1 + a_2)!\,(b_1 + b_2)!}{N!\,a_1!\,b_1!\,a_2!\,b_2!}.$$

---

[4] For a critical discussion of Yates' correction when used with 2 x 2 tables, see "Yates' Correction and the Statisticians," by Franz Adler, in *Journal of the American Statistical Association*, December 1951, pp. 490–501.

In order to give as complete an explanation as possible all the combinations of cell frequencies producing the marginal totals of Table 11.3 are shown in the first column of Table 11.4. Eight such combinations exist, and they are identified in Table 11.4 as I, II, III, $\cdots$, VIII. There are several methods of ascertaining which of the combinations show divergence equal to or greater

TABLE 11.4

The Eight Combinations Giving the Row and Column Totals of Table 11.3, Together with p_1, p_2, $p_1 - p_2$, and the Exact Probability for Each Combination

Combination		Percentage of row total in first cell and differences	Probability of this combination from $\dfrac{(a_1 + b_1)!(a_2 + b_2)!(a_1 + a_2)!(b_1 + b_2)!}{N!a_1!b_1!a_2!b_2!}$
I	5 | 8 | 13 7 | 0 | 7 12 | 8 | 20	$p_1 = 0.38$ $p_2 = 1.0$ $p_1 - p_2 = -0.62$	0.010
II	6 | 7 | 13 6 | 1 | 7 12 | 8 | 20	$p_1 = 0.46$ $p_2 = 0.86$ $p_1 - p_2 = -0.40$	0.095
III	7 | 6 | 13 5 | 2 | 7 12 | 8 | 20	$p_1 = 0.54$ $p_2 = 0.71$ $p_1 - p_2 = -0.17$	0.286
IV	8 | 5 | 13 4 | 3 | 7 12 | 8 | 20	$p_1 = 0.62$ $p_2 = 0.57$ $p_1 - p_2 = +0.05$	0.358
V	9 | 4 | 13 3 | 4 | 7 12 | 8 | 20	$p_1 = 0.69$ $p_2 = 0.43$ $p_1 - p_2 = +0.26$	0.199
VI	10 | 3 | 13 2 | 5 | 7 12 | 8 | 20	$p_1 = 0.77$ $p_2 = 0.29$ $p_1 - p_2 = +0.48$	0.048
VII	11 | 2 | 13 1 | 6 | 7 12 | 8 | 20	$p_1 = 0.85$ $p_2 = 0.14$ $p_1 - p_2 = +0.71$	0.004
VIII	12 | 1 | 13 0 | 7 | 7 12 | 8 | 20	$p_1 = 0.92$ $p_2 = 0$ $p_1 - p_2 = +0.92$	0.000
Total		$\cdots$	1.000

than that observed in Table 11.3 (combination VI). We shall proceed by computing $p_1 = \dfrac{a_1}{a_1 + b_1}$ and $p_2 = \dfrac{a_2}{a_2 + b_2}$ for each of the combinations, as shown in column 2 of Table 11.4. Then we shall ascertain[5] $p_1 - p_2$ for each of the eight combinations. All combinations having $|p_1 - p_2|$ equal to or greater than combination VI show an equal or greater divergence and are to be included when we total the probabilities for the significance test. From Table 11.4 it is clear that these combinations are I, VI, VII, and VIII. (The same conclusion would have been arrived at if we had used $p_1 = \dfrac{a_1}{a_1 + a_2}$ and $p_2 = \dfrac{b_1}{b_1 + b_2}$; that is, if we had worked with columns instead of rows.) The third column of Table 11.4 shows the probability of each of the eight combinations, so the reader may see that their total is 1.0. Combinations VI, VII, and VIII show divergences equal to or greater than that observed and in the same direction. Their probabilities total 0.052. Combination I shows a divergence greater than that observed, but in the reverse direction. Its probability is 0.010. Notice that the two tails are decidedly unequal. The sum of the probabilities of combinations I, VI, VII, and VIII is 0.062. Using the 0.05 level as a criterion, there is no clear evidence of significance here. This result contradicts the conclusion obtained by the use of uncorrected χ^2. Observe, too, that the probability given by use of Yates' correction was too large.

The exact method may be used for any 2 x 2 table, whether N, is large or small. However, when N is large, the exact method is ordinarily not required and its application involves extensive computation.

---

[5] It is not necessary to compute $|p_1 - p_2|$ for every combination. We know that VII and VIII are to be included, since they are more extreme than VI. If we begin at the other end of the series of combinations, we merely need to compute $|p_1 - p_2|$ values until we arrive at the first one (II; in this case) which shows a value smaller than the observed $|p_1 - p_2|$ value. This is true of the other methods also. They are: (1) compute $f - f_c$ for any one box for each combination, and then consider those combinations for which $|f - f_c|$ equals or exceeds $f - f_c$ for the observed combination, and (2) compute the probability for each combination and then add those probabilities which are equal to or less than the probability of the observed combination.

The 1 x 3 Table

Attention was previously called to Dahlberg's data of right or left thumb on top when hands are clasped. It is argued that, if this trait is inherited, we should expect twins, particularly one-egg (identical) twins to behave alike. For a group of 69 pairs of one-egg twins, 17 pairs both placed the left thumb on top, 34 pairs did not behave alike (one placing the right thumb on top, the other placing the left thumb on top), and 18 pairs both placed the right thumb on top. It is believed that the proportions placing the right or left thumb on top are evenly distributed in the population. Dahlberg cites figures for 854 school children of whom 426 placed the right thumb on top while 428 placed the left thumb on top. Therefore (letting A represent an occurrence of the right thumb on top and B a non-occurrence), the chance distribution for pairs of people is given by $(0.50B + 0.50A)^2 = 0.25B^2 + 0.50BA + 0.25A^2$, which is to say that 25 per cent of the pairs would both be expected to have left thumbs on top, 50 per cent would differ, and 25 per cent would both have right thumbs on top. The χ^2 test may be employed to ascertain whether the observed data for one-egg twins differ significantly from a chance distribution. This is done in Table 11.5, and χ^2 is found to be 0.04. In this problem we have three categories in the sample. With the total set at 69, there

TABLE 11.5

COMPUTATION OF χ^2 FOR THUMBS ON TOP DATA FOR ONE-EGG TWINS

Thumbs on top	f	f_c 1:2:1	$f - f_c$	$(f - f_c)^2$	$\dfrac{(f - f_c)^2}{f_c}$
Both right..................	18	17.25	0.75	0.5625	0.03
One right, one left...............	34	34.5	−0.5	0.25	0.01
Both left..................	17	17.25	−0.25	0.0625	
Total.................	69	69.00	0	...	0.04

In this table we have used the expression

$$\chi^2 = \Sigma \frac{(f - f_c)^2}{f_c}.$$

When computing χ^2 for a table having $\Sigma f = \Sigma f_c = N$, we may employ the alternative form

$$\chi^2 = \Sigma \left(\frac{f^2}{f_c} \right) - N.$$

remain two degrees of freedom. The distribution of χ^2 when $n = 2$ is shown in Chart 11.1 and looks somewhat like the distribution for $n = 1$, but is not asymptotic to zero on the vertical axis. Referring to Appendix VI for $n = 2$ and $\chi^2 = 0.04$, the probability is found to be 0.98, meaning that a divergence this great or greater might be expected to occur 98 times in 100. The agreement between the sample of 69 one-egg twins and the chance distribution is remarkably close.

Had we obtained a probability of 0.02 in the preceding problem, we should doubtless have declared the difference significant. Some writers have called attention to the fact that an occurrence with a probability of 0.98 is just as unusual as one with a probability of 0.02. That is, of course, true. Some have gone on from this statement to assert that, when a probability of 0.98 is obtained, the hypothesis is just as clearly negated as when the probability is 0.02. Such a statement is hardly tenable—certainly not as a generalization. The probability of 0.98 is surprising, and, when such a high probability is obtained, one should (as always!) check to see if there are any arithmetic mistakes, check carefully to see if the observed data have been "rigged" or possibly previously smoothed by a fitting process, and perhaps even re-examine the hypothesis involved. None of these difficulties seem to be involved in the present illustration.

It is not within the scope of this book to discuss the correction for continuity or the computation of exact probabilities which may be made for situations where $n > 1$. It may be noted, however, that the values shown in the χ^2 table are based upon a continuous distribution, and that in some problems χ^2 can assume only certain discontinuous values.[6]

2 x 3 and Larger Tables

As an illustration of a 2 x 3 table, we shall consider the "thumbs on top" data for one-egg and two-egg twins. Table 11.6 shows the data for 69 pairs of one-egg twins and 123 pairs of two-egg twins. The computation of χ^2 is given in Table 11.7, which shows $\chi^2 = 0.27$. Following the procedure described in the section on 2 x 2 tables, the reader may verify that $n = 2$. The probability, from

---

[6] See W. G. Cochran, "The χ^2 Correction for Continuity," *Iowa State College Journal of Science*, Vol. XVI, No. 4, July 1942, pp. 421–436.

TABLE 11.6

Thumbs on Top When Hands are Clasped for 69 One-Egg Twins and 123 Two-Egg Twins

Thumbs on top	One-egg twins	Two-egg twins	Total
Both right..................	18	34	52
One right, one left..........	34	56	90
Both left....................	17	33	50
Total.....................	69	123	192

Source of data: Gunnar Dahlberg, *Statistical Methods for Medical and Biological Students*, Geo. Allen & Unwin, London, 1940, p. 29.

TABLE 11.7

Computation of χ^2 for Data of Table 11.6

Cell	Computation of expected frequencies, f_c		f	$f - f_c$	$(f - f_c)^2$	$\dfrac{(f - f_c)^2}{f_c}$
	Product of row and column totals	f_c Col. (2) ÷ 192				
(1)	(2)	(3)	(4)	(5)	(6)	(7)
Row 1, column 1.	69 × 52 = 3,588	18.7	18	−0.7	0.49	0.03
Row 1, column 2.	123 × 52 = 6,396	33.3	34	+0.7	0.49	0.01
Row 2, column 1.	69 × 90 = 6,210	32.3	34	+1.7	2.89	0.09
Row 2, column 2.	123 × 90 = 11,070	57.7	56	−1.7	2.89	0.05
Row 3, column 1.	69 × 50 = 3,450	18.0	17	−1.0	1.00	0.06
Row 3, column 2.	123 × 50 = 6,150	32.0	33	+1.0	1.00	0.03
Total.........	...	192.0	192	0	...	0.27

An alternative method for computing χ^2 for 2-column (or 2-row) tables and which does not involve a worksheet may be found in C. H. Goulden, *Methods of Statistical Analysis*, John Wiley & Sons, New York, 1939, p. 97.

the χ^2 table, is more than 0.80 but less than 0.90, leading to the conclusion that the observed data do not indicate a difference in the behavior of one-egg and two-egg twins in this respect.

For tables larger than 2 x 3, having the marginal totals fixed, the procedure is similar to that for the 2 x 3 table. The worksheet (Table 11.7) will, of course, be larger, having as many rows as there are cells in the original table of data. The degrees of freedom will be $n = (R - 1)(C - 1)$. The curve of the distribution of χ^2 for $n = 3$ is shown in Chart 11.2. When $n \geq 3$, the curve is skewed to the right with its mode at $\chi^2 = n - 2$ and with its mean at $\chi^2 = n$. The horizontal-scale values range from $\chi^2 = 0$ to $\chi^2 = \infty$. The foregoing statements apply also to the curve for $n = 2$, which was shown in Chart 11.1, except that the curve is "reverse J-shaped" rather than skewed.

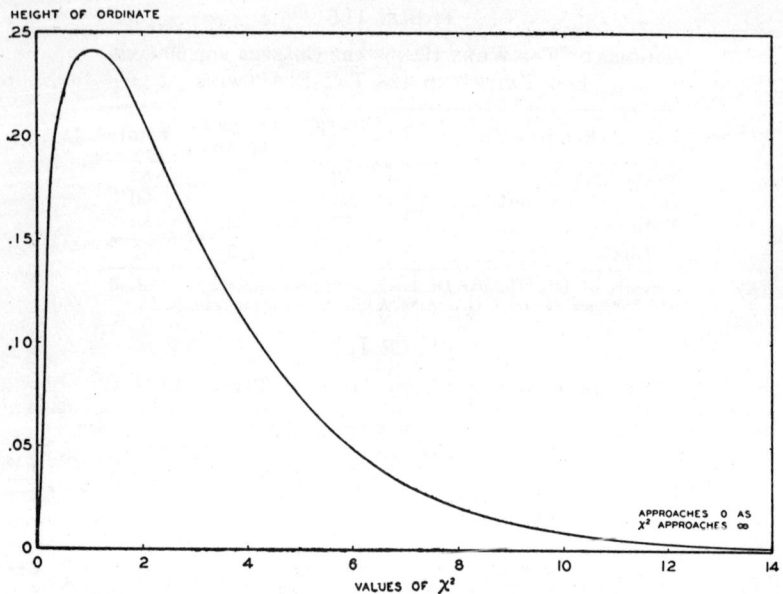

Chart 11.2. Distribution of χ^2 for Three Degrees of Freedom.

Test of "Goodness of Fit"

In Chapter 8 a normal curve was fitted to data of red blood cell counts for 137 young men. The χ^2 test may be used to test the discrepancy between the observed frequencies (f) and the frequencies obtained by the fitting process (f_c). The procedure for getting χ^2 is the same as that shown for 1 x 2 and 1 x 3 tables, and Table 11.8 shows the computations. The degrees of freedom in our problem are four. In Table 11.8 there are seven classes, and the two sets of data have been forced to agree in respect to N, $\bar{X}$, and s. Therefore, we have $n = 7 - 3 = 4$. From the χ^2 table of Appendix VI, it appears that the probability of obtaining a value of χ^2 of 1.67 or greater when $n = 4$ is about 0.80, if the underlying distribution is normal. Since such a discrepancy may occur this often because of variations due to random sampling, we conclude that our fit is satisfactory. Probabilities of 0.05 or larger are generally considered to indicate a satisfactory fit. This test is an "over-all" test, and it should be noted that, even though the individual $f - f_c$ values may be small, the presence of a number of consecutive $f - f_c$ values having the same sign may suggest that the sample was actually drawn from a non-normal population.

TABLE 11.8

χ^2 Test of "Goodness of Fit" of a Normal Curve to Data of Red Blood Cell Count for 137 Healthy Young Men

Cell count	f	f_c	$f - f_c$	$(f - f_c)^2$	$\dfrac{(f - f_c)^2}{f_c}$
4.3 or fewer		0.8	} *−1.2	1.44	0.31
4.3–4.6	3.5	3.9			
4.6–4.9	15.5	12.7	+2.8	7.84	0.62
4.9–5.2	29	27.3	+1.7	2.89	0.11
5.2–5.5	34	36.3	−2.3	5.29	0.15
5.5–5.8	32.5	31.2	+1.3	1.69	0.05
5.8–6.1	14.5	17.2	−2.7	7.29	0.42
6.1–6.4	6	6.1			
6.4–6.7	2	1.4	} *+0.3	0.09	0.01
6.7 or more		0.2			
Total	137.0	137.1	−0.1	...	1.67

Data from Tables 8.1 and 8.3.

* It is customary to group the frequencies in the end classes of a frequency distribution in order to avoid the marked effect on χ^2 of small absolute differences between f and f_c. In practical situations, it is also true that we are often not particularly interested in the f_c values for the extremes of a distribution. Upon the basis that the distribution of f values around f_c does not properly correspond to the expected distribution when f_c is small, various authorities have recommended that no class should have fewer than 5 or 10 computed frequencies. Cochran has shown, however, that, when a probability of 0.05 is used as a criterion, more latitude may be allowed. See W. G. Cochran, "The χ^2 Correction for Continuity," *Iowa State College Journal of Science*, Vol. XVI, No. 4, July 1942, pp. 421–436.

Symbols Used in

CHAPTER 12

Sample Variances

Each listed variance, s^2, $\hat{\sigma}^2$, or σ^2, has an associated standard deviation s, $\hat{\sigma}$, or σ.

$F: \dfrac{\hat{\sigma}_1^2}{\hat{\sigma}_2^2}.$

n: degrees of freedom.
n_1: degrees of freedom in sample 1.
n_2: degrees of freedom in sample 2.
N: number of items in a sample.
N_1: number of items in sample 1.
N_2: number of items in sample 2.
P: probability; varies from 0 to 1.
s^2: the variance of a sample.
s_1^2: the variance of sample 1.
s_2^2: the variance of sample 2.
σ^2: the variance of a population.
σ_1^2: the lower confidence limit of σ^2.
σ_2^2: the upper confidence limit of σ^2.
$\hat{\sigma}^2$: the estimated variance of a population obtained from a sample.
Σ: upper-case Greek sigma, meaning "take the sum of."
x: $X - \overline{X}$.
x_1: $X_1 - \overline{X}_1$.
x_2: $X_2 - \overline{X}_2$.
χ^2: chi-square. The symbol is a lower-case Greek chi.

Analysis of Variance

$F: \dfrac{\hat{\sigma}_1^2}{\hat{\sigma}_2^2}.$

k_b: the number of boxes.
k_c: the number of columns.
k_r: the number of rows.

SYMBOLS USED IN CHAPTER 12

n_1: degrees of freedom associated with $\hat{\sigma}_1^2$.
n_2: degrees of freedom associated with $\hat{\sigma}_2^2$.
N_b: number of items in a box.
N_c: number of items in a column.
N_r: number of items in a row.
$N_1, N_2, N_3, \cdots$: respectively, the number of items in columns 1, 2, 3, $\cdots$.
P: probability; varies from 0 to 1.
Σ: upper-case Greek sigma, meaning "take the sum of."
$\sum_{1}^{k_b}$: a summation over the k_b boxes.
$\sum_{1}^{k_c}$: a summation over the k_c columns.
$\sum_{1}^{k_r}$: a summation over the k_r rows.
$\sum_{1}^{N}$: a summation over all items. Same as Σ.
$\sum_{1}^{N_b}$: a summation over the N_b items in a box.
$\sum_{1}^{N_c}$: a summation over the N_c items in a column.
$\sum_{1}^{N_r}$: a summation over the N_r items in a row.
t: see Chapter 9. $t = \sqrt{F}$ when $n_1 = 1$.
X: an observed value.
$\bar{X}$: the arithmetic mean of all the items, the "grand mean."
$\bar{X}_b$: the arithmetic mean of a box.
$\bar{X}_c$: the arithmetic mean of a column.
$\bar{X}_r$: the arithmetic mean of a row.
$\bar{X}_1, \bar{X}_2, \bar{X}_3, \cdots$: respectively, the arithmetic means of columns 1, 2, 3, $\cdots$.
χ^2: chi-square; see Chapter 11. $\dfrac{\chi^2}{n} = F$ when $N_2 = \infty$.

Correlation Coefficients

b: slope of the estimating equation
$$Y_c = a + bX.$$

SYMBOLS USED IN CHAPTER 12

F: used in this section for testing $R^2_{1.234\cdots m}$ by means of the expression

$$F = \frac{R^2_{1.234\cdots m}(N-m)}{(1 - R^2_{1.234\cdots m})(m - 1)}.$$

m: number of constants in an estimating equation.
n: degrees of freedom.
N_1 and N_2: respectively, the number of pairs of items from which r_1 and r_2 were computed.
P: probability; varies from 0 to 1.
r: sample coefficient of correlation, linear correlation of two variables. When two samples are under consideration, we use r_1 and r_2.
$r_\wp$: population coefficient of correlation, linear correlation of two variables.
$r_{\wp_1}$: lower confidence limit of $r_\wp$.
$r_{\wp_2}$: upper confidence limit of $r_\wp$.
$\hat{r}^2$: estimated value of $r^2_\wp$; obtained from a sample.
$r^2_{13.2}$: coefficient of partial determination. See Chapter 7.
$r^2_{1m.234\cdots(m-1)}$: a form of the coefficient of partial determination for m variables.
$R^2_{1.234\cdots m}$: multiple coefficient of determination for m variables.
$\hat{R}^2_{1.234\cdots m}$: estimated population value of the multiple coefficient of determination, obtained from a sample.
$s^2_{Ys}: \dfrac{\Sigma y^2_s}{N}$.
$s^2_Y: \dfrac{\Sigma y^2}{N}$.
σ_Z: standard error of Z.
$\sigma_{Z_1-Z_2}$: standard error of $Z_1 - Z_2$.
Σ: upper-case Greek sigma, meaning "take the sum of."
$t: \sqrt{\dfrac{r^2(N-m)}{1-r^2}}$, where r^2 may be either a two-variable linear coefficient of determination or a partial coefficient of determination.
$x: X - \bar{X}$.
X: an observed value in the X series.
$\bar{X}$: the arithmetic mean of the X series.
$y: Y - \bar{Y}$. Σy^2 is the total variation of the Y series.
$y_s: Y - Y_c$. Σy^2_s is the unexplained variation of the Y series.
Y: an observed value in the Y series.
$\bar{Y}$: the arithmetic mean of the Y series.

Y_c: a computed Y value.

Z: $1.15129 \log \frac{1+r}{1-r}$. When two samples are under consideration, we use Z_1 and Z_2 corresponding to r_1 and r_2.

Z_φ: $1.15129 \log \frac{1+r_\varphi}{1-r_\varphi}$.

Z_{φ_1}: lower confidence limit of Z_φ.

Z_{φ_2}: upper confidence limit of Z_φ.

Skewness and Kurtosis

β_1: lower-case Greek beta; measure of skewness in a sample. See Chapter 5.

β_2: lower-case Greek beta; measure of kurtosis in a sample. See Chapter 5.

N: number of items in a sample.

Chapter 12
SIGNIFICANCE TESTS FOR VARIANCES; ANALYSIS OF VARIANCE; TESTS FOR CORRELATION COEFFICIENTS AND FOR MEASURES OF SKEWNESS AND KURTOSIS

This chapter will consider first the problems of testing the significance of the difference between a variance computed from a random sample and the known variance of the population, the confidence limits of the population variance, and the significance of the difference between two sample variances. Then it will give attention to the method of testing the differences existing between several sample means, known as *analysis of variance*. At this point there will be a brief digression to show the interrelationships between the normal, t, χ^2, and F distributions. Next it will take up the procedures for testing the significance of the difference between a two-variable linear correlation coefficient obtained from a random sample and the correlation coefficient for the population, for testing the significance of the difference between two two-variable linear correlation coefficients, for estimating the correlation in the population, and for testing the significance of partial and multiple correlation coefficients. Finally, a brief section will discuss a method for ascertaining whether significant skewness or kurtosis is present in a series.

Sample Variances

Significance of difference between $\hat{\sigma}^2$ and σ^2. It has already been pointed out that it is unusual for σ or σ^2 to be known. For that reason, we shall use the Shewhart data to illustrate the procedure for testing the significance of the difference between the variance of a random sample and the population variance. Shewhart's population of 1,000 items had $\sigma = 1.0070$, so that $\sigma^2 = 1.014$. The first sample of four items (which, it will be recalled, had a mean of

0.950) had $\hat{\sigma}^2 = 0.509$. Is there a significant difference between $\hat{\sigma}^2 = 0.509$ and $\sigma^2 = 1.014$? Our null hypothesis is that $\hat{\sigma}^2 = 0.509$ is the variance of a random sample from a population having $\sigma^2 = 1.014$. To test this hypothesis,[1] we make use of the expression

$$\chi^2 = \frac{(N-1)\hat{\sigma}^2}{\sigma^2},$$

where χ^2 is distributed according to $N - 1$ degrees of freedom. For our illustration,

$$\chi^2 = \frac{3(0.509)}{1.014} = \frac{1.527}{1.014} = 1.51,$$

with $n = 4 - 1 = 3$. Referring to the χ^2 table of Appendix VI, we find that the probability of obtaining a χ^2 value of 1.51 *or larger*, and therefore the probability of obtaining a value of $\hat{\sigma}^2 = 0.509$ *or larger*, is approximately 0.68. The probability of obtaining a value of $\chi^2 = 1.51$ *or smaller*, and therefore the probability of obtaining $\hat{\sigma}^2 = 0.509$ *or smaller*, is about 0.32. The conclusion is that there is not a significant difference between $\hat{\sigma}^2$ and σ^2.

Note that our test gave us the probability of obtaining $\hat{\sigma}^2 \leq 0.509$ and is, in effect, a one-tail test. We could also ask, what is the equally probable value of $\hat{\sigma}^2$ when $\hat{\sigma}^2 > \sigma^2$, and we could obtain this by making use of the χ^2 value for $n = 3$, which has a probability

---

[1] If one wishes to test the significance of the difference between $s^2 = \dfrac{\Sigma x^2}{N}$ and σ^2, the expression for χ^2 becomes

$$\chi^2 = \frac{(N-1)\hat{\sigma}^2}{\sigma^2} = \frac{(N-1)\dfrac{\Sigma x^2}{N-1}}{\sigma^2},$$

$$= \frac{\Sigma x^2}{\sigma^2} = \frac{N\dfrac{\Sigma x^2}{N}}{\sigma^2},$$

$$= \frac{Ns^2}{\sigma^2}.$$

Since this section on sample variances will conclude with a consideration of the significance of the difference between two sample variances using $\hat{\sigma}_1^2$ and $\hat{\sigma}_2^2$ rather than s_1^2 and s_2^2 and will lead logically to the following section on analysis of variance where two or more values of $\hat{\sigma}^2$ (estimates of σ^2) will be compared, it seems preferable that our initial approach should use $\hat{\sigma}^2$ rather than s^2.

of 0.32 in Appendix VI. This is $\chi^2 = 3.535$, which enables us to compute

$$3.535 = \frac{3\hat{\sigma}^2}{1.014}.$$

$$\hat{\sigma}^2 = \frac{(3.535)(1.014)}{3} = 1.195.$$

The test which we used did not refer to the absolute difference between $\hat{\sigma}^2$ and σ^2, but to $\frac{\hat{\sigma}^2}{\sigma^2}$. This means that, for any problem, when $N = 4$, and when $\frac{\hat{\sigma}^2}{\sigma^2} = 0.502$, the probability of obtaining the observed $\hat{\sigma}^2$ or smaller would be 0.32; and similarly that, for any problem, when $N = 4$ and $\frac{\hat{\sigma}^2}{\sigma^2} = 1.18$, the probability of obtaining the observed $\hat{\sigma}^2$ or larger would be 0.32. This situation can be made use of by determining the ratios for various lower and upper probability points of $\hat{\sigma}^2$. For example, the lower 0.01 point for $\hat{\sigma}^2$ when $N = 4$ ($n = 3$) would be obtained by using the χ^2 value having a probability of 0.99 in Appendix VI ($\chi^2 = 0.115$), while the upper 0.01 point would be computed by using the χ^2 value having a probability of 0.01 in Appendix VI ($\chi^2 = 11.345$). The desired ratios are obtained by substituting the two values for χ^2 in the expression

$$\chi^2 = \frac{(N-1)\hat{\sigma}^2}{\sigma^2}.$$

For the lower 0.01 point of $\hat{\sigma}^2$,

$$0.115 = \frac{3\hat{\sigma}^2}{\sigma^2}.$$

$$\hat{\sigma}^2 = \frac{0.115}{3}\sigma^2 = 0.038\sigma^2.$$

For the upper 0.01 point of $\hat{\sigma}^2$,

$$11.345 = \frac{3\hat{\sigma}^2}{\sigma^2}.$$

$$\hat{\sigma}^2 = \frac{11.345}{3}\sigma^2 = 3.782\sigma^2.$$

SIGNIFICANCE TESTS FOR VARIANCES

In similar fashion these, and other probability points, may be ascertained for various sample sizes. A table of $\dfrac{\hat{\sigma}^2}{\sigma^2}$ ratios[2] is given in Appendix VII.

While $\dfrac{\hat{\sigma}^2}{\sigma^2}$ is a constant value for any specified sample size and probability point, the same is not true of the difference between $\hat{\sigma}^2$ and σ^2. Our first test in this section dealt with $\sigma^2 = 1.014$, $\hat{\sigma}^2 = 0.509$, and $N = 4$, and the probability of obtaining a value of $\hat{\sigma}^2 = 0.509$ or smaller was found to be 0.32. A value of $\hat{\sigma}^2$ which differs from σ^2 by the same absolute amount as did $\hat{\sigma}^2 = 0.509$ but in the opposite direction would be $\hat{\sigma}^2 = 1.519$. If it were desired to test this value, we would compute

$$\chi^2 = \frac{3(1.519)}{1.014} = \frac{2.307}{1.014} = 2.28,$$

and the probability is a little less than 0.50. This value of $\hat{\sigma}^2$ is also not significantly different from σ^2.

The smaller probability for $\hat{\sigma}^2 = 0.509$ than for $\hat{\sigma}^2 = 1.519$ indicates that the distribution of values of $\hat{\sigma}^2$ is skewed. This, of course, does not contradict the statement in Chapter 9 that $\hat{\sigma}^2$ is an unbiased estimate of σ^2.

Confidence limits of σ^2. The expression

$$\chi^2 = \frac{(N-1)\hat{\sigma}^2}{\sigma^2}$$

also enables us to compute the confidence limits of σ^2. As an illustration, consider the data, given in Table 9.2, of the pressure, in millimeters of mercury, required to cause disruption of the abdomens of 20 unoperated rats. The value of $\hat{\sigma}$ was found to be 7.808 mm, so $\hat{\sigma}^2 = 60.96$ and $N = 20$. What are the 98 per cent confidence limits of σ^2? We need the values of χ^2 at the 0.01 and 0.99 points for $n = 19$, and these are found in Appendix VI to be 36.191

---

[2] The ratio $\dfrac{\hat{\sigma}^2}{\sigma^2} = \dfrac{\chi^2}{N-1}$ is a special case of F (see pages 293–295) when $n_2 = \infty$. The significance of the difference between $\hat{\sigma}^2$ and σ^2 may be tested by using either χ^2 or F. Chi-square was used in the preceding discussion because the reader was already familiar with that measure and because more extensive tables of χ^2 are readily available.

and 7.633. Substituting, we have

$$36.191 = \frac{19(60.96)}{\sigma_1^2}.$$

$$\sigma_1^2 = \frac{19(60.96)}{36.191},$$

$$= 32.00.$$

$$7.633 = \frac{19(60.96)}{\sigma_2^2},$$

$$\sigma_2^2 = \frac{19(60.96)}{7.633},$$

$$= 151.74.$$

The 98 per cent confidence limits of σ^2 are, therefore, 32.00 and 151.74. Notice that $\hat{\sigma}^2$ does not fall midway between the two limits. If these limits seem far removed from each other, it must be remembered that we are dealing with variances, not standard deviations. Taking the square root of each of the three values, we have:

$$\sigma_1 = 5.66 \text{ mm},$$
$$\hat{\sigma} = 7.81 \text{ mm},$$
$$\sigma_2 = 12.32 \text{ mm}.$$

Rodger P. Doyle computed the 90 per cent confidence limits[3] of σ^2 for each of Shewhart's 1,000 samples of four items. After determining the upper and lower 90 per cent confidence limits of σ^2 from a knowledge of $\hat{\sigma}^2$ and N for each sample, he checked to ascertain the number of instances in which he had succeeded in including the population value ($\sigma^2 = 1.014$) between his limits. He found that he had succeeded in 904 of the 1,000 attempts. In 96 attempts, the population variance fell outside the limits.

Just as it was possible to make a table of the probability points of $\hat{\sigma}^2$ in relation to σ^2 (Appendix VII), so one may construct a table of values of $\dfrac{\sigma^2}{\hat{\sigma}^2}$ to ascertain the confidence limits of σ^2. Consider the data of the preceding illustration. For the lower 98 per cent confidence limit of σ^2 we would have

---

[3] From unpublished material.

$$36.191 = \frac{19\hat{\sigma}^2}{\sigma_1^2},$$

$$\frac{\sigma_1^2}{\hat{\sigma}^2} = \frac{19}{36.191} = 0.525,$$

$$\sigma_1^2 = 0.525\hat{\sigma}^2,$$

and for the upper 98 per cent confidence limit

$$7.633 = \frac{19\hat{\sigma}^2}{\sigma_2^2},$$

$$\frac{\sigma_2^2}{\hat{\sigma}^2} = \frac{19}{7.633} = 2.489,$$

$$\sigma_2^2 = 2.489\hat{\sigma}^2.$$

These and other values[4] of $\dfrac{\sigma^2}{\hat{\sigma}^2}$ are shown in Appendix VIII for various confidence limits and degrees of freedom.

Significance of difference between two sample variances. The data of Table 9.3 gave the pressure in millimeters of mercury required to disrupt healing wounds, four days after the operation, for two groups of rats for which silk and wire had been used as suture material. From the information given below the table, we may compute:

for the group sutured with silk ($N_1 = 4$),

$$\hat{\sigma}_1^2 = \frac{\Sigma x_1^2}{N_1 - 1} = \frac{44.75}{3} = 14.92;$$

for the group sutured with wire ($N_2 = 5$),

$$\hat{\sigma}_2^2 = \frac{\Sigma x_2^2}{N_2 - 1} = \frac{61.2}{4} = 15.30.$$

We wish to know if there is a significant difference between $\hat{\sigma}_1^2$ and $\hat{\sigma}_2^2$, and, in order to do this, we shall consider the ratio of the two variances

$$F = \frac{\hat{\sigma}_1^2}{\hat{\sigma}_2^2} = \frac{14.92}{15.30} = 0.98.$$

---

[4] The ratio $\dfrac{\sigma^2}{\hat{\sigma}^2} = \dfrac{N-1}{\chi^2}$ is a special case of F (see pages 293–295) when $n_1 = \infty$.

The possible values of F range from 0 to ∞. If $\hat{\sigma}_1^2$ is smaller than $\hat{\sigma}_2^2$, the value of F will be less than 1; if $\hat{\sigma}_1^2$ is larger than $\hat{\sigma}_2^2$, the value of F will be greater than 1; if $\hat{\sigma}_1^2 = \hat{\sigma}_2^2$, $F = 1.0$. The distribution of $F = \dfrac{\hat{\sigma}_1^2}{\hat{\sigma}_2^2}$ (where $\hat{\sigma}_1^2$ and $\hat{\sigma}_2^2$ are independent estimates of σ^2 of a normal population) depends upon the number of degrees of freedom

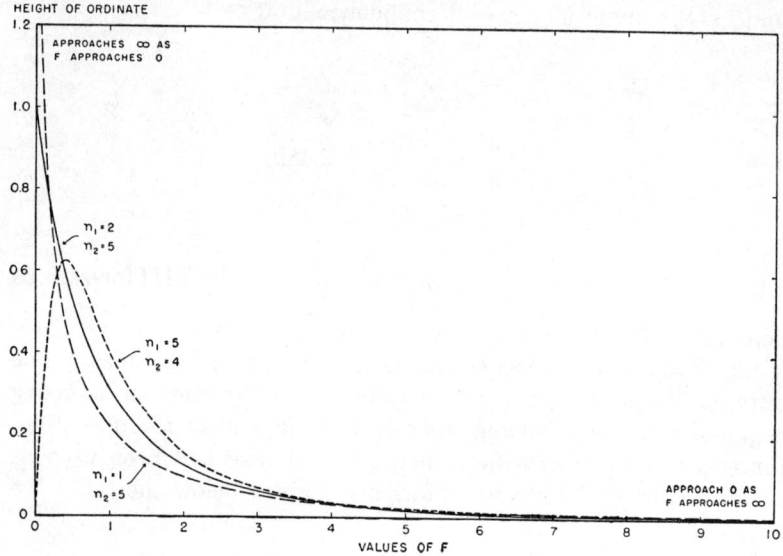

Chart 12.1. Distribution of F for $n_1 = 1$, $n_2 = 5$; $n_1 = 2$, $n_2 = 5$; and $n_1 = 5$, $n_2 = 4$. Horizontal and vertical scales extend to ∞. The ordinates of the F distribution are obtained from the expression

$$Y_c = \frac{F^{\frac{n_1-2}{2}}}{(n_1 F + n_2)^{\frac{n_1+n_2}{2}}} \cdot \frac{\left(\dfrac{n_1+n_2-2}{2}\right)! \, (n_1)^{\frac{n_1}{2}} (n_2)^{\frac{n_2}{2}}}{\left(\dfrac{n_1-2}{2}\right)! \left(\dfrac{n_2-2}{2}\right)!}$$

in the two series, $n_1 = N_1 - 1$ and $n_2 = N_2 - 1$. Except when $n_1 = 1$ or 2, the F curve will be a skewed curve with the peak of the curve above a value[5] of $F < 1$. When $n_1 = 1$ or 2, the F curve is of the "reverse J" type, similar in general shape to Chart 3.7. Sketches of the F distribution for several combinations of n_1 and n_2 are shown in Chart 12.1.

---

[5] More specifically, when $n_1 \geqq 2$, the peak is at $F = \dfrac{n_2(n_1 - 2)}{n_1(n_2 + 2)}$. When $n_1 = 1$, the peak is at $F = 0$.

An abbreviated F table, shown as Appendix IX, gives the upper and lower 0.20, 0.05, 0.01, and 0.001 points of the distribution of F for selected values of n_1 and n_2. From that table we find that, when $n_1 = 3$ and $n_2 = 4$, $F = 0.338$ is at the lower 0.20 point and $F = 0.110$ is at the lower 0.05 point. It is clear that the probability of a value of $F = 0.98$ or smaller is much more than 0.20, and, since $F = 0.98$ does not differ significantly from $F = 1.0$, $\hat{\sigma}_1^2$ is not significantly *smaller* than $\hat{\sigma}_2^2$. However, we want to know whether $\hat{\sigma}_1^2$ is significantly *different* from $\hat{\sigma}_2^2$; therefore, we test also the reciprocal of the observed F, that is,

$$F = \frac{1}{0.98} = 1.02,$$

for $n_1 = 3$ and $n_2 = 4$. From Appendix IX it appears that $F = 2.48$ is at the upper 0.20 point and $F = 6.59$ is at the upper 0.05 point. Since the probability of obtaining $F = 1.02$ or greater is much more than 0.20, we conclude that $F = 1.02$ is not significantly *larger* than 1.0. Adding the two probabilities, we may say that the probability is more than 0.40 that, when $n_1 = 3$ and $n_2 = 4$, a value of $F = 0.98$ or $F = 1.02$ may occur. Consequently, $\hat{\sigma}_1^2 = 14.92$ and $\hat{\sigma}_2^2 = 15.30$ do not differ significantly from each other.

Analysis of Variance

One criterion of classification. In Chapter 9 we tested the significance of the difference between two sample means. There are occasions in which we may be interested in testing the difference between more than two means. Consider the data of Table 12.1, which show the pressure in millimeters required to disrupt healing wounds sutured with silk as tested for varying numbers of rats 1, 2, 3, and 4 days after operation. The mean pressure for each of the columns, in order, is: $\bar{X}_1 = 77.0$ mm, $\bar{X}_2 = 98.2$ mm, $\bar{X}_3 = 40.5$ mm, and $\bar{X}_4 = 81.75$ mm. It is not desired to test $\bar{X}_1 - \bar{X}_2$, $\bar{X}_1 - \bar{X}_3$, and each of the four other differences that could be tested; we want to know whether the four means as a group differ from each other more than might be expected as a result of random sampling.

To set up the basis for such a test, we shall first recognize three sources of variation present in the data of Table 12.1.

1. *Variation between column means.* Using $\bar{X}_1$, $\bar{X}_2$, and so forth, to refer to the column means, N_1, N_2, and so forth, to refer to the

TABLE 12.1

Computation of Values Required for Analysis of Variance of Data of Pressure in Millimeters of Mercury, Required to Disrupt Healing Wounds of Rats Sutured with Silk, the Tests Having Been Made One, Two, Three, and Four Days After Operation

1		2		3		4	
X_1	X_1^2	X_2	X_2^2	X_3	X_3^2	X_4	X_4^2
63	3,969	101	10,201	40	1,600	76	5,776
79	6,241	116	13,456	42	1,764	84	7,056
79	6,241	90	8,100	40	1,600	83	6,889
82	6,724	93	8,649	41	1,681	84	7,056
82	6,724	91	8,281	40	1,600		
				40	1,600		
385	29,899	491	48,687	243	9,845	327	26,777

Data from S. A. Localio, W. Casale, and J. W. Hinton, "Wound Healing—Experimental and Statistical Study, IV. Results," *Surgery, Gynecology and Obstetrics*, October 1943, Vol. 77, pages 376–388.

$$N = 20.$$
$$\Sigma X = 385 + 491 + 243 + 327 = 1,446.$$
$$(\Sigma X)^2 = (1,446)^2 = 2,090,916.$$
$$\Sigma X^2 = 29,899 + 48,687 + 9,845 + 26,777 = 115,208.$$

$$\sum_{1}^{k_c}\left[\frac{\left(\sum_{1}^{N_c} X\right)^2}{N_c}\right] = \frac{(385)^2}{5} + \frac{(491)^2}{5} + \frac{(243)^2}{6} + \frac{(327)^2}{4} = 114,434.95.$$

number of items in the columns, and $\overline{X}$ to indicate the mean of all the items (which for brevity we shall call the "grand mean"), variation between column means may be represented by the expression

$$N_1(\overline{X}_1 - \overline{X})^2 + N_2(\overline{X}_2 - \overline{X})^2 + N_3(\overline{X}_3 - \overline{X})^2 + \cdots.$$

By using $\overline{X}_c$ to refer to the mean of a column, N_c the number in a column, and k_c the number of columns, the expression may be written more compactly:

$$\sum_{1}^{k_c}[N_c(\overline{X}_c - \overline{X})^2].$$

This says: take the difference between the mean of a column and the grand mean, square this difference, multiply by the number of items in the column; do this for all of the other columns, and add. The symbol $\sum_{1}^{k_c}$ indicates that a summation over all the k_c columns is to be made.

CHAP. 12]   ANALYSIS OF VARIANCE   297

For purposes of computation, it is not necessary to compute the column means and the grand mean. If the expression just given is expanded and simplified, the numerical value of variation between column means may be obtained from

$$\sum_{1}^{k_c}[N_c(\overline{X}_c - \overline{X})^2] = \sum_{1}^{k_c}\left[\frac{\left(\sum_{1}^{N_c}X\right)^2}{N_c}\right] - \frac{(\Sigma X)^2}{N},$$

where $\sum_{1}^{N_c}$ refers to a summation over the N_c items in a column. Using the computations given below Table 12.1,

$$\sum_{1}^{k_c}\left[\frac{\left(\sum_{1}^{N_c}X\right)^2}{N_c}\right] - \frac{(\Sigma X)^2}{N} = 114{,}434.95 - \frac{2{,}090{,}916}{20},$$
$$= 114{,}434.95 - 104{,}545.8,$$
$$= 9{,}889.15.$$

2. *Variation within columns.* This is the variation of the items in the columns about the column means, and may be written

$$\sum_{1}^{k_c}\left[\sum_{1}^{N_c}(X - \overline{X}_c)^2\right].$$

This says: square the difference between each item in a column and the mean of that column, sum these values for the column; do this for all the other columns, and add.

Again, it is not necessary to compute the column means, since

$$\sum_{1}^{k_c}\left[\sum_{1}^{N_c}(X - \overline{X}_c)^2\right] = \Sigma X^2 - \sum_{1}^{k_c}\left[\frac{\left(\sum_{1}^{N_c}X\right)^2}{N_c}\right],$$

and, by referring to figures below Table 12.1, we have

$$\Sigma X^2 - \sum_{1}^{k_c}\left[\frac{\left(\sum_{1}^{N_c}X\right)^2}{N_c}\right] = 115{,}208 - 114{,}434.95,$$
$$= 773.05.$$

3. *Total variation* is the variation of all of the items in the table from the grand mean and is the same as Ns^2 (s was discussed in

Chapter 5). It is

$$\sum_{1}^{N}(X-\bar{X})^2 = \Sigma X^2 - \frac{(\Sigma X)^2}{N},$$

and its numerical value is

$$\Sigma X^2 - \frac{(\Sigma X)^2}{N} = 115{,}208 - 104{,}545.8,$$

$$= 10{,}662.2.$$

Because total variation is the sum of variation between column means and variation within columns, it serves as a check on the two previously computed values. Symbolically:

$$\left\{\sum_{1}^{k_c}\left[\frac{\left(\sum_{1}^{N_c}X\right)^2}{N_c}\right] - \frac{(\Sigma X)^2}{N}\right\} + \left\{\Sigma X^2 - \sum_{1}^{k_c}\left[\frac{\left(\sum_{1}^{N_c}X\right)^2}{N_c}\right]\right\}$$

$$= \Sigma X^2 - \frac{(\Sigma X)^2}{N}.$$

Numerically:

$$9{,}889.15 + 773.05 = 10{,}662.2.$$

The variation within columns may be regarded as the variation due to chance, since this variation is not affected by the fact that the various column means differ. We cannot, however, make a test comparing variation between column means and variation within columns because the two variations have different degrees of freedom. Variation between column means was based upon the deviations of each of four column means from the grand mean, and therefore three degrees of freedom are present. Variation within columns involved the deviations of five items from $\bar{X}_1$, five items from $\bar{X}_2$, six items from $\bar{X}_3$, and four items from $\bar{X}_4$, giving $(5-1) + (5-1) + (6-1) + (4-1) = 16$ degrees of freedom. We are now in a position to compute the *estimated variance between column means* and the *estimated variance within columns* as follows:

Estimated variance between column means $= \dfrac{9{,}889.15}{3} = 3{,}296.38$;

Estimated variance within columns $= \dfrac{773.05}{16} = 48.32.$

The computations up to this point are summarized in Table 12.2.

To ascertain whether the estimated variance between column means is significantly larger than the estimated variance within columns, we compute

$$F = \frac{3{,}296.38}{48.32} = 68.22.$$

As just noted, there are three degrees of freedom for the numerator and 16 for the denominator, so that $n_1 = 3$ and $n_2 = 16$. Referring to the F table of Appendix X for $n_1 = 3$ and $n_2 = 16$, it is found that $F = 9.00$ is at the 0.001 point, and consequently a value of $F = 68.22$ or larger would have a probability much smaller than 0.001. Therefore, we conclude that the estimated variance between column means is significantly larger than the estimated variance within columns, or, more briefly, that the four column means differ significantly.

The hypothesis which we tested was that the estimated variance between column means and the estimated variance within columns were from the same population in respect to σ^2, and we found that hypothesis to be not tenable. When a sample is drawn from a normal population and when the population is homogeneous, we could expect the estimated variance between column means, the estimated variance within columns, or total variance $\hat{\sigma}^2$ to be a satisfactory estimate of σ^2. However, when heterogeneity is present, as it is in Table 12.1, both the estimated variances between column

TABLE 12.2

SUMMARY OF COMPUTATIONS FOR ANALYSIS OF VARIANCE OF DATA OF PRESSURE REQUIRED TO DISRUPT HEALING WOUNDS OF RATS SUTURED WITH SILK

Source of variation	Amount of variation	Degrees of freedom	Estimated variance
Between column means	9,889.15	3	3,296.38
Within columns	773.05	16	48.32
Total	10,662.20	19	...

means and $\hat{\sigma}^2$ are affected by that heterogeneity, but estimated variance within columns is not. In our example, we recognized the heterogeneity by classifying the data into columns representing the number of days after operation and measured it by the estimated variance between column means. We then compared the two independent estimates of σ^2, the estimated variance between column means and the estimated variance within columns.

The F table of Appendix X differs from the F table of Appendix IX in that the former shows only *upper* probability points of F, and also in that more n_2 values are listed. Appendix X is therefore most useful for testing whether one variance exceeds another. If *lower* probability points of F are wanted, they may be had from Appendix IX or they may be obtained from Appendix X by inverting the F value and reversing the degrees of freedom. Thus, if one had

$$F = 0.0966, n_1 = 11, n_2 = 4,$$

he would change this to

$$F = \frac{1}{0.0966} = 10.32, n_1 = 4, n_2 = 11.$$

When $n_1 = 4$ and $n_2 = 11$, $F = 10.32$ is almost exactly at the upper 0.001 point. The probability of obtaining $F = 0.0966$ or less, when $n_1 = 11$ and $n_2 = 4$, is the same.

Two criteria of classification, one entry in each box. The data in the first two columns of Table 12.3 show the percentage reduction in blood sugar for each of 26 rabbits given insulin at two different times. We now want to know whether there is significant variance between column means (that is, between dates) and between row means (that is, between rabbits). To enable us to make the necessary tests, we require several symbols not used in the preceding section. These are:

$\bar{X}_r$ the mean of a row,
N_r the number of items in a row,
k_r the number of rows,
$\sum_1^{N_r}$ a sum over the N_r items in a row, and
$\sum_1^{k_r}$ a sum over the k_r rows.

There will be four sources of variation.
Total variation, as before, is

$$\sum X^2 - \frac{(\sum X)^2}{N},$$

TABLE 12.3

Computation of Values Required for Analysis of Variance of Data of Per Cent Reduction in Blood Sugar Over a 5-hour Period, on Two Different Occasions, for 26 Rabbits Each of which Received 0.8 cc of an Insulin Solution Containing 1.25 Units of Insulin per cc

Rabbit number	Per cent reduction in blood sugar		Squares of observed data		$\overset{N_r}{\underset{1}{\Sigma}} X$	$\left(\overset{N_r}{\underset{1}{\Sigma}} X\right)^2$
	June 4	June 11	June 4	June 11		
1	47.8	43.4	2,284.84	1,883.56	91.2	8,317.44
2	28.9	37.2	835.21	1,383.84	66.1	4,369.21
3	40.9	20.0	1,672.81	400.00	60.9	3,708.81
4	59.8	55.3	3,576.04	3,058.09	115.1	13,248.01
5	45.8	44.7	2,097.64	1,998.09	90.5	8,190.25
6	36.6	15.6	1,339.56	243.36	52.2	2,724.84
7	42.4	43.6	1,797.76	1,900.96	86.0	7,396.00
8	18.6	32.1	345.96	1,030.41	50.7	2,570.49
9	31.5	46.5	992.25	2,162.25	78.0	6,084.00
10	44.8	45.6	2,007.04	2,079.36	90.4	8,172.16
11	50.0	51.1	2,500.00	2,611.21	101.1	10,221.21
12	34.1	30.6	1,162.81	936.36	64.7	4,186.09
13	40.0	37.5	1,600.00	1,406.25	77.5	6,006.25
14	37.2	52.2	1,383.84	2,724.84	89.4	7,992.36
15	31.9	46.5	1,017.61	2,162.25	78.4	6,146.56
16	31.8	37.2	1,011.24	1,383.84	69.0	4,761.00
17	41.5	50.5	1,722.25	2,550.25	92.0	8,464.00
18	28.3	23.2	800.89	538.24	51.5	2,652.25
19	30.9	33.3	954.81	1,108.89	64.2	4,121.64
20	61.4	50.5	3,769.96	2,550.25	111.9	12,521.61
21	75.0	63.8	5,625.00	4,070.44	138.8	19,265.44
22	31.1	25.5	967.21	650.25	56.6	3,203.56
23	43.2	54.2	1,866.24	2,937.64	97.4	9,486.76
24	46.8	48.9	2,190.24	2,391.21	95.7	9,158.49
25	22.2	33.3	492.84	1,108.89	55.5	3,080.25
26	49.3	37.6	2,430.49	1,413.76	86.9	7,551.61
$\overset{N_c}{\underset{1}{\Sigma}} X$	1,051.8	1,059.9	...	...	2,111.7 ΣX	183,600.29 $\overset{k_r}{\underset{1}{\Sigma}}\left(\overset{N_r}{\underset{1}{\Sigma}} X\right)^2$
$\overset{N_c}{\underset{1}{\Sigma}} X^2$	...	...	46,444.54	46,684.49	93,129.03 ΣX^2	

Data from Sharp & Dohme, Inc. In addition to the information shown above, the weight of each rabbit and its initial blood sugar were known. It is of interest that there was not significant correlation between weight and reduction in blood sugar or between initial blood sugar and reduction in blood sugar for either date.

$$N_c = 26, \; N_r = 2, \; N = 52.$$
$$\Sigma X = 2,111.7.$$
$$(\Sigma X)^2 = (2,111.7)^2 = 4,459,276.89.$$
$$\overset{k_c}{\underset{1}{\Sigma}}\left(\overset{N_c}{\underset{1}{\Sigma}} X\right)^2 = (1,051.8)^2 + (1,059.9)^2 = 2,229,671.25.$$

and, using the values given in Table 12.3, we have

$$\Sigma X^2 - \frac{(\Sigma X)^2}{N} = 93{,}129.03 - \frac{4{,}459{,}276.89}{52},$$
$$= 93{,}129.03 - 85{,}755.328,$$
$$= 7{,}373.70.$$

Variation between column means may be computed from the expression previously used,

$$\sum_{1}^{k_c} \left[\frac{\left(\sum_{1}^{N_c} X\right)^2}{N_c} \right] - \frac{(\Sigma X)^2}{N}.$$

However, the number of items in the various columns must always be equal when there is but one entry in a box[6] (or cell), and so we may write

$$\frac{\sum_{1}^{k_c}\left(\sum_{1}^{N_c} X\right)^2}{N_c} - \frac{(\Sigma X)^2}{N},$$

and its numerical value is

$$\frac{2{,}229{,}671.25}{26} - \frac{4{,}459{,}276.89}{52} = 85{,}756.587 - 85{,}755.328,$$
$$= 1.26,$$

Variation between row means is computed by use of an expression similar to that just used, the number of items in the various rows being the same,

$$\frac{\sum_{1}^{k_r}\left(\sum_{1}^{N_r} X\right)^2}{N_r} - \frac{(\Sigma X)^2}{N},$$

and its value is found to be

$$\frac{183{,}600.29}{2} - \frac{4{,}459{,}276.89}{52} = 91{,}800.145 - 85{,}755.328,$$
$$= 6{,}044.82.$$

---

[6] The term "box" rather than "cell" is used in this book since we have used $\bar{X}_c$ to refer to the mean of a column and in the following section we shall use $\bar{X}_b$ to refer to the mean of a box.

Residual variation. It will be observed that the variation between column means plus the variation between row means fails to equal total variation. The difference is

$$(7{,}373.70) - (1.26 + 6{,}044.82) = 1{,}327.62.$$

Because this value is usually obtained in this manner, it is often referred to as "residual variation." Alternatively (and more laboriously), it may be computed from the expression

$$\Sigma(X + \bar{X} - \bar{X}_r - \bar{X}_c)^2,$$

and, for the data of Table 12.3,

$$\Sigma(X + \bar{X} - \bar{X}_r - \bar{X}_c)^2 = 1{,}327.62,$$

which, of course, agrees with the value obtained by subtraction.

We are now in a position to summarize our findings in Table 12.4. Since there are but two column means, and their variation was computed in relation to $\bar{X}$, variation between column means has one degree of freedom. There are 26 row means, and their variation was also computed in relation to $\bar{X}$. Therefore, variation between row means has 25 degrees of freedom. Since total variation has $N - 1 = 52 - 1 = 51$ degrees of freedom, residual variation has $51 - (25 + 1) = 25$ degrees of freedom. Dividing each of the three component variations by the appropriate number of degrees of freedom gives the values shown in the last column of Table 12.4 for estimated variance between column means, estimated variance between row means, and estimated residual variance.

TABLE 12.4

SUMMARY OF COMPUTATIONS FOR ANALYSIS OF VARIANCE OF DATA OF REDUCTION IN BLOOD SUGAR

Source of variation	Amount of variation	Degrees of freedom	Estimated variance
Between column means	1.26	1	1.26
Between row means	6,044.82	25	241.79
Residual	1,327.62	25	53.10
Total	7,373.70	51	...

Each of the first two estimated variances may now be compared with estimated residual variance. Thus, for column means we have

$$F = \frac{1.26}{53.10} = 0.024; \; n_1 = 1, \; n_2 = 25.$$

Since F is less than one, it is obvious that there is no significant difference between the two column means. Parenthetically, it may be noted that F is not significantly less than one. This is ascertained by referring to Appendix IX.

For row means,

$$F = \frac{241.79}{53.10} = 4.55; n_1 = 25, n_2 = 25.$$

From Appendix X it may be seen that this value of F is significant at the 0.001 point, indicating that the difference between row means (means for individual rabbits) is real.

The difference between the two column means could have been tested by means of a t test, using the method described in Chapter 9 for non-independent samples. This procedure gives

$$t = \frac{0.312}{2.02} = 0.154, \text{ with } n = 25,$$

and indicates that the means for June 4 and June 11 do not differ significantly. It will be seen that $t^2 = F$, and this is always true when $n_1 = 1$, but not when $n_1 > 1$.

Two criteria of classification, more than one entry in each box. The data of Table 12.5 show the amount of pressure in millimeters of mercury required to disrupt healing wounds of rats sutured with cotton, wire, and nylon at periods one, two, three, and four days after operation. Here we have, not one, but five entries in each box, and we shall be able to distinguish five sources of variation: total, between column means (between sutures), between row means (between days), interaction between columns and rows, and within boxes.

Total variation is computed by the usual formula $\Sigma X^2 - \frac{(\Sigma X)^2}{N}$, and, from the data given in Table 12.5 its value is

$$281{,}530 - \frac{16{,}418{,}704}{60} = 281{,}530 - 273{,}645.07,$$
$$= 7{,}884.93.$$

Variation between column means will be obtained from the expression previously used when the number of items in the various

TABLE 12.5

COMPUTATION OF VALUES REQUIRED FOR ANALYSIS OF VARIANCE OF DATA OF PRESSURE, IN MILLIMETERS OF MERCURY REQUIRED TO DISRUPT HEALING WOUNDS OF RATS SUTURED WITH COTTON, WIRE, AND NYLON, THE TESTS HAVING BEEN MADE ONE, TWO, THREE, AND FOUR DAYS AFTER OPERATION

A. Observed data and sums for columns and rows

Day	Cotton	Wire	Nylon	$N_r \atop \sum_1 X$
1	67	67	47	
	67	67	70	
	66	65	71	
	60	65	67	
	60	61	68	968
2	71	70	55	
	71	65	73	
	71	70	69	
	80	53	49	
	77	63	46	983
3	61	53	66	
	59	50	96	
	61	53	69	
	61	50	66	
	60	53	97	955
4	70	71	106	
	84	70	75	
	65	77	82	
	67	76	75	
	69	79	80	1,146
$N_c \atop \sum_1 X$	1,347	1,278	1,427	4,052 = $\sum X$

B. Squares and sums for columns and rows

Day	Cotton	Wire	Nylon	$N_r \atop \sum_1 X^2$
1	4,489	4,489	2,209	
	4,489	4,489	4,900	
	4,356	4,225	5,041	
	3,600	4,225	4,489	
	3,600	3,721	4,624	62,946
2	5,041	4,900	3,025	
	5,041	4,225	5,329	
	5,041	4,900	4,761	
	6,400	2,809	2,401	
	5,929	3,969	2,116	65,887
3	3,721	2,809	4,356	
	3,481	2,500	9,216	
	3,721	2,809	4,761	
	3,721	2,500	4,356	
	3,600	2,809	9,409	63,769
4	4,900	5,041	11,236	
	7,056	4,900	5,625	
	4,225	5,929	6,724	
	4,489	5,776	5,625	
	4,761	6,241	6,400	88,928
$N_c \atop \sum_1 X^2$	91,661	83,266	106,603	281,530 = $\sum X^2$

$(\sum X)^2 = (4,052)^2 = 16,418,704.$

C. Sums and squares of sums for boxes

Box		$N_b \atop \sum_1 X$	$\left(\sum_1^{N_b} X\right)^2$
Row 1,	Col. 1	320	102,400
	Col. 2	325	105,625
	Col. 3	323	104,329
Row 2,	Col. 1	370	136,900
	Col. 2	321	103,041
	Col. 3	292	85,264
Row 3,	Col. 1	302	91,204
	Col. 2	259	67,081
	Col. 3	394	155,236
Row 4,	Col. 1	355	126,025
	Col. 2	373	139,129
	Col. 3	418	174,724
Total		4,052	1,390,958 = $\sum_1^{k_b}\left(\sum_1^{N_b} X\right)^2$

$\sum_1^{k_c}\left(\sum_1^{N_c} X\right)^2 = (1,347)^2 + (1,278)^2 + (1,427)^2$
$= 5,484,022.$

$\sum_1^{k_r}\left(\sum_1^{N_r} X\right)^2 = (968)^2 + (983)^2 + (955)^2 + (1,146)^2$
$= 4,128,654.$

Data from S. A. Localio, W. Casale, and J. W. Hinton, "Wound Healing—Experimental and Statistical Study. IV. Results," *Surgery, Gynecology and Obstetrics,* October 1943, Vol. 77, pages 376–388.

columns is the same, and, using figures from Table 12.5,

$$\frac{\overset{k_c}{\underset{1}{\Sigma}}\left(\overset{N_c}{\underset{1}{\Sigma}}X\right)^2}{N_c} - \frac{(\Sigma X)^2}{N} = \frac{5{,}484{,}022}{20} - \frac{16{,}418{,}704}{60},$$
$$= 274{,}201.1 - 273{,}645.07,$$
$$= 556.03.$$

Variation between row means. Since the number of items in the several columns is the same, this expression is also identical with that previously used.

$$\frac{\overset{k_r}{\underset{1}{\Sigma}}\left(\overset{N_r}{\underset{1}{\Sigma}}X\right)^2}{N_r} - \frac{(\Sigma X)^2}{N} = \frac{4{,}128{,}654}{15} - \frac{16{,}418{,}704}{60},$$
$$= 275{,}243.60 - 273{,}645.07,$$
$$= 1{,}598.53.$$

Variation within boxes is the variation of the items within each box around the mean of the box. Using the symbols

$\bar{X}_b$ the mean of a box,
N_b the number of items in a box,
k_b the number of boxes,

$\overset{N_b}{\underset{1}{\Sigma}}$ a sum over the N_b items in a box, and

$\overset{k_b}{\underset{1}{\Sigma}}$ a sum over the k_b boxes,

variation within boxes is

$$\overset{k_b}{\underset{1}{\Sigma}}\left[\overset{N_b}{\underset{1}{\Sigma}}(X - \bar{X}_b)^2\right].$$

This expression reduces to

$$\Sigma X^2 - \overset{k_b}{\underset{1}{\Sigma}}\left[\frac{\left(\overset{N_b}{\underset{1}{\Sigma}}X\right)^2}{N_b}\right]$$

or, since there is the same number of items in each box,

$$\Sigma X^2 - \frac{\overset{k_b}{\underset{1}{\Sigma}}\left(\overset{N_b}{\underset{1}{\Sigma}}X\right)^2}{N_b}.$$

For the illustration under consideration,

$$\Sigma X^2 - \frac{\overset{k_b}{\underset{1}{\Sigma}}\left(\overset{N_b}{\underset{1}{\Sigma}} X\right)^2}{N_b} = 281{,}530 - \frac{1{,}390{,}958}{5},$$
$$= 281{,}530 - 278{,}191.6,$$
$$= 3{,}338.4.$$

Interaction may be computed from the expression

$$\overset{k_b}{\underset{1}{\Sigma}}[N_b(\bar{X}_b + \bar{X} - \bar{X}_r - \bar{X}_c)^2],$$

but it is much more easily obtained by subtracting variation between column means, variation between row means, and variation within boxes from total variation. This gives

$$7{,}884.93 - (556.03 + 1{,}598.53 + 3{,}338.4) = 2{,}391.97.$$

Estimated variances. Following the reasoning previously used, there are two degrees of freedom between column means and three degrees of freedom between row means. When computing the variation within boxes, the deviation of each item was taken from the mean of the box in which the item occurred, and the number of degrees of freedom is, therefore, $12(5 - 1) = 48$. Degrees of freedom for total variation are $N - 1 = 59$, and, therefore, the number of degrees of freedom for interaction is given by

$$59 - (2 + 3 + 48) = 6.$$

Table 12.6 summarizes the values obtained for variation and degrees of freedom and shows also the four estimated variances which are of concern to us.

TABLE 12.6

SUMMARY OF COMPUTATIONS FOR ANALYSIS OF VARIANCE OF DATA OF PRESSURE REQUIRED TO DISRUPT HEALING WOUNDS OF RATS SUTURED WITH COTTON, WIRE, AND NYLON

Source of variation	Amount of variation	Degrees of freedom	Estimated variance
Between column means	556.03	2	278.02
Between row means	1,598.53	3	532.84
Interaction	2,391.97	6	398.66
Within boxes	3,338.40	48	69.55
Total	7,884.93	59	...

Using the estimated variances shown in Table 12.6, we first test interaction for significance, computing

$$F = \frac{398.66}{69.55} = 5.73,$$

with $n_1 = 6$ and $n_2 = 48$. From Appendix X it is seen that the probability of obtaining a value of $F \geqq 5.73$ is less than 0.001. We conclude that interaction is significant.

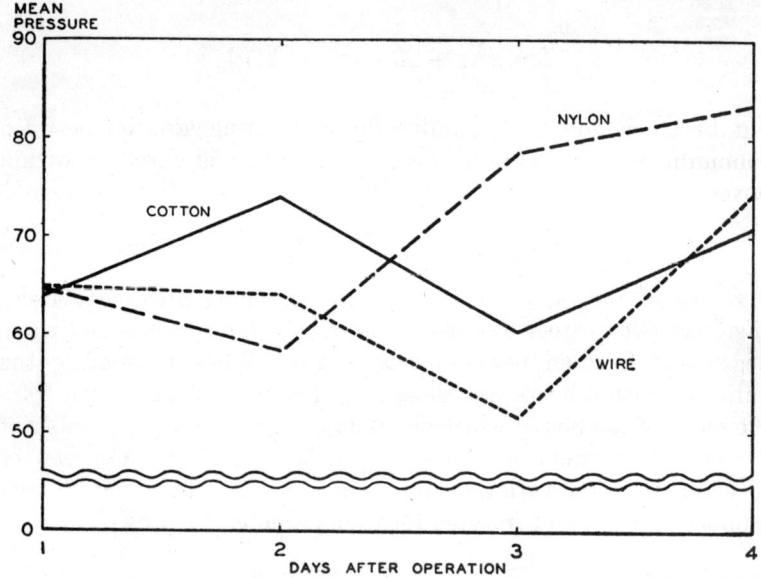

Chart 12.2. Mean Pressure, in Millimeters of Mercury, Required to Disrupt Healing Wounds of Rats Sutured with Cotton, Wire, and Nylon, the Tests Having Been Made One, Two, Three, and Four Days After Operation.

We are now in a position to test the difference between the column means (between the different kinds of suture materials) and the difference between the row means (between days). Considering first the estimated variance of the column means, we use as the denominator for our F test, not the estimated variance within boxes, but the estimated variance of the interaction. Interaction, which has already been shown to be significant, refers to the fact that the sutures which produce the strongest and weakest wounds after one day do not consistently produce the strongest and weakest wounds after 2, 3, or 4 days. That this is true may be seen by a glance at Chart 12.2, which shows the mean strength of the wounds sutured with cotton, wire, and nylon when tests were made one, two, three, and four days after operation. Wounds sutured with cotton were weakest after one day, strongest after two days, intermediate after 3 days, and weakest after four days. Considering the four time periods in order, wounds sutured with wire were strongest, intermediate, weakest, and intermediate, while wounds sutured with nylon were intermediate, weakest, strongest, and strongest. It is clear, then, that while one suture may give the strongest wound after a certain lapse of time it may, after a different lapse of time, yield a wound which is not the strongest and may even be the weakest. The estimated variance between column means cannot be considered significant unless it is large in relation to the estimated variance of the interaction.[7] Consequently, we compute

$$F = \frac{278.02}{398.66} = 0.697,$$

with $n_1 = 2$ and $n_2 = 6$. Since $F < 1$ the estimated variance between column means is not greater than the estimated variance of the interaction, and no test is necessary. (Reference to Appendix IX shows that F is not significantly *less* than one.)

Similarly, the estimated variance between row means (between days) is tested by using the same denominator for F, giving

$$F = \frac{532.84}{398.66} = 1.34,$$

with $n_1 = 3$ and $n_2 = 6$. This value of F is not significantly greater than 1.0, as may be ascertained by referring to Appendix IX or X.

If our test of the estimated variance of the interaction had shown that it was not significantly greater than the estimated variance within boxes, we might then proceed by testing the estimated variance of column means and the estimated variance of row means against an estimated variance obtained by combining the variation within boxes with the variation attributable to interaction and then dividing by their combined degrees of freedom. Alternatively, the denominator sometimes used for the F test may be the larger of the

---

[7] For a more extended discussion, see W. J. Dixon and Frank J. Massey Jr., *An Introduction to Statistical Analysis*, McGraw-Hill Book Co., New York, 1951, pp. 134–138.

two variances attributable to interaction or within boxes. When the estimated variance due to interaction is the larger, this procedure allows for possible small effects of interaction which were not revealed by the initial test; it might, of course, also serve to increase the number of Type II errors.

Interrelationships Between the Normal Distribution, t, χ^2, and F

It has already been pointed out (in Chapter 9) that the t distribution approaches the normal distribution as n approaches infinity. The normal distribution is, therefore, a special case of the t distribution when $n = \infty$ and the values of t given in the last row of the t table of Appendix V are the same as the values which may be had, by proper interpolation, from the normal table of Appendix IV for any selected P value.

In an earlier part of the present chapter it was pointed out that, when $n_1 = 1$, a t test could be used in place of an F test, the degrees of freedom for the t test being the same as n_2. More specifically, $t^2 = F$, as was shown on page 304 for a particular case. Reference to Appendix V, the t table, and to Appendix X, the F table, will show that, when n for t is the same as n_2 for F, $t^2 = F$ for any selected P value in the $n_1 = 1$ portion of the F table.

When $n_2 = \infty$, the F test and the χ^2 test may be interchanged, with the degrees of freedom for χ^2 being the same as n_1. To be more specific, we already know that

$$\chi^2 = \frac{n\hat{\sigma}^2}{\sigma^2},$$

and, therefore,

$$\frac{\chi^2}{n} = \frac{\hat{\sigma}^2}{\sigma^2}.$$

But
$$F = \frac{\hat{\sigma}^2}{\sigma^2}, \text{ with } n_2 = \infty,$$

and we have

$$F = \frac{\chi^2}{n}, \text{ when } n_2 = \infty.$$

Referring to the χ^2 table of Appendix VI and the F table of Appendix X, it may be seen that, when n for χ^2 is the same as n_1 for F, $\dfrac{\chi^2}{n} = F$ for any selected P value in the $n_2 = \infty$ row of the F table.

In addition to the relationships just mentioned, the normal distribution is a special case of χ^2 when $n = 1$. Examining the normal table of Appendix IV and the χ^2 table of Appendix VI, it

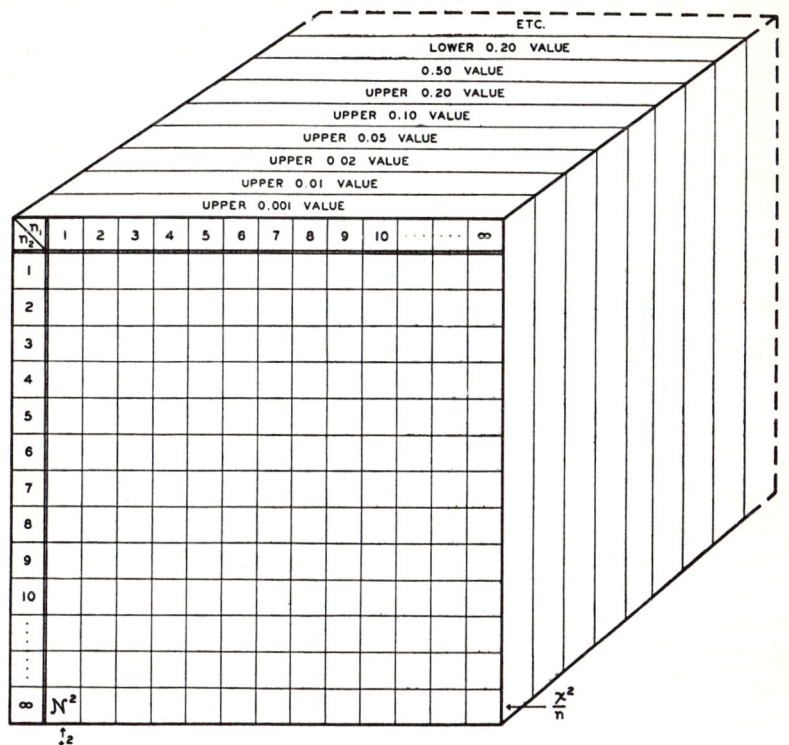

Chart 12.3. Relationship Between the Normal, t, χ^2, and F Distributions. Each box within the double rules may be thought of as the end of a drawer which, when pulled out, reveals the F values and, in some instances, the squared normal ($\mathcal{N}^2$), t^2, and $\frac{\chi^2}{n}$ values for the indicated probabilities. The entire diagram is F. The box at the extreme lower left is $\mathcal{N}^2$. The left column is t^2. The bottom row is $\frac{\chi^2}{n}$. This chart is an elaboration of one given in K. Mather, *Statistical Analysis in Biology*, p. 47, Interscience Publishers, New York, 1943.

will be found that, for any selected P value, the normal deviate is the square root of χ^2 when $n = 1$. This was noted in Chapter 11.

The statements of the four preceding paragraphs have been brought together to form Chart 12.3, which shows the interrelationships of the normal, t, χ^2, and F distributions.

Correlation Coefficients

Simple correlation. *Does r differ significantly from zero?* To ascertain whether a two-variable linear correlation coefficient, r, differs significantly from zero, we make use of a t test, our null hypotheses being that the value obtained for r is that of a random sample from a population of paired variables having a correlation coefficient of zero. We obtain the value of t from the expression

$$t = \sqrt{\frac{r^2(N-2)}{1-r^2}},$$

and, by referring to the t table of Appendix V with $N-2$ degrees of freedom, evaluate the probability of obtaining a value of t equal to or greater than that computed.

Consider the results obtained in Chapter 6 for the correlation of the glucose data of Table 6.1. For 18 pairs of items, r^2 was found to be 0.9319 and r was $+0.9653$.

Therefore,

$$t = \sqrt{\frac{r^2(N-2)}{1-r^2}} = \sqrt{\frac{0.9319(18-2)}{1-0.9319}},$$

$$= \sqrt{\frac{14.9104}{0.0681}} = \sqrt{218.95} = 14.8,$$

with $n = N - 2 = 18 - 2 = 16$. This value of t is far beyond the 0.001 level, and we conclude that the value obtained for r is significant.

In Chapter 6 an illustration of low correlation was given in Chart 6.4, which was a scatter plot of the IQ's of 26 pairs of twins of different sex. The value of r was $+0.29$. Is this value of r significant? Computing t, we have

$$t = \sqrt{\frac{0.084(26-2)}{1-0.084}} = 1.48$$

and $n = 24$. Referring to Appendix V, the associated probability is between 0.10 and 0.20, and we conclude that the correlation is not significant.

One occasionally encounters a test made to ascertain whether b is significantly greater than zero. This is accomplished by computing

$$t = b\sqrt{\frac{(N-2)\Sigma x^2}{\Sigma y_s^2}}$$

for $n = N - 2$ degrees of freedom. For the glucose data of Table 6.1, b was found to be 0.804, and therefore

$$t = 0.804\sqrt{\frac{(18-2)7.026768}{0.332160}},$$
$$= 0.804(18.40) = 14.8.$$

For $N = 16$, this value of t is far beyond the 0.001 level. The value of b is significant. Note that the value obtained here for t is exactly the same as the value of t based upon r. The two expressions are, of course, algebraic equivalents.[8] When one has tested r, he has also tested b, and vice versa.

Does r differ significantly from some value other than zero? When sample r's are from a population having $r_\varphi = 0$, it is clear that the sample correlation coefficients can range from 0 to $+1.0$ on one side of r_φ and from 0 to -1.0 on the other side of r_φ. Actually, when $r_\varphi = 0$, the probability of getting (say) $r = +0.90$ is exactly the same as the probability of getting $r = -0.90$ from random samples of the same size. If the distribution of sample r's around r_φ had not been symmetrical, the t test could not have been used. When $r_\varphi = +0.80$, for example, sample r's may range up to $+1.0$ on one side of r_φ and from $+0.80$ through 0 to -1.0 on the other side of r_φ. The distribution of sample r's around $r_\varphi = +0.80$ is far from symmetrical.

---

[8] This may be demonstrated as follows:

$$t = b\sqrt{\frac{(N-2)\Sigma x^2}{\Sigma y_s^2}} = \sqrt{\frac{(\Sigma xy)^2}{(\Sigma x^2)^2}\frac{(N-2)\Sigma x^2}{\Sigma y_s^2}},$$
$$= \sqrt{\frac{(\Sigma xy)^2(N-2)}{\Sigma x^2 \Sigma y_s^2}}.$$

From footnote 14 of Chapter 6, we know that $r^2 = 1 - \frac{\Sigma y_s^2}{\Sigma y^2}$; so that

$$\Sigma y_s^2 = \Sigma y^2(1-r^2).$$

Substituting,

$$t = \sqrt{\frac{(\Sigma xy)^2(N-2)}{\Sigma x^2 \Sigma y^2(1-r^2)}} = \sqrt{\frac{r^2(N-2)}{1-r^2}}.$$

To ascertain whether a sample correlation coefficient differs significantly from $r_\wp \neq 0$, we compute[9]

$$Z = 1.15129 \log \frac{1+r}{1-r}.$$

The distribution of values of Z is approximately normal around

$$Z_\wp = 1.15129 \log \frac{1+r_\wp}{1-r_\wp},$$

with the standard error given approximately by

$$\sigma_z = \frac{1}{\sqrt{N-m-1}},$$

where m is the number of constants in the estimating equation.

Suppose that a value of $r = +0.90$ has been obtained for a linear correlation problem involving 28 pairs of items and it is desired to know whether this value of r differs significantly from $r_\wp = +0.84$. We compute

$$Z = 1.15129 \log \frac{1+0.90}{1-0.90} = 1.472,$$

$$Z_\wp = 1.15129 \log \frac{1+0.84}{1-0.84} = 1.221,$$

$$\sigma_z = \frac{1}{\sqrt{28-2-1}} = 0.20.$$

Since the distribution of Z around $Z_\wp$ is approximately normal, we use

$$\frac{Z - Z_\wp}{\sigma_z} = \frac{1.472 - 1.221}{0.20} = \frac{0.251}{0.20} = 1.26$$

and, referring to the table of areas of the normal curve, conclude that the observed value of $r = +0.90$ does not differ significantly from $r_\wp = +0.84$.

Do two r values differ significantly from each other? To ascertain whether two sample correlation coefficients r_1 and r_2 differ signifi-

---

[9] For a discussion, see R. A. Fisher, *Statistical Methods for Research Workers*, Hafner Publishing Co., New York, 1950, 11th ed., pp. 197–204.

cantly from each other, we may make an approximate test by computing

$$Z_1 = 1.15129 \log \frac{1 + r_1}{1 - r_1},$$

$$\sigma_{Z_1} = \frac{1}{\sqrt{N_1 - m - 1}},$$

$$Z_2 = 1.15129 \log \frac{1 + r_2}{1 - r_2},$$

$$\sigma_{Z_2} = \frac{1}{\sqrt{N_2 - m - 1}}, \text{ and}$$

$$\sigma_{Z_1 - Z_2} = \sqrt{\sigma_{Z_1}^2 + \sigma_{Z_2}^2},$$

after which we determine the significance ratio

$$\frac{Z_1 - Z_2}{\sigma_{Z_1 - Z_2}},$$

the distribution of which is approximately normal.

Estimates of correlation in the population. In Chapter 9 we made use of an estimate of σ^2, which we called $\hat{\sigma}^2$. In similar fashion, an estimate of the coefficient of determination in the population may be had from[10]

$$\hat{r}^2 = 1 - (1 - r^2) \frac{N - 1}{N - m}.$$

---

[10] This expression is general for linear, non-linear, and multiple correlation. It is developed from the expression given in Chapter 6, note 14,

$$r^2 = 1 - \frac{\Sigma y_s^2}{\Sigma y^2},$$

which may also be written

$$r^2 = 1 - \frac{\Sigma y_s^2 \div N}{\Sigma y^2 \div N} = 1 - \frac{s_{Y.X}^2}{s_Y^2}.$$

If allowance is made for degrees of freedom in the numerator and denominator, we have

$$\hat{r}^2 = 1 - \frac{\hat{\sigma}_{Y.X}^2}{\hat{\sigma}_Y^2} = 1 - \frac{\Sigma y_s^2 \div (N - m)}{\Sigma y^2 \div (N - 1)},$$

$$= 1 - (1 - r^2) \frac{N - 1}{N - m}.$$

For the glucose data referred to before,

$$\hat{r}^2 = 1 - (1 - 0.9319)\frac{18-1}{18-2},$$
$$= 0.9276.$$

Instead of a single estimate of r_φ^2, confidence limits may be desired. Approximate limits of r_φ may be had by computing Z for the sample correlation coefficient and, using normal curve areas, proceeding as for arithmetic means. For the 95 per cent confidence limits of r_φ for the glucose data, for which $r = +0.9653$, we compute

$$Z = 1.15129 \log \frac{1 + 0.9653}{1 - 0.9653} = 2.0183 \text{ and}$$

$$\sigma_Z = \frac{1}{\sqrt{18 - 2 - 1}} = \frac{1}{\sqrt{15}} = 0.2582.$$

Then we obtain Z_{φ_1} and Z_{φ_2} from the expression

$$Z = Z_\varphi \pm 1.960\sigma_Z.$$
$$2.0183 = Z_\varphi \pm 1.960(0.2582).$$
$$Z_\varphi = 2.0183 \pm 0.5061.$$
$$Z_{\varphi_1} = 1.5122.$$
$$Z_{\varphi_2} = 2.5244.$$

Converting Z_{φ_1} to r_{φ_1} and Z_{φ_2} to r_{φ_2} gives

$$r_{\varphi_1} = +0.9073 \text{ and}$$
$$r_{\varphi_2} = +0.9872.$$

Partial correlation. As far as a partial coefficient of determination is concerned, we are primarily interested in knowing whether the additional explained variation attributable to an added independent variable is significant. That is to say, we want to know whether the partial coefficient of determination is significantly greater than zero. For the data of Table 7.2, which dealt with height (X_1), femur length (X_2), and radius length (X_3) for 18 young adult females, it was found that $r_{13.2}^2 = 0.119$. The significance of this is ascertained by computing

$$t = \sqrt{\frac{r_{13.2}^2(N-3)}{1-r_{13.2}^2}},$$

$$= \sqrt{\frac{(0.119)(18-3)}{1-0.119}} = 1.4,$$

and referring to the t table for $n = N - 3 = 15$. Since the associated probability is less than 0.20 but greater than 0.10, we must conclude that $r_{13.2}^2$ is not significant. Upon the basis of the sample of 18 individuals, we have no evidence that X_3 supplies a significant added amount of explained variation. If a larger sample were to be used, significance might appear.

In general, for any partial coefficient of determination,

$$t = \sqrt{\frac{r_{1m.234\cdots(m-1)}^2(N-m)}{1-r_{1m.234\cdots(m-1)}^2}},$$

and the appropriate degrees of freedom are $n = N - m$.

Multiple correlation. To ascertain whether a multiple coefficient of determination differs significantly from zero, we employ an F test, writing[11]

$$F = \frac{R_{1.234\cdots m}^2(N-m)}{(1-R_{1.234\cdots m}^2)(m-1)},$$

with $n_1 = m - 1$ and $n_2 = N - m$.

For the data of Table 7.2 it was found, for $N = 18$, that $R_{1.23}^2 = 0.742$. Making the F test, we have

$$F = \frac{0.742(18-3)}{(1-0.742)(3-1)} = 21.6,$$

$n_1 = 3 - 1 = 2$, and $n_2 = 18 - 3 = 15$. Referring to the F table of Appendix X it is seen that the probability is much less than 0.001, and we conclude that $R_{1.23}^2$ is significant.

---

[11] This is the algebraic equivalent of the usual form

$$F = \frac{\Sigma x_{c1.234\cdots m}^2 \div (m-1)}{\Sigma x_{s1.234\cdots m}^2 \div (N-m)}.$$

However, it is more convenient, since $R_{1.234\cdots m}^2$ may be obtained by a procedure which does not involve explained variation, unexplained variation, or total variation.

It was previously found that $r^2_{13.2}$ was not significant. The conclusion that $R^2_{1.23}$ is significant is not contradictory. It merely indicates that the significance of X_2 (which may be ascertained by testing $r^2_{12.3}$) is so marked as to offset the lack of significance of $r^2_{13.2}$.

To ascertain whether $R^2_{1.234\cdots m}$ differs significantly from a value other than zero, an approximate test may be made using Z and σ_Z, as described for r. These expressions may also be used to obtain approximate confidence limits of the multiple correlation in the population. For a single population estimate, use

$$\hat{R}^2_{1.234\cdots m} = 1 - (1 - R^2_{1.234\cdots m})\frac{N-1}{N-m}.$$

Skewness and Kurtosis

To test the significance of the measures of skewness and kurtosis, β_1 and β_2, described in Chapter 5, special tables are required.

When no skewness is present, $\beta_1 = 0$. The table in Appendix XI has been computed on the assumption that random samples were drawn from a normal population. It will be remembered that a normal population has no skewness. The exact shape of the sampling distribution of β_1 depends upon the size of the sample, but in general it resembles the curve accompanying Appendix XI. To illustrate the use of this table, consider the value $\beta_1 = 0.424$ obtained for the weights of 2,266 white selectees shown in Table 5.6. Sample values of β_1, computed from samples drawn from a normal population, may vary from 0 to ∞. Appendix XI shows that, for samples of 2,000, β_1 could be expected to equal or exceed 0.008 ten times out of 100 and to equal or exceed 0.016 two times out of 100; for samples of 2,500, β_1, could be expected to equal or exceed 0.006 ten times out of 100 and to equal or exceed 0.013 two times out of 100. It is clear that the observed value of $\beta_1 = 0.424$ is significant. The reader may wish to test the values of β_1 obtained for the data of Tables 5.5 and 5.7.

A normal distribution is not only free of skewness but is mesokurtic, having $\beta_2 = 3.0$. The table shown as Appendix XII indicates the behavior of values of β_2 computed from random samples from a normal population. Again the sampling distribution depends upon N, but in general it describes a curve skewed to the right, as shown with Appendix XII. For the data of heights of white boys, shown in Table 5.8, β_2 was found to be 4.60 (or 4.74, using Sheppard's corrections). When samples are drawn from a normal population, the values of β_2 computed for those samples may range from 0 to ∞. Since a value of $\beta_2 = 3.0$ indicates no kurtosis, we are interested in knowing whether values of β_2 which are less than 3.0 are significantly less than 3.0; and whether values of β_2 which are greater than 3.0 are significantly greater than 3.0. For the data of Table 5.8, having $\beta_2 = 4.60$ and $N = 1.575$, it is clear that β_2 is significantly greater than 3.0, since Appendix XII shows that 4.60 is far beyond the 1 per cent upper limits of β_2 for either $N = 1,400$ or $N = 1,600$.

Appendix I
ORDINATES OF THE NORMAL CURVE
Erected at Distances $\frac{x}{s}$ from $\bar{X}$, Expressed as Decimal Fractions of the Maximum Ordinate Y_0

The maximum ordinate is computed from $Y_0 = \dfrac{Ni}{s\sqrt{2\pi}} = \dfrac{Ni}{2.5066s}$. The values below result from solving the expression $e^{\frac{-x^2}{2s^2}}$.

The proportional height of an ordinate to be erected at any given value on the X axis can be read from the table by determining x (the deviation of the given value from the mean) and computing $\dfrac{x}{s}$. Thus, if $\bar{X} = \$25.00$, $s = \$4.00$, $Y_0 = 1950$, and it is desired to ascertain the height of an ordinate to be erected at $\$23.00$, $x = \$2.00$ and $\dfrac{x}{s} = \dfrac{\$2.00}{\$4.00} = .50$. From the table, the ordinate is found to be 0.88250 of the maximum ordinate Y_0 or $0.88250 \times 1950 = 1721$.

$\frac{x}{s}$	0	.01	.02	.03	.04	.05	.06	.07	.08	.09
0.0	1.00000	.99995	.99980	.99955	.99920	.99875	.99820	.99755	.99685	.99596
0.1	.99501	.99396	.99283	.99158	.99025	.98881	.98728	.98565	.98393	.98211
0.2	.98020	.97819	.97609	.97390	.97161	.96923	.96676	.96420	.96156	.95882
0.3	.95600	.95309	.95010	.94702	.94387	.94055	.93723	.93382	.93024	.92677
0.4	.92312	.91939	.91558	.91169	.90774	.90371	.89961	.89543	.89119	.88688
0.5	.88250	.87805	.87353	.86896	.86432	.85962	.85489	.85006	.84519	.84025
0.6	.83527	.83023	.82514	.82000	.81481	.80957	.80429	.79896	.79359	.78817
0.7	.78270	.77721	.77167	.76610	.76048	.75484	.74916	.74342	.73769	.73193
0.8	.72615	.72033	.71448	.70861	.70272	.69681	.69087	.68493	.67896	.67298
0.9	.66698	.66097	.65494	.64891	.64287	.63683	.63077	.62472	.61865	.61259
1.0	.60653	.60047	.59440	.58834	.58228	.57623	.57017	.56414	.55810	.55209
1.1	.54607	.54007	.53409	.52812	.52214	.51620	.51027	.50437	.49848	.49260
1.2	.48675	.48092	.47511	.46933	.46357	.45783	.45212	.44644	.44078	.43516
1.3	.42956	.42399	.41845	.41294	.40747	.40202	.39661	.39123	.38569	.38058
1.4	.37531	.37007	.36487	.35971	.35459	.34950	.34445	.33944	.33447	.32954
1.5	.32465	.31980	.31500	.31023	.30550	.30082	.29618	.29158	.28702	.28251
1.6	.27804	.27361	.26923	.26489	.26059	.25634	.25213	.24797	.24385	.23978
1.7	.23575	.23176	.22782	.22392	.22008	.21627	.21251	.20879	.20511	.20148
1.8	.19790	.19436	.19086	.18741	.18400	.18064	.17732	.17404	.17081	.16762
1.9	.16448	.16137	.15831	.15530	.15232	.14939	.14650	.14364	.14083	.13806
2.0	.13534	.13265	.13000	.12740	.12483	.12230	.11981	.11737	.11496	.11259
2.1	.11025	.10795	.10570	.10347	.10129	.09914	.09702	.09495	.09290	.09090
2.2	.08892	.08698	.08507	.08320	.08136	.07956	.07778	.07604	.07433	.07265
2.3	.07100	.06939	.06780	.06624	.06471	.06321	.06174	.06029	.05888	.05750
2.4	.05614	.05481	.05350	.05222	.05096	.04973	.04852	.04734	.04618	.04505
2.5	.04394	.04285	.04179	.04074	.03972	.03873	.03775	.03680	.03586	.03494
2.6	.03405	.03317	.03232	.03148	.03066	.02986	.02908	.02831	.02757	.02684
2.7	.02612	.02542	.02474	.02408	.02343	.02280	.02218	.02157	.02098	.02040
2.8	.01984	.01929	.01876	.01823	.01772	.01723	.01674	.01627	.01581	.01536
2.9	.01492	.01449	.01408	.01367	.01328	.01288	.01252	.01215	.01179	.01145

$\frac{x}{s}$	0	.1	.2	.3	.4	.5	.6	.7	.8	.9
3.	.01111	.00819	.00598	.00432	.00309	.00219	.00153	.00106	.00073	.00050
4.	.00034	.00022	.00015	.00010	.00006	.00004	.00003	.00002	.00001	.00001
5.	.00000									

From Rugg's *Statistical Methods Applied to Education*, reprinted by arrangement with the publishers, Houghton Mifflin Company. More detailed tables of normal-curve ordinates may be found in Karl Pearson, *Tables for Statisticians and Biometricians*, The University Press, Cambridge, England, 1914, pp. 4–8, and in Federal Works Agency, Work Projects Administration for the City of New York, *Tables of Probability Functions*, National Bureau of Standards, New York, 1942, Vol. II, pp. 2–238. The values shown in these tables should be multiplied by $\sqrt{2\pi} = 2.5066$ to agree with those shown above.

Appendix II
AREAS UNDER THE NORMAL CURVE

From the Arithmetic Mean to Distances $\frac{x}{s}$ or $\frac{x}{\sigma}$ from the Arithmetic Mean,

Expressed as Decimal Fractions of the Total Area 1.0000

This table shows: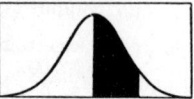

$\frac{x}{s}$ or $\frac{x}{\sigma}$	.00	.01	.02	.03	.04	.05	.06	.07	.08	.09
0.0	.0000	.0040	.0080	.0120	.0160	.0199	.0239	.0279	.0319	.0359
0.1	.0398	.0438	.0478	.0517	.0557	.0596	.0636	.0675	.0714	.0753
0.2	.0793	.0832	.0871	.0910	.0948	.0987	.1026	.1064	.1103	.1141
0.3	.1179	.1217	.1255	.1293	.1331	.1368	.1406	.1443	.1480	.1517
0.4	.1554	.1591	.1628	.1664	.1700	.1736	.1772	.1808	.1844	.1879
0.5	.1915	.1950	.1985	.2019	.2054	.2088	.2123	.2157	.2190	.2224
0.6	.2257	.2291	.2324	.2357	.2389	.2422	.2454	.2486	.2518	.2549
0.7	.2580	.2612	.2642	.2673	.2704	.2734	.2764	.2794	.2823	.2852
0.8	.2881	.2910	.2939	.2967	.2995	.3023	.3051	.3078	.3106	.3133
0.9	.3159	.3186	.3212	.3238	.3264	.3289	.3315	.3340	.3365	.3389
1.0	.3413	.3438	.3461	.3485	.3508	.3531	.3554	.3577	.3599	.3621
1.1	.3643	.3665	.3686	.3708	.3729	.3749	.3770	.3790	.3810	.3830
1.2	.3849	.3869	.3888	.3907	.3925	.3944	.3962	.3980	.3997	.4015
1.3	.4032	.4049	.4066	.4082	.4099	.4115	.4131	.4147	.4162	.4177
1.4	.4192	.4207	.4222	.4236	.4251	.4265	.4279	.4292	.4306	.4319
1.5	.4332	.4345	.4357	.4370	.4382	.4394	.4406	.4418	.4429	.4441
1.6	.4452	.4463	.4474	.4484	.4495	.4505	.4515	.4525	.4535	.4545
1.7	.4554	.4564	.4573	.4582	.4591	.4599	.4608	.4616	.4625	.4633
1.8	.4641	.4649	.4656	.4664	.4671	.4678	.4686	.4693	.4699	.4706
1.9	.4713	.4719	.4726	.4732	.4738	.4744	.4750	.4756	.4761	.4767
2.0	.4772	.4778	.4783	.4788	.4793	.4798	.4803	.4808	.4812	.4817
2.1	.4821	.4826	.4830	.4834	.4838	.4842	.4846	.4850	.4854	.4857
2.2	.4861	.4864	.4868	.4871	.4875	.4878	.4881	.4884	.4887	.4890
2.3	.4893	.4896	.4898	.4901	.4904	.4906	.4909	.4911	.4913	.4916
2.4	.4918	.4920	.4922	.4925	.4927	.4929	.4931	.4932	.4934	.4936
2.5	.4938	.4940	.4941	.4943	.4945	.4946	.4948	.4949	.4951	.4952
2.6	.4953	.4955	.4956	.4957	.4959	.4960	.4961	.4962	.4963	.4964
2.7	.4965	.4966	.4967	.4968	.4969	.4970	.4971	.4972	.4973	.4974
2.8	.4974	.4975	.4976	.4977	.4977	.4978	.4979	.4979	.4980	.4981
2.9	.4981	.4982	.4982	.4983	.4984	.4984	.4985	.4985	.4986	.4986
3.0	.49865	.4987	.4987	.4988	.4988	.4989	.4989	.4989	.4990	.4990
3.1	.49903	.4991	.4991	.4991	.4992	.4992	.4992	.4992	.4993	.4993
3.2	.4993129									
3.3	.4995166									
3.4	.4996631									
3.5	.4997674									
3.6	.4998409									
3.7	.4998922									
3.8	.4999277									
3.9	.4999519									
4.0	.4999683									
4.5	.4999966									
5.0	.4999997133									

From Rugg's *Statistical Methods Applied to Education* (with corrections), reprinted by arrangement with the publishers, Houghton Mifflin Company. A more detailed table of normal-curve areas, but in two directions from the arithmetic mean, is given in Federal Works Agency, Work Projects Administration for the City of New York, *Tables of Probability Functions*, National Bureau of Standards, New York, 1942, Vol. II, pp. 2–338.

Appendix III

AREAS IN ONE TAIL OF THE NORMAL CURVE AT SELECTED VALUES OF $\frac{x}{s}$ OR $\frac{x}{\sigma}$ FROM THE ARITHMETIC MEAN

This table shows:

$\frac{x}{s}$ or $\frac{x}{\sigma}$	.00	.01	.02	.03	.04	.05	.06	.07	.08	.09
0.0	.5000	.4960	.4920	.4880	.4840	.4801	.4761	.4721	.4681	.4641
0.1	.4602	.4562	.4522	.4483	.4443	.4404	.4364	.4325	.4286	.4247
0.2	.4207	.4168	.4129	.4090	.4052	.4013	.3974	.3936	.3897	.3859
0.3	.3821	.3783	.3745	.3707	.3669	.3632	.3594	.3557	.3520	.3483
0.4	.3446	.3409	.3372	.3336	.3300	.3264	.3228	.3192	.3156	.3121
0.5	.3085	.3050	.3015	.2981	.2946	.2912	.2877	.2843	.2810	.2776
0.6	.2743	.2709	.2676	.2643	.2611	.2578	.2546	.2514	.2483	.2451
0.7	.2420	.2389	.2358	.2327	.2296	.2266	.2236	.2206	.2177	.2148
0.8	.2119	.2090	.2061	.2033	.2005	.1977	.1949	.1922	.1894	.1867
0.9	.1841	.1814	.1788	.1762	.1736	.1711	.1685	.1660	.1635	.1611
1.0	.1587	.1562	.1539	.1515	.1492	.1469	.1446	.1423	.1401	.1379
1.1	.1357	.1335	.1314	.1292	.1271	.1251	.1230	.1210	.1190	.1170
1.2	.1151	.1131	.1112	.1093	.1075	.1056	.1038	.1020	.1003	.0985
1.3	.0968	.0951	.0934	.0918	.0901	.0885	.0869	.0853	.0838	.0823
1.4	.0808	.0793	.0778	.0764	.0749	.0735	.0721	.0708	.0694	.0681
1.5	.0668	.0655	.0643	.0630	.0618	.0606	.0594	.0582	.0571	.0559
1.6	.0548	.0537	.0526	.0516	.0505	.0495	.0485	.0475	.0465	.0455
1.7	.0446	.0436	.0427	.0418	.0409	.0401	.0392	.0384	.0375	.0367
1.8	.0359	.0351	.0344	.0336	.0329	.0322	.0314	.0307	.0301	.0294
1.9	.0287	.0281	.0274	.0268	.0262	.0256	.0250	.0244	.0239	.0233
2.0	.0228	.0222	.0217	.0212	.0207	.0202	.0197	.0192	.0188	.0183
2.1	.0179	.0174	.0170	.0166	.0162	.0158	.0154	.0150	.0146	.0143
2.2	.0139	.0136	.0132	.0129	.0125	.0122	.0119	.0116	.0113	.0110
2.3	.0107	.0104	.0102	.00990	.00964	.00939	.00914	.00889	.00866	.00842
2.4	.00820	.00798	.00776	.00755	.00734	.00714	.00695	.00676	.00657	.00639
2.5	.00621	.00604	.00587	.00570	.00554	.00539	.00523	.00508	.00494	.00480
2.6	.00466	.00453	.00440	.00427	.00415	.00402	.00391	.00379	.00368	.00357
2.7	.00347	.00336	.00326	.00317	.00307	.00298	.00289	.00280	.00272	.00264
2.8	.00256	.00248	.00240	.00233	.00226	.00219	.00212	.00205	.00199	.00193
2.9	.00187	.00181	.00175	.00169	.00164	.00159	.00154	.00149	.00144	.00139

$\frac{x}{s}$ or $\frac{x}{\sigma}$	.0	.1	.2	.3	.4	.5	.6	.7	.8	.9
3	.00135	$.0^3968$	$.0^3687$	$.0^3483$	$.0^3337$	$.0^3233$	$.0^3159$	$.0^3108$	$.0^4723$	$.0^4481$
4	$.0^4317$	$.0^4207$	$.0^4133$	$.0^5854$	$.0^5541$	$.0^5340$	$.0^5211$	$.0^5130$	$.0^6793$	$.0^6479$
5	$.0^6287$	$.0^6170$	$.0^796$	$.0^7579$	$.0^7333$	$.0^7190$	$.0^7107$	$.0^8599$	$.0^8332$	$.0^8182$
6	$.0^9987$	$.0^9530$	$.0^9282$	$.0^9149$	$.0^{10}777$	$.0^{10}402$	$.0^{10}206$	$.0^{10}104$	$.0^{11}523$	$.0^{11}260$

From *Tables of Areas in Two Tails and in One Tail of the Normal Curve*, by Frederick E. Croxton. Copyright, 1949, by Prentice-Hall, Inc. Permission is given to reproduce this table provided credit is given to the author and provided the Prentice-Hall copyright line is included.

Appendix IV

AREAS IN TWO TAILS OF THE NORMAL CURVE AT SELECTED VALUES OF $\frac{x}{s}$ OR $\frac{x}{\sigma}$ FROM THE ARITHMETIC MEAN

This table shows:

$\frac{x}{s}$ or $\frac{x}{\sigma}$	.00	.01	.02	.03	.04	.05	.06	.07	.08	.09
0.0	1.0000	.9920	.9840	.9761	.9681	.9601	.9522	.9442	.9362	.9283
0.1	.9203	.9124	.9045	.8966	.8887	.8808	.8729	.8650	.8572	.8493
0.2	.8415	.8337	.8259	.8181	.8103	.8026	.7949	.7872	.7795	.7718
0.3	.7642	.7566	.7490	.7414	.7339	.7263	.7188	.7114	.7039	.6965
0.4	.6892	.6818	.6745	.6672	.6599	.6527	.6455	.6384	.6312	.6241
0.5	.6171	.6101	.6031	.5961	.5892	.5823	.5755	.5687	.5619	.5552
0.6	.5485	.5419	.5353	.5287	.5222	.5157	.5093	.5029	.4965	.4902
0.7	.4839	.4777	.4715	.4654	.4593	.4533	.4473	.4413	.4354	.4295
0.8	.4237	.4179	.4122	.4065	.4009	.3953	.3898	.3843	.3789	.3735
0.9	.3681	.3628	.3576	.3524	.3472	.3421	.3371	.3320	.3271	.3222
1.0	.3173	.3125	.3077	.3030	.2983	.2937	.2891	.2846	.2801	.2757
1.1	.2713	.2670	.2627	.2585	.2543	.2501	.2460	.2420	.2380	.2340
1.2	.2301	.2263	.2225	.2187	.2150	.2113	.2077	.2041	.2005	.1971
1.3	.1936	.1902	.1868	.1835	.1802	.1770	.1738	.1707	.1676	.1645
1.4	.1615	.1585	.1556	.1527	.1499	.1471	.1443	.1416	.1389	.1362
1.5	.1336	.1310	.1285	.1260	.1236	.1211	.1188	.1164	.1141	.1118
1.6	.1096	.1074	.1052	.1031	.1010	.0989	.0969	.0949	.0930	.0910
1.7	.0891	.0873	.0854	.0836	.0819	.0801	.0784	.0767	.0751	.0735
1.8	.0719	.0703	.0688	.0672	.0658	.0643	.0629	.0615	.0601	.0588
1.9	.0574	.0561	.0549	.0536	.0524	.0512	.0500	.0488	.0477	.0466
2.0	.0455	.0444	.0434	.0424	.0414	.0404	.0394	.0385	.0375	.0366
2.1	.0357	.0349	.0340	.0332	.0324	.0316	.0308	.0300	.0293	.0285
2.2	.0278	.0271	.0264	.0257	.0251	.0244	.0238	.0232	.0226	.0220
2.3	.0214	.0209	.0203	.0198	.0193	.0188	.0183	.0178	.0173	.0168
2.4	.0164	.0160	.0155	.0151	.0147	.0143	.0139	.0135	.0131	.0128
2.5	.0124	.0121	.0117	.0114	.0111	.0108	.0105	.0102	.00988	.00960
2.6	.00932	.00905	.00879	.00854	.00829	.00805	.00781	.00759	.00736	.00715
2.7	.00693	.00673	.00653	.00633	.00614	.00596	.00578	.00561	.00544	.00527
2.8	.00511	.00495	.00480	.00465	.00451	.00437	.00424	.00410	.00398	.00385
2.9	.00373	.00361	.00350	.00339	.00328	.00318	.00308	.00298	.00288	.00279

$\frac{x}{s}$ or $\frac{x}{\sigma}$	.0	.1	.2	.3	.4	.5	.6	.7	.8	.9
3	.00270	.00194	.00137	$.0^3967$	$.0^3674$	$.0^3465$	$.0^3318$	$.0^3216$	$.0^3145$	$.0^4962$
4	$.0^4633$	$.0^4413$	$.0^4267$	$.0^4171$	$.0^4108$	$.0^6680$	$.0^5422$	$.0^5260$	$.0^5159$	$.0^5958$
5	$.0^6573$	$.0^6340$	$.0^6199$	$.0^6116$	$.0^7666$	$.0^7380$	$.0^7214$	$.0^7120$	$.0^8663$	$.0^8364$
6	$.0^8197$	$.0^8106$	$.0^9565$	$.0^9298$	$.0^9155$	$.0^{10}803$	$.0^{10}411$	$.0^{10}208$	$.0^{10}105$	$.0^{11}520$

From *Tables of Areas in Two Tails and in One Tail of the Normal Curve*, by Frederick E. Croxton. Copyright, 1949, by Prentice-Hall, Inc. Permission is given to reproduce this table provided credit is given to the author and provided the Prentice-Hall copyright line is included.

Appen
VALUES
For Given Degrees of Freedom (n) and

This table

n	Level of significance (P)							
	.90	.80	.70	.60	.50	.40	.30	.25
1	.158	.325	.510	.727	1.000	1.376	1.963	2.414
2	.142	.289	.445	.617	.816	1.061	1.386	1.604
3	.137	.277	.424	.584	.765	.978	1.250	1.423
4	.134	.271	.414	.569	.741	.941	1.190	1.344
5	.132	.267	.408	.559	.727	.920	1.156	1.301
6	.131	.265	.404	.553	.718	.906	1.134	1.273
7	.130	.263	.402	.549	.711	.896	1.119	1.254
8	.130	.262	.399	.546	.706	.889	1.108	1.240
9	.129	.261	.398	.543	.703	.883	1.100	1.230
10	.129	.260	.397	.542	.700	.879	1.093	1.221
11	.129	.260	.396	.540	.697	.876	1.088	1.214
12	.128	.259	.395	.539	.695	.873	1.083	1.209
13	.128	.259	.394	.538	.694	.870	1.079	1.204
14	.128	.258	.393	.537	.692	.868	1.076	1.200
15	.128	.258	.393	.536	.691	.866	1.074	1.197
16	.128	.258	.392	.535	.690	.865	1.071	1.194
17	.128	.257	.392	.534	.689	.863	1.069	1.191
18	.127	.257	.392	.534	.688	.862	1.067	1.189
19	.127	.257	.391	.533	.688	.861	1.066	1.187
20	.127	.257	.391	.533	.687	.860	1.064	1.185
21	.127	.257	.391	.532	.686	.859	1.063	1.183
22	.127	.256	.390	.532	.686	.858	1.061	1.182
23	.127	.256	.390	.532	.685	.858	1.060	1.180
24	.127	.256	.390	.531	.685	.857	1.059	1.179
25	.127	.256	.390	.531	.684	.856	1.058	1.178
26	.127	.256	.390	.531	.684	.856	1.058	1.177
27	.127	.256	.389	.531	.684	.855	1.057	1.176
28	.127	.256	.389	.530	.683	.855	1.056	1.175
29	.127	.256	.389	.530	.683	.854	1.055	1.174
30	.127	.256	.389	.530	.683	.854	1.055	1.173
40	.126	.255	.388	.529	.681	.851	1.050	1.167
60	.126	.254	.387	.527	.679	.848	1.046	1.162
120	.126	.254	.386	.526	.677	.845	1.041	1.156
∞	.126	.253	.385	.524	.674	.842	1.036	1.150

The values in this table were taken, by permission, from *Statistical Tables for Biological, Agricultural, and Medical Research*, by R. A. Fisher and F. Yates, published by Oliver and Boyd, Edinburgh, and from *Bio-*

dix V
OF t
at Specified Levels of Significance (P)

shows: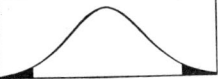

Level of significance (P)								n
.20	.10	.05	.025	.02	.01	.005	.001	
3.078	6.314	12.706	25.452	31.821	63.657	127.32	636.619	1
1.886	2.920	4.303	6.205	6.965	9.925	14.089	31.598	2
1.638	2.353	3.182	4.176	4.541	5.841	7.453	12.941	3
1.533	2.132	2.776	3.495	3.747	4.604	5.598	8.610	4
1.476	2.015	2.571	3.163	3.365	4.032	4.773	6.859	5
1.440	1.943	2.447	2.969	3.143	3.707	4.317	5.959	6
1.415	1.895	2.365	2.841	2.998	3.499	4.029	5.405	7
1.397	1.860	2.306	2.752	2.896	3.355	3.832	5.041	8
1.383	1.833	2.262	2.685	2.821	3.250	3.690	4.781	9
1.372	1.812	2.228	2.634	2.764	3.169	3.581	4.587	10
1.363	1.796	2.201	2.593	2.718	3.106	3.497	4.437	11
1.356	1.782	2.179	2.560	2.681	3.055	3.428	4.318	12
1.350	1.771	2.160	2.533	2.650	3.012	3.372	4.221	13
1.345	1.761	2.145	2.510	2.624	2.977	3.326	4.140	14
1.341	1.753	2.131	2.490	2.602	2.947	3.286	4.073	15
1.337	1.746	2.120	2.473	2.583	2.921	3.252	4.015	16
1.333	1.740	2.110	2.458	2.567	2.898	3.222	3.965	17
1.330	1.734	2.101	2.445	2.552	2.878	3.197	3.922	18
1.328	1.729	2.093	2.433	2.539	2.861	3.174	3.883	19
1.325	1.725	2.086	2.423	2.528	2.845	3.153	3.850	20
1.323	1.721	2.080	2.414	2.518	2.831	3.135	3.819	21
1.321	1.717	2.074	2.406	2.508	2.819	3.119	3.792	22
1.319	1.714	2.069	2.398	2.500	2.807	3.104	3.767	23
1.318	1.711	2.064	2.391	2.492	2.797	3.090	3.745	24
1.316	1.708	2.060	2.385	2.485	2.787	3.078	3.725	25
1.315	1.706	2.056	2.379	2.479	2.779	3.067	3.707	26
1.314	1.703	2.052	2.373	2.473	2.771	3.056	3.690	27
1.313	1.701	2.048	2.368	2.467	2.763	3.047	3.674	28
1.311	1.699	2.045	2.364	2.462	2.756	3.038	3.659	29
1.310	1.697	2.042	2.360	2.457	2.750	3.030	3.646	30
1.303	1.684	2.021	2.329	2.423	2.704	2.971	3.551	40
1.296	1.671	2.000	2.299	2.390	2.660	2.915	3.460	60
1.289	1.658	1.980	2.270	2.358	2.617	2.860	3.373	120
1.282	1.645	1.960	2.241	2.326	2.576	2.807	3.291	∞

metrika, Vol. XXXII, April 1942, p. 300, "Table of Percentage Points of the t-distribution," by Maxine Merrington.

Appendix
VALUES

For Given Degrees of Freedom

This table shows 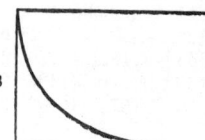 for $n = 1$ and $n = 2$,

n	Value of P									
	.995	.99	.98	.975	.95	.90	.80	.75	.70	.50
1	.0⁴393	.0³157	.0³628	.0³982	.00393	.0158	.0642	.102	.148	.455
2	.0100	.0201	.0404	.0506	.103	.211	.446	.575	.713	1.386
3	.0717	.115	.185	.216	.352	.584	1.005	1.213	1.424	2.366
4	.207	.297	.429	.484	.711	1.064	1.649	1.923	2.195	3.357
5	.412	.554	.752	.831	1.145	1.610	2.343	2.675	3.000	4.351
6	.676	.872	1.134	1.237	1.635	2.204	3.070	3.455	3.828	5.348
7	.989	1.239	1.564	1.690	2.167	2.833	3.822	4.255	4.671	6.346
8	1.344	1.646	2.032	2.180	2.733	3.490	4.594	5.071	5.527	7.344
9	1.735	2.088	2.532	2.700	3.325	4.168	5.380	5.899	6.393	8.343
10	2.156	2.558	3.059	3.247	3.940	4.865	6.179	6.737	7.267	9.342
11	2.603	3.053	3.609	3.816	4.575	5.578	6.989	7.584	8.148	10.341
12	3.074	3.571	4.178	4.404	5.226	6.304	7.807	8.438	9.034	11.340
13	3.565	4.107	4.765	5.009	5.892	7.042	8.634	9.299	9.926	12.340
14	4.075	4.660	5.368	5.629	6.571	7.790	9.467	10.165	10.821	13.339
15	4.601	5.229	5.985	6.262	7.261	8.547	10.307	11.036	11.721	14.339
16	5.142	5.812	6.614	6.908	7.962	9.312	11.152	11.912	12.624	15.338
17	5.697	6.408	7.255	7.564	8.672	10.085	12.002	12.792	13.531	16.338
18	6.265	7.015	7.906	8.231	9.390	10.865	12.857	13.675	14.440	17.338
19	6.844	7.633	8.567	8.907	10.117	11.651	13.716	14.562	15.352	18.338
20	7.434	8.260	9.237	9.591	10.851	12.443	14.578	15.452	16.266	19.337
21	8.034	8.897	9.915	10.283	11.591	13.240	15.445	16.344	17.182	20.337
22	8.643	9.542	10.600	10.982	12.338	14.041	16.314	17.240	18.101	21.337
23	9.260	10.196	11.293	11.688	13.091	14.848	17.187	18.137	19.021	22.337
24	9.886	10.856	11.992	12.401	13.848	15.659	18.062	19.037	19.943	23.337
25	10.520	11.524	12.697	13.120	14.611	16.473	18.940	19.939	20.867	24.337
26	11.160	12.198	13.409	13.844	15.379	17.292	19.820	20.843	21.792	25.336
27	11.808	12.879	14.125	14.573	16.151	18.114	20.703	21.749	22.719	26.336
28	12.461	13.565	14.847	15.308	16.928	18.939	21.588	22.657	23.647	27.336
29	13.121	14.256	15.574	16.047	17.708	19.768	22.475	23.567	24.577	28.336
30	13.787	14.953	16.306	16.791	18.493	20.599	23.364	24.478	25.508	29.336

For values of $n > 30$, approximate values for χ^2 may be obtained from the expression $n \left[1 - \frac{2}{9n} \pm \frac{x}{\sigma} \sqrt{\frac{2}{9n}} \right]^3$, where $\frac{x}{\sigma}$ is the normal deviate cutting off the corresponding tails of a normal distribution. If $\frac{x}{\sigma}$ is taken at the 0.02 level, so that 0.01 of the normal distribution is in each tail, the expression yields χ^2 at the 0.99 and 0.01 points. For very large values of n, it

VI
OF χ^2

(n) and for Specified Values of P

and 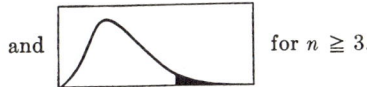 for $n \geq 3$.

				Value of P						n
.30	.25	.20	.10	.05	.025	.02	.01	.005	.001	
1.074	1.323	1.642	2.706	3.841	5.024	5.412	6.635	7.879	10.827	1
2.408	2.773	3.219	4.605	5.991	7.378	7.824	9.210	10.597	13.815	2
3.665	4.108	4.642	6.251	7.815	9.348	9.837	11.345	12.838	16.268	3
4.878	5.385	5.989	7.779	9.488	11.143	11.668	13.277	14.860	18.465	4
6.064	6.626	7.289	9.236	11.070	12.832	13.388	15.086	16.750	20.517	5
7.231	7.841	8.558	10.645	12.592	14.449	15.033	16.812	18.548	22.457	6
8.383	9.037	9.803	12.017	14.067	16.013	16.622	18.475	20.278	24.322	7
9.524	10.219	11.030	13.362	15.507	17.535	18.168	20.090	21.955	26.125	8
10.656	11.389	12.242	14.684	16.919	19.023	19.679	21.666	23.589	27.877	9
11.781	12.549	13.442	15.987	18.307	20.483	21.161	23.209	25.188	29.588	10
12.899	13.701	14.631	17.275	19.675	21.920	22.618	24.725	26.757	31.264	11
14.011	14.845	15.812	18.549	21.026	23.337	24.054	26.217	28.300	32.909	12
15.119	15.984	16.985	19.812	22.362	24.736	25.472	27.688	29.819	34.528	13
16.222	17.117	18.151	21.064	23.685	26.119	26.873	29.141	31.319	36.123	14
17.322	18.245	19.311	22.307	24.996	27.488	28.259	30.578	32.801	37.697	15
18.418	19.369	20.465	23.542	26.296	28.845	29.633	32.000	34.267	39.252	16
19.511	20.489	21.615	24.769	27.587	30.191	30.995	33.409	35.718	40.790	17
20.601	21.605	22.760	25.989	28.869	31.526	32.346	34.805	37.156	42.312	18
21.689	22.718	23.900	27.204	30.144	32.852	33.687	36.191	38.582	43.820	19
22.775	23.828	25.038	28.412	31.410	34.170	35.020	37.566	39.997	45.315	20
23.858	24.935	26.171	29.615	32.671	35.479	36.343	38.932	41.401	46.797	21
24.939	26.039	27.301	30.813	33.924	36.781	37.659	40.289	42.796	48.268	22
26.018	27.141	28.429	32.007	35.172	38.076	38.968	41.638	44.181	49.728	23
27.096	28.241	29.553	33.196	36.415	39.364	40.270	42.980	45.558	51.179	24
28.172	29.339	30.675	34.382	37.652	40.646	41.566	44.314	46.928	52.620	25
29.246	30.434	31.795	35.563	38.885	41.923	42.856	45.642	48.290	54.052	26
30.319	31.528	32.912	36.741	40.113	43.194	44.140	46.963	49.645	55.476	27
31.391	32.620	34.027	37.916	41.337	44.461	45.419	48.278	50.993	56.893	28
32.461	33.711	35.139	39.087	42.557	45.722	46.693	49.588	52.336	58.302	29
33.530	34.800	36.250	40.256	43.773	46.979	47.962	50.892	53.672	59.703	30

is sufficiently accurate to compute $\sqrt{2\chi^2}$, the distribution of which is approximately normal around a mean of $\sqrt{2n-1}$ and with a standard deviation of 1.

This table is taken by consent from *Statistical Tables for Biological, Agricultural, and Medical Research*, by R. A. Fisher and F. Yates, published by Oliver and Boyd, Edinburgh, and from *Biometrika*, Vol. XXXII, Part II, October 1941, pp. 187–191, "Table of Percentage Points of the χ^2 Distribution," by Catherine M. Thompson.

Appen

VALUES OF $\dfrac{\hat{\sigma}^2}{\sigma^2}$ FOR USE IN DETER

This table shows:

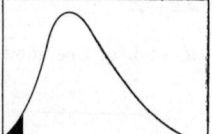

n	Lower points						.50
	.005	.01	.025	.05	.10	.25	
1	.0⁴3927	.0³1571	.0³9821	.003932	.01579	.1015	.4549
2	.005013	.01005	.02532	.05129	.1054	.2877	.6931
3	.02391	.03828	.07193	.1173	.1948	.4042	.7887
4	.05175	.07428	.1211	.1777	.2659	.4806	.8392
5	.08235	.1109	.1662	.2291	.3221	.5349	.8703
6	.1126	.1453	.2062	.2726	.3674	.5758	.8914
7	.1413	.1770	.2414	.3096	.4047	.6078	.9065
8	.1681	.2058	.2725	.3416	.4362	.6338	.9180
9	.1928	.2320	.3000	.3695	.4631	.6554	.9270
10	.2156	.2558	.3247	.3940	.4865	.6737	.9342
11	.2367	.2776	.3469	.4159	.5071	.6895	.9401
12	.2562	.2975	.3670	.4355	.5253	.7032	.9450
13	.2742	.3159	.3853	.4532	.5417	.7153	.9492
14	.2910	.3329	.4021	.4693	.5564	.7261	.9528
15	.3067	.3486	.4175	.4841	.5698	.7358	.9559
16	.3214	.3633	.4317	.4976	.5820	.7445	.9587
17	.3351	.3769	.4450	.5101	.5932	.7525	.9611
18	.3480	.3897	.4573	.5217	.6036	.7597	.9632
19	.3602	.4017	.4688	.5325	.6132	.7664	.9651
20	.3717	.4130	.4795	.5425	.6221	.7726	.9669
21	.3826	.4237	.4897	.5520	.6305	.7783	.9684
22	.3929	.4337	.4992	.5608	.6382	.7836	.9699
23	.4026	.4433	.5082	.5692	.6456	.7886	.9712
24	.4119	.4524	.5167	.5770	.6524	.7932	.9724
25	.4208	.4610	.5248	.5845	.6589	.7976	.9735
26	.4292	.4692	.5325	.5915	.6651	.8017	.9745
27	.4373	.4770	.5398	.5982	.6709	.8055	.9754
28	.4450	.4845	.5467	.6046	.6764	.8092	.9763
29	.4525	.4916	.5533	.6106	.6816	.8126	.9771
30	.4596	.4984	.5597	.6164	.6866	.8159	.9779
40	.5177	.5541	.6108	.6627	.7263	.8415	.9834
50	.5598	.5941	.6471	.6953	.7538	.8588	.9867
60	.5922	.6247	.6747	.7198	.7743	.8716	.9889
70	.6182	.6492	.6965	.7391	.7904	.8814	.9905
80	.6396	.6692	.7144	.7549	.8035	.8893	.9917
90	.6577	.6862	.7294	.7681	.8143	.8958	.9926
100	.6733	.7006	.7422	.7793	.8236	.9013	.9933
∞	1.0000	1.0000	1.0000	1.0000	1.0000	1.0000	1.0000
$\dfrac{x}{\sigma}$*	−2.5758	−2.3263	−1.9600	−1.6449	−1.2816	−.6745	0

The values in this table were computed from values of χ^2 given in *Biometrika*, Vol. XXXII, Part II, October 1941, pp. 187–191, "Tables of Percentage Points of the χ^2 Distribution," by Catherine M. Thompson, by use of the expression $\hat{\sigma}^2 = \dfrac{\chi^2}{n}\sigma^2$.

* When $n > 30$, values of $\dfrac{\hat{\sigma}^2}{\sigma^2}$ may be approximated by use of the expression

dix VII

MINING SAMPLING LIMITS OF $\hat{\sigma}^2$

and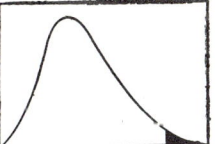

Upper points						n
.25	.10	.05	.025	.01	.005	
1.323	2.706	3.841	5.024	6.635	7.879	1
1.336	2.303	2.996	3.689	4.605	5.298	2
1.369	2.084	2.605	3.116	3.782	4.279	3
1.346	1.945	2.372	2.786	3.319	3.715	4
1.325	1.847	2.214	2.566	3.017	3.350	5
1.307	1.774	2.099	2.408	2.802	3.091	6
1.291	1.717	2.010	2.288	2.639	2.897	7
1.277	1.670	1.938	2.192	2.511	2.744	8
1.265	1.632	1.880	2.114	2.407	2.621	9
1.255	1.599	1.831	2.048	2.321	2.519	10
1.246	1.570	1.789	1.993	2.248	2.432	11
1.237	1.546	1.752	1.945	2.185	2.358	12
1.230	1.524	1.720	1.903	2.130	2.294	13
1.223	1.505	1.692	1.866	2.082	2.237	14
1.216	1.487	1.666	1.833	2.039	2.187	15
1.211	1.471	1.644	1.803	2.000	2.142	16
1.205	1.457	1.623	1.776	1.965	2.101	17
1.200	1.444	1.604	1.751	1.934	2.064	18
1.196	1.432	1.586	1.729	1.905	2.031	19
1.191	1.421	1.571	1.708	1.878	2.000	20
1.187	1.410	1.556	1.689	1.854	1.971	21
1.184	1.401	1.542	1.672	1.831	1.945	22
1.180	1.392	1.529	1.655	1.810	1.921	23
1.177	1.383	1.517	1.640	1.791	1.898	24
1.174	1.375	1.506	1.626	1.773	1.877	25
1.171	1.368	1.496	1.612	1.755	1.857	26
1.168	1.361	1.486	1.600	1.739	1.839	27
1.165	1.354	1.476	1.588	1.724	1.821	28
1.162	1.348	1.467	1.577	1.710	1.805	29
1.160	1.342	1.459	1.566	1.696	1.789	30
1.140	1.295	1.394	1.484	1.592	1.669	40
1.127	1.263	1.350	1.428	1.523	1.590	50
1.116	1.240	1.318	1.388	1.473	1.533	60
1.108	1.222	1.293	1.357	1.435	1.489	70
1.102	1.207	1.273	1.333	1.404	1.454	80
1.096	1.195	1.257	1.313	1.379	1.426	90
1.091	1.185	1.243	1.296	1.358	1.402	100
1.000	1.000	1.000	1.000	1.000	1.000	∞
+ .6745	+1.2816	+1.6449	+1.9600	+2.3263	+2.5758	$\frac{x}{\sigma}*$

$$\left(\frac{9n - 2 + \frac{x}{\sigma}\sqrt{18n}}{9n}\right)^3,$$

where $\frac{x}{\sigma}$ is the normal deviate cutting off the corresponding tail of a normal distribution.

Appen

VALUES OF $\dfrac{\sigma^2}{\hat{\sigma}^2}$ FOR USE IN DETER

This table shows:

n	Lower limits						.50
	.005	.01	.025	.05	.10	.25	
1	.1269	.1507	.1990	.2603	.3696	.7557	2.198
2	.1887	.2171	.2711	.3338	.4343	.7213	1.443
3	.2337	.2644	.3209	.3839	.4799	.7302	1.268
4	.2692	.3013	.3590	.4216	.5142	.7428	1.192
5	.2985	.3314	.3896	.4517	.5413	.7546	1.149
6	.3235	.3569	.4152	.4765	.5637	.7652	1.122
7	.3452	.3789	.4372	.4976	.5825	.7746	1.103
8	.3644	.3982	.4562	.5159	.5987	.7829	1.089
9	.3815	.4154	.4731	.5319	.6129	.7903	1.079
10	.3970	.4309	.4882	.5462	.6255	.7969	1.070
11	.4111	.4449	.5018	.5591	.6368	.8029	1.064
12	.4240	.4577	.5142	.5707	.6469	.8083	1.058
13	.4360	.4695	.5256	.5813	.6562	.8133	1.054
14	.4470	.4804	.5360	.5911	.6646	.8179	1.050
15	.4573	.4906	.5457	.6001	.6724	.8221	1.046
16	.4669	.5000	.5547	.6085	.6796	.8261	1.043
17	.4759	.5088	.5631	.6162	.6863	.8297	1.041
18	.4844	.5172	.5710	.6235	.6926	.8331	1.038
19	.4925	.5250	.5783	.6303	.6984	.8363	1.036
20	.5000	.5324	.5853	.6367	.7039	.8394	1.034
21	.5072	.5394	.5919	.6428	.7091	.8422	1.033
22	.5141	.5460	.5981	.6485	.7140	.8449	1.031
23	.5206	.5524	.6041	.6539	.7186	.8474	1.030
24	.5268	.5584	.6097	.6591	.7230	.8498	1.028
25	.5327	.5642	.6151	.6640	.7271	.8521	1.027
26	.5384	.5697	.6202	.6686	.7311	.8543	1.026
27	.5439	.5749	.6251	.6731	.7349	.8564	1.025
28	.5491	.5800	.6298	.6774	.7385	.8584	1.024
29	.5542	.5848	.6343	.6814	.7419	.8603	1.023
30	.5590	.5895	.6386	.6854	.7452	.8621	1.023
40	.5991	.6280	.6741	.7174	.7721	.8769	1.017
50	.6290	.6566	.7001	.7407	.7916	.8876	1.013
60	.6525	.6789	.7203	.7587	.8065	.8958	1.011
70	.6717	.6970	.7367	.7732	.8185	.9023	1.010
80	.6878	.7122	.7503	.7852	.8283	.9077	1.008
90	.7015	.7251	.7618	.7954	.8367	.9123	1.007
100	.7134	.7363	.7718	.8042	.8439	.9162	1.007
∞	1.0000	1.0000	1.0000	1.0000	1.0000	1.0000	1.000
$\dfrac{x_*}{\sigma}$	+2.5758	+2.3263	+1.9600	+1.6449	+1.2816	+ .6745	0

The values in this table were computed from values of χ^2 given in *Biometrika*, Vol. XXXII, Part II, October 1941, pp. 187–191, "Tables of Percentage Points of the χ^2 Distribution," by Catherine M. Thompson, by use of the expression $\sigma^2 = \dfrac{n}{\chi^2}\hat{\sigma}^2$.

* When $n > 30$, values of $\dfrac{\sigma^2}{\hat{\sigma}^2}$ may be approximated by use of the expression

dix VIII

MINING CONFIDENCE LIMITS OF σ^2

and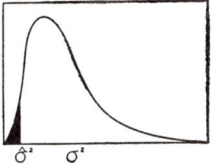

Upper limits						n
.25	.10	.05	.025	.01	.005	
9.849	63.328	254.32	1,018.3	6,366.0	25,465	1
3.476	9.491	19.496	39.498	99.501	199.51	2
2.474	5.134	8.526	13.902	26.125	41.829	3
2.081	3.761	5.628	8.257	13.463	19.325	4
1.869	3.105	4.365	6.015	9.020	12.144	5
1.737	2.722	3.669	4.849	6.880	8.879	6
1.645	2.471	3.230	4.142	5.650	7.076	7
1.578	2.293	2.928	3.670	4.859	5.951	8
1.526	2.159	2.707	3.333	4.311	5.188	9
1.484	2.055	2.538	3.080	3.909	4.639	10
1.450	1.972	2.404	2.883	3.602	4.226	11
1.422	1.904	2.296	2.725	3.361	3.904	12
1.398	1.846	2.206	2.595	3.165	3.647	13
1.377	1.797	2.131	2.487	3.004	3.436	14
1.359	1.755	2.066	2.395	2.868	3.260	15
1.343	1.718	2.010	2.316	2.753	3.111	16
1.329	1.686	1.960	2.247	2.653	2.984	17
1.316	1.657	1.917	2.187	2.566	2.873	18
1.305	1.631	1.878	2.133	2.489	2.776	19
1.294	1.607	1.843	2.085	2.421	2.690	20
1.285	1.586	1.812	2.042	2.360	2.614	21
1.276	1.567	1.783	2.003	2.305	2.545	22
1.268	1.549	1.757	1.968	2.256	2.484	23
1.261	1.533	1.733	1.935	2.211	2.428	24
1.254	1.518	1.711	1.906	2.169	2.376	25
1.247	1.504	1.691	1.878	2.131	2.330	26
1.241	1.491	1.672	1.853	2.097	2.287	27
1.236	1.478	1.654	1.829	2.064	2.247	28
1.231	1.467	1.638	1.807	2.034	2.210	29
1.226	1.456	1.622	1.787	2.006	2.176	30
1.188	1.377	1.509	1.637	1.805	1.932	40
1.164	1.327	1.438	1.545	1.683	1.786	50
1.147	1.291	1.389	1.482	1.601	1.688	60
1.135	1.265	1.353	1.436	1.540	1.618	70
1.124	1.245	1.325	1.400	1.494	1.563	80
1.116	1.228	1.302	1.371	1.457	1.520	90
1.109	1.214	1.283	1.347	1.427	1.485	100
1.000	1.000	1.000	1.000	1.000	1.000	∞
− .6745	−1.2816	−1.6449	−1.9600	−2.3263	−2.5758	$\frac{x_*}{\sigma}$

$$1 \div \left(\frac{9n - 2 + \frac{x}{\sigma}\sqrt{18n}}{9n} \right)^3,$$

where $\frac{x}{\sigma}$ is the corresponding normal deviate.

Appen

VALUES

For Given Degrees of Freedom (n_1 and n_2)

This table

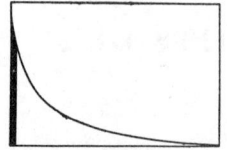

and

for $n_1 = 1$ and $n_1 = 2$

n_2	Lower Points				Upper Points			
	.001	.01	.05	.20	.20	.05	.01	.001
				$n_1 = 1$				
1	$.0^2247$	$.0^2247$	.00619	.106	9.47	161.45	4,052.2	405,284
2	$.0^2200$	$.0^2200$	.00501	.0833	3.56	18.51	98.50	998.5
3	$.0^5185$	$.0^3185$	.00464	.0766	2.68	10.13	34.12	167.5
4	$.0^5178$	$.0^3178$	.00445	.0728	2.35	7.71	21.20	74.14
5	$.0^5173$	$.0^3173$	.00434	.0714	2.18	6.61	16.26	47.04
6	$.0^5171$	$.0^3171$	.00427	.0701	2.07	5.99	13.74	35.51
8	$.0^5167$	$.0^3167$	.00419	.0685	1.95	5.32	11.26	25.42
12	$.0^5164$	$.0^3164$	.00410	.0671	1.84	4.75	9.33	18.64
24	$.0^5160$	$.0^3160$	.00402	.0656	1.74	4.26	7.82	14.03
∞	$.0^5157$	$.0^3157$	.00393	.0642	1.64	3.84	6.63	10.83
				$n_1 = 2$				
1	.00100	.0102	.0540	.281	12.00	190.50	4,999.5	500,000
2	.00100	.0101	.0526	.250	4.00	19.00	99.00	999.0
3	.00100	.0101	.0522	.240	2.89	9.55	30.82	148.5
4	.00100	.0101	.0520	.236	2.47	6.94	18.00	61.25
5	.00100	.0101	.0518	.234	2.26	5.79	13.27	36.61
6	.00100	.0101	.0517	.231	2.13	5.14	10.92	27.00
8	.00100	.0101	.0516	.229	1.98	4.46	8.65	18.49
12	.00100	.0101	.0515	.227	1.85	3.89	6.93	12.97
24	.00100	.0101	.0514	.225	1.72	3.40	5.61	9.34
∞	.00100	.0101	.0513	.223	1.61	3.00	4.61	6.91
				$n_1 = 3$				
1	.00597	.0293	.0987	.373	13.06	215.71	5,403.3	540,379
2	.00673	.0324	.105	.346	4.16	19.16	99.17	999.2
3	.00709	.0339	.108	.340	2.94	9.28	29.46	141.1
4	.00729	.0348	.110	.338	2.48	6.59	16.69	56.18
5	.00743	.0354	.111	.337	2.25	5.41	12.06	33.20
6	.00753	.0358	.112	.337	2.11	4.76	9.78	23.70
8	.00766	.0364	.113	.336	1.95	4.07	7.59	15.83
12	.00779	.0370	.114	.336	1.80	3.49	5.95	10.80
24	.00794	.0376	.116	.336	1.67	3.01	4.72	7.55
∞	.00810	.0383	.117	.335	1.55	2.60	3.78	5.42
				$n_1 = 4$				
1	.0135	.0472	.130	.426	13.73	224.58	5,624.6	562,500
2	.0163	.0556	.144	.405	4.24	19.25	99.25	999.2
3	.0178	.0599	.152	.403	2.96	9.12	28.71	137.1
4	.0187	.0626	.157	.403	2.48	6.39	15.98	53.44
5	.0193	.0644	.160	.403	2.24	5.19	11.39	31.09
6	.0198	.0658	.162	.405	2.09	4.53	9.15	21.90
8	.0204	.0676	.166	.405	1.92	3.84	7.01	14.39
12	.0211	.0696	.169	.407	1.77	3.26	5.41	9.63
24	.0218	.0718	.173	.410	1.63	2.78	4.22	6.59
∞	.0227	.0743	.178	.412	1.50	2.37	3.32	4.62
				$n_1 = 5$				
1	.0213	.0615	.151	.459	14.01	230.16	5,763.7	576,405
2	.0273	.0753	.173	.442	4.28	19.30	99.30	999.3
3	.0301	.0829	.185	.444	2.97	9.01	28.24	134.6
4	.0322	.0878	.193	.446	2.48	6.26	15.52	51.71
5	.0336	.0912	.198	.448	2.23	5.05	10.97	29.75
6	.0347	.0937	.202	.45	2.08	4.39	8.75	20.81
8	.0362	.0972	.208	.45	1.90	3.69	6.63	13.49
12	.0379	.101	.214	.46	1.74	3.11	5.06	8.89
24	.0398	.106	.221	.46	1.59	2.62	3.90	5.98
∞	.0420	.111	.229	.469	1.46	2.21	3.02	4.10

Taken (with minor changes in some of the upper 0.001 points) from *Two Extensions of the F*

dix IX
OF F
and at Selected Upper and Lower Points

shows:

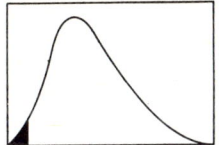 and 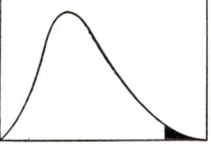 for $n_1 \geqq 3$.

n_2	Lower Points				Upper Points			
	.001	.01	.05	.20	.20	.05	.01	.001
				$n_1 = 6$				
1	.0282	.0728	.167	.483	14.26	233.99	5,859.0	585,937
2	.0370	.0915	.194	.47	4.32	19.33	99.33	999.3
3	.0422	.102	.210	.47	2.97	8.94	27.91	132.8
4	.0457	.109	.221	.48	2.47	6.16	15.21	50.53
5	.0481	.114	.228	.48	2.22	4.95	10.67	28.84
6	.0499	.118	.233	.49	2.06	4.28	8.47	20.03
8	.0526	.123	.241	.49	1.88	3.58	6.37	12.86
12	.0556	.130	.250	.50	1.72	3.00	4.82	8.38
24	.0592	.137	.260	.50	1.57	2.51	3.67	5.55
∞	.0635	.145	.273	.512	1.43	2.10	2.80	3.74
				$n_1 = 8$				
1	.0393	.0888	.188	.513	14.59	238.88	5,981.6	598,144
2	.0541	.116	.224	.51	4.36	19.37	99.37	999.4
3	.0632	.132	.246	.51	2.98	8.85	27.49	130.6
4	.0695	.143	.261	.52	2.47	6.04	14.80	49.00
5	.0742	.151	.271	.53	2.20	4.82	10.29	27.64
6	.0778	.157	.279	.53	2.04	4.15	8.10	19.03
8	.0830	.166	.291	.54	1.86	3.44	6.03	12.04
12	.0893	.176	.305	.55	1.69	2.85	4.50	7.71
24	.0971	.189	.321	.56	1.53	2.36	3.36	4.99
∞	.107	.206	.342	.574	1.38	1.94	2.51	3.27
				$n_1 = 12$				
1	.0536	.107	.211	.543	14.90	243.91	6,106.3	610,667
2	.0771	.144	.257	.54	4.40	19.41	99.42	999.4
3	.0925	.168	.287	.56	2.98	8.74	27.05	128.3
4	.104	.185	.307	.56	2.46	5.91	14.37	47.41
5	.112	.197	.322	.57	2.18	4.68	9.89	26.42
6	.119	.207	.334	.58	2.02	4.00	7.72	17.99
8	.130	.222	.351	.59	1.83	3.28	5.67	11.19
12	.143	.241	.372	.61	1.65	2.69	4.16	7.00
24	.160	.265	.399	.62	1.48	2.18	3.03	4.39
∞	.185	.298	.436	.651	1.32	1.75	2.18	2.74
				$n_1 = 24$				
1	.0713	.128	.235	.575	15.24	249.05	6,234.6	623,497
2	.107	.178	.294	.58	4.44	19.45	99.46	999.5
3	.132	.212	.332	.60	2.98	8.64	26.60	125.9
4	.152	.237	.360	.61	2.44	5.77	13.93	45.77
5	.167	.257	.382	.63	2.16	4.53	9.47	25.14
6	.180	.273	.399	.64	1.99	3.84	7.31	16.89
8	.200	.297	.425	.65	1.79	3.12	5.28	10.30
12	.228	.330	.458	.68	1.60	2.51	3.78	6.25
24	.268	.376	.504	.70	1.42	1.98	2.66	3.74
∞	.337	.452	.577	.753	1.23	1.52	1.79	2.13
				$n_1 = \infty$				
1	.0924	.151	.260	.610	15.58	254.32	6,366.0	636,619
2	.145	.217	.334	.62	4.48	19.50	99.50	999.5
3	.184	.264	.384	.65	2.98	8.53	26.12	123.5
4	.217	.301	.422	.67	2.43	5.63	13.46	44.05
5	.244	.331	.452	.69	2.13	4.36	9.02	23.78
6	.267	.357	.477	.70	1.95	3.67	6.88	15.75
8	.306	.398	.516	.73	1.74	2.93	4.86	9.34
12	.365	.458	.571	.76	1.54	2.30	3.36	5.42
24	.469	.558	.659	.81	1.33	1.73	2.21	2.97
∞	1.000	1.000	1.000	1.00	1.00	1.00	1.00	1.00

Table, by F. E. Croxton and D. J. Cowden, Prentice-Hall, Inc., New York, 1945.

Appendix X

VALUES OF F

For Given Degrees of Freedom (n_1 and n_2) and at Selected Upper Points

Values of F for corresponding lower points may be obtained by transposing the values of n_1 and n_2 and computing $\frac{1}{F}$.

This table shows for $n_1 = 1$ and $n_1 = 2$ for $n_1 \geqq 3$.

n_2	$n_1 = 1$					$n_1 = 2$				
	.10	.05	.025	.01	.001	.10	.05	.025	.01	.001
1	39.864	161.45	647.79	4,052.2	405,284	49.500	199.50	799.50	4,999.5	500,000
2	8.526	18.513	38.506	98.503	998.5	9.000	19.000	39.000	99.000	999.0
3	5.538	10.128	17.443	34.116	167.0	5.462	9.552	16.044	30.817	148.5
4	4.545	7.709	12.218	21.198	74.14	4.325	6.944	10.649	18.000	61.25
5	4.060	6.608	10.007	16.258	47.18	3.780	5.786	8.434	13.274	37.12
6	3.776	5.987	8.813	13.745	35.51	3.463	5.143	7.260	10.925	27.00
7	3.589	5.591	8.073	12.246	29.25	3.257	4.737	6.542	9.547	21.69
8	3.458	5.318	7.571	11.259	25.42	3.113	4.459	6.060	8.649	18.49
9	3.360	5.117	7.209	10.561	22.86	3.006	4.256	5.715	8.022	16.39
10	3.285	4.965	6.937	10.044	21.04	2.924	4.103	5.456	7.559	14.91
11	3.225	4.844	6.724	9.646	19.69	2.860	3.982	5.256	7.206	13.81
12	3.176	4.747	6.554	9.330	18.64	2.807	3.885	5.096	6.927	12.97
13	3.136	4.667	6.414	9.074	17.81	2.763	3.806	4.965	6.701	12.31
14	3.102	4.600	6.298	8.862	17.14	2.726	3.739	4.857	6.515	11.78
15	3.073	4.543	6.200	8.683	16.59	2.695	3.682	4.765	6.359	11.34
16	3.048	4.494	6.115	8.531	16.12	2.668	3.634	4.687	6.226	10.97
17	3.026	4.451	6.042	8.400	15.72	2.645	3.592	4.619	6.112	10.66
18	3.007	4.414	5.978	8.285	15.38	2.624	3.555	4.560	6.013	10.39
19	2.990	4.381	5.922	8.185	15.08	2.606	3.522	4.508	5.926	10.16
20	2.975	4.351	5.872	8.096	14.82	2.589	3.493	4.461	5.849	9.95
21	2.961	4.325	5.827	8.017	14.59	2.575	3.467	4.420	5.780	9.77
22	2.949	4.301	5.786	7.945	14.38	2.561	3.443	4.383	5.719	9.61
23	2.937	4.279	5.750	7.881	14.19	2.549	3.422	4.349	5.664	9.47
24	2.927	4.260	5.717	7.823	14.03	2.538	3.403	4.319	5.614	9.34
25	2.918	4.242	5.686	7.770	13.88	2.528	3.385	4.291	5.568	9.22
26	2.909	4.225	5.659	7.721	13.74	2.519	3.369	4.266	5.526	9.12
27	2.901	4.210	5.633	7.677	13.61	2.511	3.354	4.242	5.488	9.02
28	2.894	4.196	5.610	7.636	13.50	2.503	3.340	4.220	5.453	8.93
29	2.887	4.183	5.588	7.598	13.39	2.496	3.328	4.201	5.421	8.85
30	2.881	4.171	5.568	7.563	13.29	2.489	3.316	4.182	5.390	8.77
40	2.835	4.085	5.424	7.314	12.61	2.440	3.232	4.051	5.178	8.25
60	2.791	4.001	5.286	7.077	11.97	2.393	3.150	3.925	4.977	7.76
120	2.748	3.920	5.152	6.851	11.38	2.347	3.072	3.805	4.786	7.32
∞	2.706	3.841	5.024	6.635	10.83	2.303	2.996	3.689	4.605	6.91

Values of F at the 0.10, 0.05, 0.025, and 0.01 points were taken, by permission, from *Biometrika*, Vol. XXXIII, April 1943, pp. 73–78, "Tables of Percentage Points of the Inverted Beta (F) Distribution," by Maxine Merrington and Catherine M. Thompson. Values of F at the 0.001 point were taken from Table V of R. A. Fisher and

Appendix X—Continued
VALUES OF F

For Given Degrees of Freedom (n_1 and n_2) and at Selected Upper Points

Values of F for corresponding lower points may be obtained by transposing the values of n_1 and n_2 and computing $\frac{1}{F}$.

n_2	$n_1 = 3$					$n_1 = 4$				
	.10	.05	.025	.01	.001	.10	.05	.025	.01	.001
1	53.593	215.71	864.16	5,403.3	540,379	55.833	224.58	899.58	5,624.6	562,500
2	9.162	19.164	39.165	99.166	999.2	9.243	19.247	39.248	99.249	999.2
3	5.391	9.277	15.439	29.457	141.1	5.343	9.117	15.101	28.710	137.1
4	4.191	6.591	9.979	16.694	56.18	4.107	6.388	9.604	15.977	53.44
5	3.620	5.410	7.764	12.060	33.20	3.520	5.192	7.388	11.392	31.09
6	3.289	4.757	6.599	9.779	23.70	3.181	4.534	6.227	9.148	21.92
7	3.074	4.347	5.890	8.451	18.77	2.960	4.120	5.523	7.847	17.19
8	2.924	4.066	5.416	7.591	15.83	2.806	3.838	5.053	7.006	14.39
9	2.813	3.863	5.078	6.992	13.90	2.693	3.633	4.718	6.422	12.56
10	2.728	3.708	4.826	6.552	12.55	2.605	3.478	4.468	5.994	11.28
11	2.660	3.587	4.630	6.217	11.56	2.536	3.357	4.275	5.668	10.35
12	2.606	3.490	4.474	5.953	10.80	2.480	3.259	4.121	5.412	9.63
13	2.560	3.410	4.347	5.739	10.21	2.434	3.179	3.996	5.205	9.07
14	2.522	3.344	4.242	5.564	9.73	2.395	3.112	3.892	5.035	8.62
15	2.490	3.287	4.153	5.417	9.34	2.361	3.056	3.804	4.893	8.25
16	2.462	3.239	4.077	5.292	9.00	2.333	3.007	3.729	4.773	7.94
17	2.437	3.197	4.011	5.185	8.73	2.308	2.965	3.665	4.669	7.68
18	2.416	3.160	3.954	5.092	8.49	2.286	2.928	3.608	4.579	7.46
19	2.397	3.127	3.903	5.010	8.28	2.266	2.895	3.559	4.500	7.26
20	2.380	3.098	3.859	4.938	8.10	2.249	2.866	3.515	4.431	7.10
21	2.365	3.072	3.819	4.874	7.94	2.233	2.840	3.475	4.369	6.95
22	2.351	3.049	3.783	4.817	7.80	2.219	2.817	3.440	4.313	6.81
23	2.339	3.028	3.750	4.765	7.67	2.206	2.795	3.408	4.264	6.69
24	2.327	3.009	3.721	4.718	7.55	2.195	2.776	3.379	4.218	6.59
25	2.317	2.991	3.694	4.676	7.45	2.184	2.759	3.353	4.177	6.49
26	2.308	2.975	3.670	4.637	7.36	2.174	2.743	3.329	4.140	6.41
27	2.299	2.960	3.647	4.601	7.27	2.166	2.728	3.307	4.106	6.33
28	2.291	2.947	3.626	4.568	7.19	2.157	2.714	3.286	4.074	6.25
29	2.283	2.934	3.607	4.538	7.12	2.149	2.701	3.267	4.045	6.19
30	2.276	2.922	3.589	4.510	7.05	2.142	2.690	3.250	4.018	6.12
40	2.226	2.839	3.463	4.313	6.60	2.091	2.606	3.126	3.828	5.70
60	2.177	2.758	3.342	4.126	6.17	2.041	2.525	3.008	3.649	5.31
120	2.130	2.680	3.227	3.949	5.79	1.992	2.447	2.894	3.480	4.95
∞	2.084	2.605	3.116	3.782	5.42	1.945	2.372	2.786	3.319	4.62

F. Yates, *Statistical Tables for Biological, Agricultural, and Medical Research*, Oliver and Boyd, Ltd., Edinburgh, 1949, by permission of the authors and publishers.

Appendix X—Continued
VALUES OF F

For Given Degrees of Freedom (n_1 and n_2) and at Selected Upper Points
Values of F for corresponding lower points may be obtained by transposing the values of n_1 and n_2 and computing $\frac{1}{F}$.

n_2	$n_1 = 5$					$n_1 = 6$				
	.10	.05	.025	.01	.001	.10	.05	.025	.01	.001
1	57.241	230.16	921.85	5,763.7	576,405	58.204	233.99	937.11	5,859.0	585,937
2	9.293	19.296	39.298	99.299	999.3	9.326	19.330	39.331	99.332	999.3
3	5.309	9.014	14.885	28.237	134.6	5.285	8.941	14.735	27.911	132.8
4	4.051	6.256	9.364	15.522	51.71	4.010	6.163	9.197	15.207	50.53
5	3.453	5.050	7.146	10.967	29.75	3.404	4.950	6.978	10.672	28.84
6	3.108	4.387	5.988	8.746	20.81	3.055	4.284	5.820	8.466	20.03
7	2.883	3.972	5.285	7.460	16.21	2.827	3.866	5.119	7.191	15.52
8	2.726	3.688	4.817	6.632	13.49	2.668	3.581	4.652	6.371	12.86
9	2.611	3.482	4.484	6.057	11.71	2.551	3.374	4.320	5.802	11.13
10	2.522	3.326	4.236	5.636	10.48	2.461	3.217	4.072	5.386	9.92
11	2.451	3.204	4.044	5.316	9.58	2.389	3.095	3.881	5.069	9.05
12	2.394	3.106	3.891	5.064	8.89	2.331	2.996	3.728	4.821	8.38
13	2.347	3.025	3.767	4.862	8.35	2.283	2.915	3.604	4.620	7.86
14	2.307	2.958	3.663	4.695	7.92	2.243	2.848	3.501	4.456	7.43
15	2.273	2.901	3.576	4.556	7.57	2.208	2.790	3.415	4.318	7.09
16	2.244	2.852	3.502	4.437	7.27	2.178	2.741	3.341	4.202	6.81
17	2.218	2.810	3.438	4.336	7.02	2.152	2.699	3.277	4.102	6.56
18	2.196	2.773	3.382	4.248	6.81	2.130	2.661	3.221	4.015	6.35
19	2.176	2.740	3.333	4.171	6.62	2.109	2.628	3.172	3.939	6.18
20	2.158	2.711	3.289	4.103	6.46	2.091	2.599	3.128	3.871	6.02
21	2.142	2.685	3.250	4.042	6.32	2.075	2.573	3.090	3.812	5.88
22	2.128	2.661	3.215	3.988	6.19	2.060	2.549	3.055	3.758	5.76
23	2.115	2.640	3.184	3.939	6.08	2.047	2.528	3.023	3.710	5.65
24	2.103	2.621	3.155	3.895	5.98	2.035	2.508	2.995	3.667	5.55
25	2.092	2.603	3.129	3.855	5.88	2.024	2.490	2.969	3.627	5.46
26	2.082	2.587	3.105	3.818	5.80	2.014	2.474	2.945	3.591	5.38
27	2.073	2.572	3.083	3.785	5.73	2.004	2.459	2.923	3.558	5.31
28	2.064	2.558	3.062	3.754	5.66	1.996	2.445	2.903	3.528	5.24
29	2.057	2.545	3.044	3.725	5.59	1.988	2.432	2.884	3.499	5.18
30	2.049	2.534	3.026	3.699	5.53	1.980	2.421	2.867	3.474	5.12
40	1.997	2.450	2.904	3.514	5.13	1.927	2.336	2.744	3.291	4.73
60	1.946	2.368	2.786	3.339	4.76	1.875	2.254	2.627	3.119	4.37
120	1.896	2.290	2.674	3.174	4.42	1.824	2.175	2.515	2.956	4.04
∞	1.847	2.214	2.566	3.017	4.10	1.774	2.099	2.408	2.802	3.74

Appendix X—Continued
VALUES OF F

For Given Degrees of Freedom (n_1 and n_2) and at Selected Upper Points

Values of F for corresponding lower points may be obtained by transposing the values of n_1 and n_2 and computing $\frac{1}{F}$.

n_2	$n_1 = 8$					$n_1 = 12$				
	.10	.05	.025	.01	.001	.10	.05	.025	.01	.001
1	59.439	238.88	956.66	5,981.6	598,144	60.705	243.91	976.71	6,106.3	610,667
2	9.367	19.371	39.373	99.374	999.4	9.408	19.413	39.415	99.416	999.4
3	5.252	8.845	14.540	27.489	130.6	5.216	8.745	14.337	27.052	128.3
4	3.955	6.041	8.980	14.799	49.00	3.896	5.912	8.751	14.374	47.41
5	3.339	4.818	6.757	10.289	27.64	3.268	4.678	6.525	9.888	26.42
6	2.983	4.147	5.600	8.102	19.03	2.905	4.000	5.366	7.718	17.99
7	2.752	3.726	4.899	6.840	14.63	2.668	3.575	4.666	6.469	13.71
8	2.589	3.438	4.433	6.029	12.04	2.502	3.284	4.200	5.667	11.19
9	2.469	3.230	4.102	5.467	10.37	2.379	3.073	3.868	5.111	9.57
10	2.377	3.072	3.855	5.057	9.20	2.284	2.913	3.621	4.706	8.45
11	2.304	2.948	3.664	4.745	8.35	2.209	2.788	3.430	4.397	7.63
12	2.245	2.849	3.512	4.499	7.71	2.147	2.687	3.277	4.155	7.00
13	2.195	2.767	3.388	4.302	7.21	2.097	2.604	3.153	3.960	6.52
14	2.154	2.699	3.285	4.140	6.80	2.054	2.534	3.050	3.800	6.13
15	2.118	2.641	3.199	4.004	6.47	2.017	2.475	2.963	3.666	5.81
16	2.088	2.591	3.125	3.890	6.19	1.985	2.425	2.889	3.553	5.55
17	2.061	2.548	3.061	3.791	5.96	1.958	2.381	2.825	3.455	5.32
18	2.038	2.510	3.005	3.705	5.76	1.933	2.342	2.769	3.371	5.13
19	2.017	2.477	2.956	3.631	5.59	1.912	2.308	2.720	3.296	4.97
20	1.998	2.447	2.913	3.564	5.44	1.892	2.278	2.676	3.231	4.82
21	1.982	2.421	2.874	3.506	5.31	1.875	2.250	2.637	3.173	4.70
22	1.967	2.397	2.839	3.453	5.19	1.859	2.226	2.602	3.121	4.58
23	1.953	2.375	2.808	3.406	5.09	1.845	2.204	2.570	3.074	4.48
24	1.941	2.355	2.779	3.363	4.99	1.832	2.183	2.541	3.032	4.39
25	1.929	2.337	2.753	3.324	4.91	1.820	2.165	2.515	2.993	4.31
26	1.919	2.321	2.729	3.288	4.83	1.809	2.148	2.491	2.958	4.24
27	1.909	2.305	2.707	3.256	4.76	1.799	2.132	2.469	2.926	4.17
28	1.900	2.291	2.687	3.226	4.69	1.790	2.118	2.448	2.896	4.11
29	1.892	2.278	2.669	3.198	4.64	1.781	2.104	2.430	2.869	4.05
30	1.884	2.266	2.651	3.173	4.58	1.773	2.092	2.412	2.843	4.00
40	1.829	2.180	2.529	2.993	4.21	1.715	2.004	2.288	2.665	3.64
60	1.775	2.097	2.412	2.823	3.87	1.657	1.917	2.169	2.496	3.31
120	1.722	2.016	2.299	2.663	3.55	1.601	1.834	2.055	2.336	3.02
∞	1.670	1.938	2.192	2.511	3.27	1.546	1.752	1.945	2.185	2.74

Appendix X—Concluded
VALUES OF F

For Given Degrees of Freedom (n_1 and n_2) and at Selected Upper Points

Values of F for corresponding lower points may be obtained by transposing the values of n_1 and n_2 and computing $\frac{1}{F}$.

n_2	$n_1 = 24$					$n_1 = \infty$				
	.10	.05	.025	.01	.001	.10	.05	.025	.01	.001
1	62.002	249.05	997.25	6,234.6	623,497	63.328	254.32	1,018.3	6,366.0	636,619
2	9.450	19.454	39.456	99.458	999.5	9.491	19.496	39.498	99.501	999.5
3	5.176	8.638	14.124	26.598	125.9	5.134	8.527	13.902	26.125	123.5
4	3.831	5.774	8.511	13.929	45.77	3.761	5.628	8.257	13.463	44.05
5	3.190	4.527	6.278	9.467	25.14	3.105	4.365	6.015	9.020	23.79
6	2.818	3.841	5.117	7.313	16.89	2.722	3.669	4.849	6.880	15.75
7	2.575	3.410	4.415	6.074	12.73	2.471	3.230	4.142	5.650	11.70
8	2.404	3.115	3.947	5.279	10.30	2.293	2.928	3.670	4.859	9.33
9	2.277	2.900	3.614	4.729	8.72	2.159	2.707	3.333	4.311	7.81
10	2.178	2.737	3.365	4.327	7.64	2.055	2.538	3.080	3.909	6.76
11	2.100	2.609	3.172	4.021	6.85	1.972	2.405	2.883	3.602	6.00
12	2.036	2.505	3.019	3.780	6.25	1.904	2.296	2.725	3.361	5.42
13	1.983	2.420	2.893	3.587	5.78	1.846	2.206	2.596	3.165	4.97
14	1.938	2.349	2.789	3.427	5.41	1.797	2.131	2.487	3.004	4.60
15	1.899	2.288	2.701	3.294	5.10	1.755	2.066	2.395	2.868	4.31
16	1.866	2.235	2.625	3.181	4.85	1.718	2.010	2.316	2.753	4.06
17	1.836	2.190	2.560	3.083	4.63	1.686	1.960	2.247	2.653	3.85
18	1.810	2.150	2.503	2.999	4.45	1.657	1.917	2.187	2.566	3.67
19	1.787	2.114	2.452	2.925	4.29	1.631	1.878	2.133	2.489	3.51
20	1.767	2.083	2.408	2.859	4.15	1.607	1.843	2.085	2.421	3.38
21	1.748	2.054	2.368	2.801	4.03	1.586	1.812	2.042	2.360	3.26
22	1.731	2.028	2.332	2.749	3.92	1.567	1.783	2.003	2.305	3.15
23	1.716	2.005	2.299	2.702	3.82	1.549	1.757	1.968	2.256	3.05
24	1.702	1.984	2.269	2.659	3.74	1.533	1.733	1.935	2.211	2.97
25	1.689	1.964	2.242	2.620	3.66	1.518	1.711	1.906	2.169	2.89
26	1.677	1.946	2.217	2.585	3.59	1.504	1.691	1.878	2.132	2.82
27	1.666	1.930	2.195	2.552	3.52	1.491	1.672	1.853	2.096	2.75
28	1.656	1.915	2.174	2.522	3.46	1.478	1.654	1.829	2.064	2.69
29	1.646	1.901	2.154	2.495	3.41	1.467	1.638	1.807	2.034	2.64
30	1.638	1.887	2.136	2.469	3.36	1.456	1.622	1.787	2.006	2.59
40	1.574	1.793	2.007	2.288	3.01	1.377	1.509	1.637	1.805	2.23
60	1.511	1.700	1.882	2.115	2.69	1.292	1.389	1.482	1.601	1.89
120	1.447	1.608	1.760	1.950	2.40	1.193	1.254	1.310	1.380	1.54
∞	1.383	1.517	1.640	1.791	2.13	1.000	1.000	1.000	1.000	1.00

Appendix XI

UPPER 0.10 AND 0.02 LIMITS OF β_1 WHEN COMPUTED FROM RANDOM SAMPLES FROM A NORMAL POPULATION

This table shows:

N	0.10	0.02
50	.285	.619
75	.198	.424
100	.152	.321
125	.123	.258
150	.103	.216
175	.089	.185
200	.078	.162
250	.063	.130
300	.053	.108
350	.045	.093
400	.040	.081
450	.035	.072
500	.032	.065
550	.029	.059
600	.027	.054
650	.025	.050
700	.023	.046
750	.021	.043
800	.020	.041
850	.019	.038
900	.018	.036
950	.017	.034
1000	.016	.032
1200	.013	.027
1400	.012	.023
1600	.010	.020
1800	.009	.018
2000	.008	.016
2500	.006	.013
3000	.005	.011
3500	.005	.009
4000	.004	.008
4500	.004	.007
5000	.003	.006

Taken, by permission, from a table given by Egon S. Pearson in his article "A Further Development of Tests of Normality," *Biometrika*, Vol. XXII, pages 239 ff.

Appendix XII

UPPER AND LOWER 0.05 AND 0.01 LIMITS OF β_2 WHEN COMPUTED FROM RANDOM SAMPLES FROM A NORMAL POPULATION

This table shows: 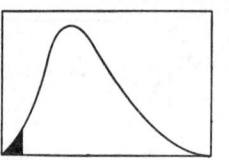 and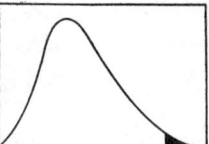

N	Lower limits		Upper limits	
	0.01	0.05	0.05	0.01
100	2.18	2.35	3.77	4.39
125	2.24	2.40	3.70	4.24
150	2.29	2.45	3.65	4.14
175	2.33	2.48	3.61	4.05
200	2.37	2.51	3.57	3.98
250	2.42	2.55	3.52	3.87
300	2.46	2.59	3.47	3.79
350	2.50	2.62	3.44	3.72
400	2.52	2.64	3.41	3.67
450	2.55	2.66	3.39	3.63
500	2.57	2.67	3.37	3.60
550	2.58	2.69	3.35	3.57
600	2.60	2.70	3.34	3.54
650	2.61	2.71	3.33	3.52
700	2.62	2.72	3.31	3.50
750	2.64	2.73	3.30	3.48
800	2.65	2.74	3.29	3.46
850	2.66	2.74	3.28	3.45
900	2.66	2.75	3.28	3.43
950	2.67	2.76	3.27	3.42
1000	2.68	2.76	3.26	3.41
1200	2.71	2.78	3.24	3.37
1400	2.72	2.80	3.22	3.34
1600	2.74	2.81	3.21	3.32
1800	2.76	2.82	3.20	3.30
2000	2.77	2.83	3.18	3.28
2500	2.79	2.85	3.16	3.25
3000	2.81	2.86	3.15	3.22
3500	2.82	2.87	3.14	3.21
4000	2.83	2.88	3.13	3.19
4500	2.84	2.88	3.12	3.18
5000	2.85	2.89	3.12	3.17

Taken, by permission, from a table given by Egon S. Pearson in his article "A Further Development of Tests of Normality," *Biometrika*, Vol. XXII, pages 239 ff.

Appendix XIII

SQUARES, SQUARE ROOTS, AND RECIPROCALS

1 to 1,000

No.	Square	Square Root	Reciprocal	No.	Square	Square Root	Reciprocal
1	1	1.0000000	1.000000000	51	26 01	7.1414284	.019607843
2	4	1.4142136	0.500000000	52	27 04	7.2111026	.019230769
3	9	1.7320508	.333333333	53	28 09	7.2801099	.018867925
4	16	2.0000000	.250000000	54	29 16	7.3484692	.018518519
5	25	2.2360680	.200000000	55	30 25	7.4161985	.018181818
6	36	2.4494897	.166666667	56	31 36	7.4833148	.017857143
7	49	2.6457513	.142857143	57	32 49	7.5498344	.017543860
8	64	2.8284271	.125000000	58	33 64	7.6157731	.017241379
9	81	3.0000000	.111111111	59	34 81	7.6811457	.016949153
10	1 00	3.1622777	.100000000	60	36 00	7.7459667	.016666667
11	1 21	3.3166248	.090909091	61	37 21	7.8102497	.016393443
12	1 44	3.4641016	.083333333	62	38 44	7.8740079	.016129032
13	1 69	3.6055513	.076923077	63	39 69	7.9372539	.015873016
14	1 96	3.7416574	.071428571	64	40 96	8.0000000	.015625000
15	2 25	3.8729833	.066666667	65	42 25	8.0622577	.015384615
16	2 56	4.0000000	.062500000	66	43 56	8.1240384	.015151515
17	2 89	4.1231056	.058823529	67	44 89	8.1853528	.014925373
18	3 24	4.2426407	.055555556	68	46 24	8.2462113	.014705882
19	3 61	4.3588989	.052631579	69	47 61	8.3066239	.014492754
20	4 00	4.4721360	.050000000	70	49 00	8.3666003	.014285714
21	4 41	4.5825757	.047619048	71	50 41	8.4261498	.014084507
22	4 84	4.6904158	.045454545	72	51 84	8.4852814	.013888889
23	5 29	4.7958315	.043478261	73	53 29	8.5440037	.013698630
24	5 76	4.8989795	.041666667	74	54 76	8.6023253	.013513514
25	6 25	5.0000000	.040000000	75	56 25	8.6602540	.013333333
26	6 76	5.0990195	.038461538	76	57 76	8.7177979	.013157895
27	7 29	5.1961524	.037037037	77	59 29	8.7749644	.012987013
28	7 84	5.2915026	.035714286	78	60 84	8.8317609	.012820513
29	8 41	5.3851648	.034482759	79	62 41	8.8881944	.012658228
30	9 00	5.4772256	.033333333	80	64 00	8.9442719	.012500000
31	9 61	5.5677644	.032258065	81	65 61	9.0000000	.012345679
32	10 24	5.6568542	.031250000	82	67 24	9.0553851	.012195122
33	10 89	5.7445626	.030303030	83	68 89	9.1104336	.012048193
34	11 56	5.8309519	.029411765	84	70 56	9.1651514	.011904762
35	12 25	5.9160798	.028571429	85	72 25	9.2195445	.011764706
36	12 96	6.0000000	.027777778	86	73 96	9.2736185	.011627907
37	13 69	6.0827625	.027027027	87	75 69	9.3273791	.011494253
38	14 44	6.1644140	.026315789	88	77 44	9.3808315	.011363636
39	15 21	6.2449980	.025641026	89	79 21	9.4339811	.011235955
40	16 00	6.3245553	.025000000	90	81 00	9.4868330	.011111111
41	16 81	6.4031242	.024390244	91	82 81	9.5393920	.010989011
42	17 64	6.4807407	.023809524	92	84 64	9.5916630	.010869565
43	18 49	6.5574385	.023255814	93	86 49	9.6436508	.010752688
44	19 36	6.6332496	.022727273	94	88 36	9.6953597	.010638298
45	20 25	6.7082039	.022222222	95	90 25	9.7467943	.010526316
46	21 16	6.7823300	.021739130	96	92 16	9.7979590	.010416667
47	22 09	6.8556546	.021276596	97	94 09	9.8488578	.010309278
48	23 04	6.9282032	.020833333	98	96 04	9.8994949	.010204082
49	24 01	7.0000000	.020408163	99	98 01	9.9498744	.010101010
50	25 00	7.0710678	.020000000	100	1 00 00	10.0000000	.010000000

No.	Square	Square Root	Reciprocal .00	No.	Square	Square Root	Reciprocal .00
101	1 02 01	10.0498756	9900990	151	2 28 01	12.2882057	6622517
102	1 04 04	10.0995049	9803922	152	2 31 04	12.3288280	6578947
103	1 06 09	10.1488916	9708738	153	2 34 09	12.3693169	6535948
104	1 08 16	10.1980390	9615385	154	2 37 16	12.4096736	6493506
105	1 10 25	10.2469508	9523810	155	2 40 25	12.4498996	6451613
106	1 12 36	10.2956301	9433962	156	2 43 36	12.4899960	6410256
107	1 14 49	10.3440804	9345794	157	2 46 49	12.5299641	6369427
108	1 16 64	10.3923048	9259259	158	2 49 64	12.5698051	6329114
109	1 18 81	10.4403065	9174312	159	2 52 81	12.6095202	6289308
110	1 21 00	10.4880885	9090909	160	2 56 00	12.6491106	6250000
111	1 23 21	10.5356538	9009009	161	2 59 21	12.6885775	6211180
112	1 25 44	10.5830052	8928571	162	2 62 44	12.7279221	6172840
113	1 27 69	10.6301458	8849558	163	2 65 69	12.7671453	6134969
114	1 29 96	10.6770783	8771930	164	2 68 96	12.8062485	6097561
115	1 32 25	10.7238053	8695652	165	2 72 25	12.8452326	6060606
116	1 34 56	10.7703296	8620690	166	2 75 56	12.8840987	6024096
117	1 36 89	10.8166538	8547009	167	2 78 89	12.9228480	5988024
118	1 39 24	10.8627805	8474576	168	2 82 24	12.9614814	5952381
119	1 41 61	10.9087121	8403361	169	2 85 61	13.0000000	5917160
120	1 44 00	10.9544512	8333333	170	2 89 00	13.0384048	5882353
121	1 46 41	11.0000000	8264463	171	2 92 41	13.0766968	5847953
122	1 48 84	11.0453610	8196721	172	2 95 84	13.1148770	5813953
123	1 51 29	11.0905365	8130081	173	2 99 29	13.1529464	5780347
124	1 53 76	11.1355287	8064516	174	3 02 76	13.1909060	5747126
125	1 56 25	11.1803399	8000000	175	3 06 25	13.2287566	5714286
126	1 58 76	11.2249722	7936508	176	3 09 76	13.2664992	5681818
127	1 61 29	11.2694277	7874016	177	3 13 29	13.3041347	5649718
128	1 63 84	11.3137085	7812500	178	3 16 84	13.3416641	5617978
129	1 66 41	11.3578167	7751938	179	3 20 41	13.3790882	5586592
130	1 69 00	11.4017543	7692308	180	3 24 00	13.4164079	5555556
131	1 71 61	11.4455231	7633588	181	3 27 61	13.4536240	5524862
132	1 74 24	11.4891253	7575758	182	3 31 24	13.4907376	5494505
133	1 76 89	11.5325626	7518797	183	3 34 89	13.5277493	5464481
134	1 79 56	11.5758369	7462687	184	3 38 56	13.5646600	5434783
135	1 82 25	11.6189500	7407407	185	3 42 25	13.6014705	5405405
136	1 84 96	11.6619038	7352941	186	3 45 96	13.6381817	5376344
137	1 87 69	11.7046999	7299270	187	3 49 69	13.6747943	5347594
138	1 90 44	11.7473401	7246377	188	3 53 44	13.7113092	5319149
139	1 93 21	11.7898261	7194245	189	3 57 21	13.7477271	5291005
140	1 96 00	11.8321596	7142857	190	3 61 00	13.7840488	5263158
141	1 98 81	11.8743422	7092199	191	3 64 81	13.8202750	5235602
142	2 01 64	11.9163753	7042254	192	3 68 64	13.8564065	5208333
143	2 04 49	11.9582607	6993007	193	3 72 49	13.8924440	5181347
144	2 07 36	12.0000000	6944444	194	3 76 36	13.9283883	5154639
145	2 10 25	12.0415946	6896552	195	3 80 25	13.9642400	5128205
146	2 13 16	12.0830460	6849315	196	3 84 16	14.0000000	5102041
147	2 16 09	12.1243557	6802721	197	3 88 09	14.0356688	5076142
148	2 19 04	12.1655251	6756757	198	3 92 04	14.0712473	5050505
149	2 22 01	12.2065556	6711409	199	3 96 01	14.1067360	5025126
150	2 25 00	12.2474487	6666667	200	4 00 00	14.1421356	5000000

No.	Square	Square Root	Reciprocal .00	No.	Square	Square Root	Reciprocal .00
201	4 04 01	14.1774469	4975124	251	6 30 01	15.8429795	3984064
202	4 08 04	14.2126704	4950495	252	6 35 04	15.8745079	3968254
203	4 12 09	14.2478068	4926108	253	6 40 09	15.9059737	3952569
204	4 16 16	14.2828569	4901961	254	6 45 16	15.9373775	3937008
205	4 20 25	14.3178211	4878049	255	6 50 25	15.9687194	3921569
206	4 24 36	14.3527001	4854369	256	6 55 36	16.0000000	3906250
207	4 28 49	14.3874946	4830918	257	6 60 49	16.0312195	3891051
208	4 32 64	14.4222051	4807692	258	6 65 64	16.0623784	3875969
209	4 36 81	14.4568323	4784689	259	6 70 81	16.0934769	3861004
210	4 41 00	14.4913767	4761905	260	6 76 00	16.1245155	3846154
211	4 45 21	14.5258390	4739336	261	6 81 21	16.1554944	3831418
212	4 49 44	14.5602198	4716981	262	6 86 44	16.1864141	3816794
213	4 53 69	14.5945195	4694836	263	6 91 69	16.2172747	3802281
214	4 57 96	14.6287388	4672897	264	6 96 96	16.2480768	3787879
215	4 62 25	14.6628783	4651163	265	7 02 25	16.2788206	3773585
216	4 66 56	14.6969385	4629630	266	7 07 56	16.3095064	3759398
217	4 70 89	14.7309199	4608295	267	7 12 89	16.3401346	3745318
218	4 75 24	14.7648231	4587156	268	7 18 24	16.3707055	3731343
219	4 79 61	14.7986486	4566210	269	7 23 61	16.4012195	3717472
220	4 84 00	14.8323970	4545455	270	7 29 00	16.4316767	3703704
221	4 88 41	14.8660687	4524887	271	7 34 41	16.4620776	3690037
222	4 92 84	14.8996644	4504505	272	7 39 84	16.4924225	3676471
223	4 97 29	14.9331845	4484305	273	7 45 29	16.5227116	3663004
224	5 01 76	14.9666295	4464286	274	7 50 76	16.5529454	3649635
225	5 06 25	15.0000000	4444444	275	7 56 25	16.5831240	3636364
226	5 10 76	15.0332964	4424779	276	7 61 76	16.6132477	3623188
227	5 15 29	15.0665192	4405286	277	7 67 29	16.6433170	3610108
228	5 19 84	15.0996689	4385965	278	7 72 84	16.6733320	3597122
229	5 24 41	15.1327460	4366812	279	7 78 41	16.7032931	3584229
230	5 29 00	15.1657509	4347826	280	7 84 00	16.7332005	3571429
231	5 33 61	15.1986842	4329004	281	7 89 61	16.7630546	3558719
232	5 38 24	15.2315462	4310345	282	7 95 24	16.7928556	3546099
233	5 42 89	15.2643375	4291845	283	8 00 89	16.8226038	3533569
234	5 47 56	15.2970585	4273504	284	8 06 56	16.8522995	3521127
235	5 52 25	15.3297097	4255319	285	8 12 25	16.8819430	3508772
236	5 56 96	15.3622915	4237288	286	8 17 96	16.9115345	3496503
237	5 61 69	15.3948043	4219409	287	8 23 69	16.9410743	3484321
238	5 66 44	15.4272486	4201681	288	8 29 44	16.9705627	3472222
239	5 71 21	15.4596248	4184100	289	8 35 21	17.0000000	3460208
240	5 76 00	15.4919334	4166667	290	8 41 00	17.0293864	3448276
241	5 80 81	15.5241747	4149378	291	8 46 81	17.0587221	3436426
242	5 85 64	15.5563492	4132231	292	8 52 64	17.0880075	3424658
243	5 90 49	15.5884573	4115226	293	8 58 49	17.1172428	3412969
244	5 95 36	15.6204994	4098361	294	8 64 36	17.1464282	3401361
245	6 00 25	15.6524758	4081633	295	8 70 25	17.1755640	3389831
246	6 05 16	15.6843871	4065041	296	8 76 16	17.2046505	3378378
247	6 10 09	15.7162336	4048583	297	8 82 09	17.2336879	3367003
248	6 15 04	15.7480157	4032258	298	8 88 04	17.2626765	3355705
249	6 20 01	15.7797338	4016064	299	8 94 01	17.2916165	3344482
250	6 25 00	15.8113883	4000000	300	9 00 00	17.3205081	3333333

No.	Square	Square Root	Reciprocal .00	No.	Square	Square Root	Reciprocal .00
301	9 06 01	17.3493516	3322259	351	12 32 01	18.7349940	2849003
302	9 12 04	17.3781472	3311258	352	12 39 04	18.7616630	2840909
303	9 18 09	17.4068952	3300330	353	12 46 09	18.7882942	2832861
304	9 24 16	17.4355958	3289474	354	12 53 16	18.8148877	2824859
305	9 30 25	17.4642492	3278689	355	12 60 25	18.8414437	2816901
306	9 36 36	17.4928557	3267974	356	12 67 36	18.8679623	2808989
307	9 42 49	17.5214155	3257329	357	12 74 49	18.8944436	2801120
308	9 48 64	17.5499288	3246753	358	12 81 64	18.9208879	2793296
309	9 54 81	17.5783958	3236246	359	12 88 81	18.9472953	2785515
310	9 61 00	17.6068169	3225806	360	12 96 00	18.9736660	2777778
311	9 67 21	17.6351921	3215434	361	13 03 21	19.0000000	2770083
312	9 73 44	17.6635217	3205128	362	13 10 44	19.0262976	2762431
313	9 79 69	17.6918060	3194888	363	13 17 69	19.0525589	2754821
314	9 85 96	17.7200451	3184713	364	13 24 96	19.0787840	2747253
315	9 92 25	17.7482393	3174603	365	13 32 25	19.1049732	2739726
316	9 98 56	17.7763888	3164557	366	13 39 56	19.1311265	2732240
317	10 04 89	17.8044938	3154574	367	13 46 89	19.1572441	2724796
318	10 11 24	17.8325545	3144654	368	13 54 24	19.1833261	2717391
319	10 17 61	17.8605711	3134796	369	13 61 61	19.2093727	2710027
320	10 24 00	17.8885438	3125000	370	13 69 00	19.2353841	2702703
321	10 30 41	17.9164729	3115265	371	13 76 41	19.2613603	2695418
322	10 36 84	17.9443584	3105590	372	13 83 84	19.2873015	2688172
323	10 43 29	17.9722008	3095975	373	13 91 29	19.3132079	2680965
324	10 49 76	18.0000000	3086420	374	13 98 76	19.3390796	2673797
325	10 56 25	18.0277564	3076923	375	14 06 25	19.3649167	2666667
326	10 62 76	18.0554701	3067485	376	14 13 76	19.3907194	2659574
327	10 69 29	18.0831413	3058104	377	14 21 29	19.4164878	2652520
328	10 75 84	18.1107703	3048780	378	14 28 84	19.4422221	2645503
329	10 82 41	18.1383571	3039514	379	14 36 41	19.4679223	2638522
330	10 89 00	18.1659021	3030303	380	14 44 00	19.4935887	2631579
331	10 95 61	18.1934054	3021148	381	14 51 61	19.5192213	2624672
332	11 02 24	18.2208672	3012048	382	14 59 24	19.5448203	2617801
333	11 08 89	18.2482876	3003003	383	14 66 89	19.5703858	2610966
334	11 15 56	18.2756669	2994012	384	14 74 56	19.5959179	2604167
335	11 22 25	18.3030052	2985075	385	14 82 25	19.6214169	2597403
336	11 28 96	18.3303028	2976190	386	14 89 96	19.6468827	2590674
337	11 35 69	18.3575598	2967359	387	14 97 69	19.6723156	2583979
338	11 42 44	18.3847763	2958580	388	15 05 44	19.6977156	2577320
339	11 49 21	18.4119526	2949853	389	15 13 21	19.7230829	2570694
340	11 56 00	18.4390889	2941176	390	15 21 00	19.7484177	2564103
341	11 62 81	18.4661853	2932551	391	15 28 81	19.7737199	2557545
342	11 69 64	18.4932420	2923977	392	15 36 64	19.7989899	2551020
343	11 76 49	18.5202592	2915452	393	15 44 49	19.8242276	2544529
344	11 83 36	18.5472370	2906977	394	15 52 36	19.8494332	2538071
345	11 90 25	18.5741756	2898551	395	15 60 25	19.8746069	2531646
346	11 97 16	18.6010752	2890173	396	15 68 16	19.8997487	2525253
347	12 04 09	18.6279360	2881844	397	15 76 09	19.9248588	2518892
348	12 11 04	18.6547581	2873563	398	15 84 04	19.9499373	2512563
349	12 18 01	18.6815417	2865330	399	15 92 01	19.9749844	2506266
350	12 25 00	18.7082869	2857143	400	16 00 00	20.0000000	2500000

No.	Square	Square Root	Reciprocal .00	No	Square	Square Root	Reciprocal .00
401	16 08 01	20.0249844	2493766	451	20 34 01	21.2367606	2217295
402	16 16 04	20.0499377	2487562	452	20 43 04	21.2602916	2212389
403	16 24 09	20.0748599	2481390	453	20 52 09	21.2837967	2207506
404	16 32 16	20.0997512	2475248	454	20 61 16	21.3072758	2202643
405	16 40 25	20.1246118	2469136	455	20 70 25	21.3307290	2197802
406	16 48 36	20.1494417	2463054	456	20 79 36	21.3541565	2192982
407	16 56 49	20.1742410	2457002	457	20 88 49	21.3775583	2188184
408	16 64 64	20.1990099	2450980	458	20 97 64	21.4009346	2183406
409	16 72 81	20.2237484	2444988	459	21 06 81	21.4242853	2178649
410	16 81 00	20.2484567	2439024	460	21 16 00	21.4476106	2173913
411	16 89 21	20.2731349	2433090	461	21 25 21	21.4709106	2169197
412	16 97 44	20.2977831	2427184	462	21 34 44	21.4941853	2164502
413	17 05 69	20.3224014	2421308	463	21 43 69	21.5174348	2159827
414	17 13 96	20.3469899	2415459	464	21 52 96	21.5406592	2155172
415	17 22 25	20.3715488	2409639	465	21 62 25	21.5638587	2150538
416	17 30 56	20.3960781	2403846	466	21 71 56	21.5870331	2145923
417	17 38 89	20.4205779	2398082	467	21 80 89	21.6101828	2141328
418	17 47 24	20.4450483	2392344	468	21 90 24	21.6333077	2136752
419	17 55 61	20.4694895	2386635	469	21 99 61	21.6564078	2132196
420	17 64 00	20.4939015	2380952	470	22 09 00	21.6794834	2127660
421	17 72 41	20.5182845	2375297	471	22 18 41	21.7025344	2123142
422	17 80 84	20.5426386	2369668	472	22 27 84	21.7255610	2118644
423	17 89 29	20.5669638	2364066	473	22 37 29	21.7485632	2114165
424	17 97 76	20.5912603	2358491	474	22 46 76	21.7715411	2109705
425	18 06 25	20.6155281	2352941	475	22 56 25	21.7944947	2105263
426	18 14 76	20.6397674	2347418	476	22 65 76	21.8174242	2100840
427	18 23 29	20.6639783	2341920	477	22 75 29	21.8403297	2096436
428	18 31 84	20.6881609	2336449	478	22 84 84	21.8632111	2092050
429	18 40 41	20.7123152	2331002	479	22 94 41	21.8860686	2087683
430	18 49 00	20.7364414	2325581	480	23 04 00	21.9089023	2083333
431	18 57 61	20.7605395	2320186	481	23 13 61	21.9317122	2079002
432	18 66 24	20.7846097	2314815	482	23 23 24	21.9544984	2074689
433	18 74 89	20.8086520	2309469	483	23 32 89	21.9772610	2070393
434	18 83 56	20.8326667	2304147	484	23 42 56	22.0000000	2066116
435	18 92 25	20.8566536	2298851	485	23 52 25	22.0227155	2061856
436	19 00 96	20.8806130	2293578	486	23 61 96	22.0454077	2057613
437	19 09 69	20.9045450	2288330	487	23 71 69	22.0680765	2053388
438	19 18 44	20.9284495	2283105	488	23 81 44	22.0907220	2049180
439	19 27 21	20.9523268	2277904	489	23 91 21	22.1133444	2044990
440	19 36 00	20.9761770	2272727	490	24 01 00	22.1359436	2040816
441	19 44 81	21.0000000	2267574	491	24 10 81	22.1585198	2036660
442	19 53 64	21.0237960	2262443	492	24 20 64	22.1810730	2032520
443	19 62 49	21.0475652	2257336	493	24 30 49	22.2036033	2028398
444	19 71 36	21.0713075	2252252	494	24 40 36	22.2261108	2024291
445	19 80 25	21.0950231	2247191	495	24 50 25	22.2485955	2020202
446	19 89 16	21.1187121	2242152	496	24 60 16	22.2710575	2016129
447	19 98 09	21.1423745	2237136	497	24 70 09	22.2934968	2012072
448	20 07 04	21.1660105	2232143	498	24 80 04	22.3159136	2008032
449	20 16 01	21.1896201	2227171	499	24 90 01	22.3383079	2004008
450	20 25 00	21.2132034	2222222	500	25 00 00	22.3606798	2000000

No.	Square	Square Root	Reciprocal .00	No.	Square	Square Root	Reciprocal .00
501	25 10 01	22.3830293	1996008	551	30 36 01	23.4733892	1814882
502	25 20 04	22.4053565	1992032	552	30 47 04	23.4946802	1811594
503	25 30 09	22.4276615	1988072	553	30 58 09	23.5159520	1808318
504	25 40 16	22.4499443	1984127	554	30 69 16	23.5372046	1805054
505	25 50 25	22.4722051	1980198	555	30 80 25	23.5584380	1801802
506	25 60 36	22.4944438	1976285	556	30 91 36	23.5796522	1798561
507	25 70 49	22.5166605	1972387	557	31 02 49	23.6008474	1795332
508	25 80 64	22.5388553	1968504	558	31 13 64	23.6220236	1792115
509	25 90 81	22.5610283	1964637	559	31 24 81	23.6431808	1788909
510	26 01 00	22.5831796	1960784	560	31 36 00	23.6643191	1785714
511	26 11 21	22.6053091	1956947	561	31 47 21	23.6854386	1782531
512	26 21 44	22.6274170	1953125	562	31 58 44	23.7065392	1779359
513	26 31 69	22.6495033	1949318	563	31 69 69	23.7276210	1776199
514	26 41 96	22.6715681	1945525	564	31 80 96	23.7486842	1773050
515	26 52 25	22.6936114	1941748	565	31 92 25	23.7697286	1769912
516	26 62 56	22.7156334	1937984	566	32 03 56	23.7907545	1766784
517	26 72 89	22.7376340	1934236	567	32 14 89	23.8117618	1763668
518	26 83 24	22.7596134	1930502	568	32 26 24	23 8327506	1760563
519	26 93 61	22.7815715	1926782	569	32 37 61	23.8537209	1757469
520	27 04 00	22.8035085	1923077	570	32 49 00	23.8746728	1754386
521	27 14 41	22.8254244	1919386	571	32 60 41	23.8956063	1751313
522	27 24 84	22.8473193	1915709	572	32 71 84	23 9165215	1748252
523	27 35 29	22.8691933	1912046	573	32 83 29	23.9374184	1745201
524	27 45 76	22.8910463	1908397	574	32 94 76	23.9582971	1742160
525	27 56 25	22.9128785	1904762	575	33 06 25	23 9791576	1739130
526	27 66 76	22.9346899	1001141	576	33 17 76	24 0000000	1736111
527	27 77 29	22.9564806	1897533	577	33 29 29	24.0208243	1733102
528	27 87 84	22.9782506	1893939	578	33 40 84	24 0416306	1730104
529	27 98 41	23.0000000	1890359	579	33 52 41	24.0624188	1727116
530	28 09 00	23.0217289	1886792	580	33 64 00	24 0831891	1724138
531	28 19 61	23.0434372	1883239	581	33 75 61	24 1039416	1721170
532	28 30 24	23.0651252	1879699	582	33 87 24	24 1246762	1718213
533	28 40 89	23.0867928	1876173	583	33 98 89	24 1453929	1715266
534	28 51 56	23.1084400	1872659	584	34 10 56	24 1660919	1712329
535	28 62 25	23.1300670	1869159	585	34 22 25	24 1867732	1709402
536	28 72 96	23.1516738	1865672	586	34 33 96	24 2074369	1706485
537	28 83 69	23.1732605	1862197	587	34 45 69	24.2280829	1703578
538	28 94 44	23.1948270	1858736	588	34 57 44	24 2487113	1700680
539	29 05 21	23.2163735	1855288	589	34 69 21	24. 2693222	1697793
540	29 16 00	23.2379001	1851852	590	34 81 00	24 2899156	1694915
541	29 26 81	23.2594067	1848429	591	34 92 81	24 3104916	1692047
542	29 37 64	23.2808935	1845018	592	35 04 64	24 3310501	1689189
543	29 48 49	23.3023604	1841621	593	35 16 49	24 3515913	1686341
544	29 59 36	23.3238076	1838235	594	35 28 36	24 3721152	1683502
545	29 70 25	23.3452351	1834862	595	35 40 25	24 3926218	1680672
546	29 81 16	23.3666429	1831502	596	35 52 16	24 4131112	1677852
547	29 92 09	23.3880311	1828154	597	35 64 09	24 4335834	1675042
548	30 03 04	23.4093998	1824818	598	35 76 04	24 4540385	1672241
549	30 14 01	23.4307490	1821494	599	35 88 01	24 4744765	1669449
550	30 25 00	23.4520788	1818182	600	36 00 00	24 4948974	1666667

No.	Square	Square Root	Reciprocal .00	No.	Square	Square Root	Reciprocal .00
601	36 12 01	24.5153013	1663894	651	42 38 01	25 5147016	1536098
602	36 24 04	24.5356883	1661130	652	42 51 04	25 5342907	1533742
603	36 36 09	24.5560583	1658375	653	42 64 09	25.5538647	1531394
604	36 48 16	24.5764115	1655629	654	42 77 16	25.5734237	1529052
605	36 60 25	24.5967478	1652893	655	42 90 25	25 5929678	1526718
606	36 72 36	24.6170673	1650165	656	43 03 36	25.6124969	1524390
607	36 84 49	24.6373700	1647446	657	43 16 49	25.6320112	1522070
608	36 96 64	24.6576560	1644737	658	43 29 64	25.6515107	1519757
609	37 08 81	24.6779254	1642036	659	43 42 81	25 6709953	1517451
610	37 21 00	24.6981781	1639344	660	43 56 00	25 6904652	1515152
611	37 33 21	24.7184142	1636661	661	43 69 21	25 7099203	1512859
612	37 45 44	24.7386338	1633987	662	43 82 44	25.7293607	1510574
613	37 57 69	24.7588368	1631321	663	43 95 69	25.7487864	1508296
614	37 69 96	24.7790234	1628664	664	44 08 96	25.7681975	1506024
615	37 82 25	24.7991935	1626016	665	44 22 25	25 7875939	1503759
616	37 94 56	24.8193473	1623377	666	44 35 56	25.8069758	1501502
617	38 06 89	24.8394847	1620746	667	44 48 89	25.8263431	1499250
618	38 19 24	24.8596058	1618123	668	44 62 24	25.8456960	1497006
619	38 31 61	24.8797106	1615509	669	44 75 61	25.8650343	1494768
620	38 44 00	24.8997992	1612903	670	44 89 00	25.8843582	1492537
621	38 56 41	24.9198716	1610306	671	45 02 41	25.9036677	1490313
622	38 68 84	24.9399278	1607717	672	45 15 84	25.9229628	1488095
623	38 81 29	24.9599679	1605136	673	45 29 29	25 9422435	1485884
624	38 93 76	24.9799920	1602564	674	45 42 76	25 9615100	1483680
625	39 06 25	25.0000000	1600000	675	45 56 25	25.9807621	1481481
626	39 18 76	25.0199920	1597444	676	45 69 76	26.0000000	1479290
627	39 31 29	25.0399681	1594896	677	45 83 29	26.0192237	1477105
628	39 43 84	25.0599282	1592357	678	45 96 84	26 0384331	1474926
629	39 56 41	25.0798724	1589825	679	46 10 41	26.0576284	1472754
630	39 69 00	25.0998008	1587302	680	46 24 00	26 0768096	1470588
631	39 81 61	25.1197134	1584786	681	46 37 61	26.0959767	1468429
632	39 94 24	25.1396102	1582278	682	46 51 24	26.1151297	1466276
633	40 06 89	25.1594913	1579779	683	46 64 89	26 1342687	1464129
634	40 19 56	25.1793566	1577287	684	46 78 56	26.1533937	1461988
635	40 32 25	25.1992063	1574803	685	46 92 25	26 1725047	1459854
636	40 44 96	25.2190404	1572327	686	47 05 96	26.1916017	1457726
637	40 57 69	25.2388589	1569859	687	47 19 69	26.2106848	1455604
638	40 70 44	25.2586619	1567398	688	47 33 44	26.2297541	1453488
639	40 83 21	25.2784493	1564945	689	47 47 21	26.2488095	1451379
640	40 96 00	25.2982213	1562500	690	47 61 00	26.2678511	1449275
641	41 08 81	25.3179778	1560062	691	47 74 81	26.2868789	1447178
642	41 21 64	25.3377189	1557632	692	47 88 64	26.3058929	1445087
643	41 34 49	25.3574447	1555210	693	48 02 49	26.3248932	1443001
644	41 47 36	25.3771551	1552795	694	48 16 36	26.3438797	1440922
645	41 60 25	25.3968502	1550388	695	48 30 25	26.3628527	1438849
646	41 73 16	25.4165301	1547988	696	48 44 16	26.3818119	1436782
647	41 86 09	25.4361947	1545595	697	48 58 09	26.4007576	1434720
648	41 99 04	25.4558441	1543210	698	48 72 04	26.4196896	1432665
649	42 12 01	25.4754784	1540832	699	48 86 01	26.4386081	1430615
650	42 25 00	25.4950976	1538462	700	49 00 00	26.4575131	1428571

No.	Square	Square Root	Reciprocal .00	No.	Square	Square Root	Reciprocal .00
701	49 14 01	26.4764046	1426534	751	56 40 01	27.4043792	1331558
702	49 28 04	26.4952826	1424501	752	56 55 04	27.4226184	1329787
703	49 42 09	26.5141472	1422475	753	56 70 09	27.4408455	1328021
704	49 56 16	26.5329983	1420455	754	56 85 16	27.4590604	1326260
705	49 70 25	26.5518361	1418440	755	57 00 25	27.4772633	1324503
706	49 84 36	26.5706605	1416431	756	57 15 36	27.4954542	1322751
707	49 98 49	26.5894716	1414427	757	57 30 49	27.5136330	1321004
708	50 12 64	26.6082694	1412429	758	57 45 64	27.5317998	1319261
709	50 26 81	26.6270539	1410437	759	57 60 81	27.5499546	1317523
710	50 41 00	26.6458252	1408451	760	57 76 00	27.5680975	1315789
711	50 55 21	26.6645833	1406470	761	57 91 21	27.5862284	1314060
712	50 69 44	26.6833281	1404494	762	58 06 44	27.6043475	1312336
713	50 83 69	26.7020598	1402525	763	58 21 69	27.6224546	1310616
714	50 97 96	26.7207784	1400560	764	58 36 96	27.6405499	1308901
715	51 12 25	26.7394839	1398601	765	58 52 25	27.6586334	1307190
716	51 26 56	26.7581763	1396648	766	58 67 56	27.6767050	1305483
717	51 40 89	26.7768557	1394700	767	58 82 89	27.6947648	1303781
718	51 55 24	26.7955220	1392758	768	58 98 24	27.7128129	1302083
719	51 69 61	26.8141754	1390821	769	59 13 61	27.7308492	1300390
720	51 84 00	26.8328157	1388889	770	59 29 00	27.7488739	1298701
721	51 98 41	26.8514432	1386963	771	59 44 41	27.7668868	1297017
722	52 12 84	26.8700577	1385042	772	59 59 84	27.7848880	1295337
723	52 27 29	26.8886593	1383126	773	59 75 29	27.8028775	1293661
724	52 41 76	26.9072481	1381215	774	59 90 76	27.8208555	1291990
725	52 56 25	26.9258240	1379310	775	60 06 25	27.8388218	1290323
726	52 70 76	26.9443872	1377410	776	60 21 76	27.8567766	1288660
727	52 85 29	26.9629375	1375516	777	60 37 29	27.8747197	1287001
728	52 99 84	26.9814751	1373626	778	60 52 84	27.8926514	1285347
729	53 14 41	27.0000000	1371742	779	60 68 41	27.9105715	1283697
730	53 29 00	27.0185122	1369863	780	60 84 00	27.9284801	1282051
731	53 43 61	27.0370117	1367989	781	60 99 61	27.9463772	1280410
732	53 58 24	27.0554985	1366120	782	61 15 24	27.9642629	1278772
733	53 72 89	27.0739727	1364256	783	61 30 89	27.9821372	1277139
734	53 87 56	27.0924344	1362398	784	61 46 56	28.0000000	1275510
735	54 02 25	27.1108834	1360544	785	61 62 25	28.0178515	1273885
736	54 16 96	27.1293199	1358696	786	61 77 96	28.0356915	1272265
737	54 31 69	27.1477439	1356852	787	61 93 69	28.0535203	1270648
738	54 46 44	27.1661554	1355014	788	62 09 44	28.0713377	1269036
739	54 61 21	27.1845544	1353180	789	62 25 21	28.0891438	1267427
740	54 76 00	27.2029410	1351351	790	62 41 00	28.1069386	1265823
741	54 90 81	27.2213152	1349528	791	62 56 81	28.1247222	1264223
742	55 05 64	27.2396769	1347709	792	62 72 64	28.1424946	1262626
743	55 20 49	27.2580263	1345895	793	62 88 49	28.1602557	1261034
744	55 35 36	27.2763634	1344086	794	63 04 36	28.1780056	1259446
745	55 50 25	27.2946881	1342282	795	63 20 25	28.1957444	1257862
746	55 65 16	27.3130006	1340483	796	63 36 16	28.2134720	1256281
747	55 80 09	27.3313007	1338688	797	63 52 09	28.2311884	1254705
748	55 95 04	27.3495887	1336898	798	63 68 04	28.2488938	1253133
749	56 10 01	27.3678644	1335113	799	63 84 01	28.2665881	1251564
750	56 25 00	27.3861279	1333333	800	64 00 00	28.2842712	1250000

No.	Square	Square Root	Reciprocal .00	No.	Square	Square Root	Reciprocal .00
801	64 16 01	28.3019434	1248439	851	72 42 01	29.1719043	1175088
802	64 32 04	28.3196045	1246883	852	72 59 04	29.1890390	1173709
803	64 48 09	28.3372546	1245330	853	72 76 09	29.2061637	1172333
804	64 64 16	28.3548938	1243781	854	72 93 16	29.2232784	1170960
805	64 80 25	28.3725219	1242236	855	73 10 25	29.2403830	1169591
806	64 96 36	28.3901391	1240695	856	73 27 36	29.2574777	1168224
807	65 12 49	28.4077454	1239157	857	73 44 49	29.2745623	1166861
808	65 28 64	28.4253408	1237624	858	73 61 64	29.2916370	1165501
809	65 44 81	28.4429253	1236094	859	73 78 81	29.3087018	1164144
810	65 61 00	28.4604989	1234568	860	73 96 00	29.3257566	1162791
811	65 77 21	28.4780617	1233046	861	74 13 21	29.3428015	1161440
812	65 93 44	28.4956137	1231527	862	74 30 44	29.3598365	1160093
813	66 09 69	28.5131549	1230012	863	74 47 69	29.3768616	1158749
814	66 25 96	28.5306852	1228501	864	74 64 96	29.3938769	1157407
815	66 42 25	28.5482048	1226994	865	74 82 25	29.4108823	1156069
816	66 58 56	28.5657137	1225490	866	74 99 56	29.4278779	1154734
817	66 74 89	28.5832119	1223990	867	75 16 89	29.4448637	1153403
818	66 91 24	28.6006993	1222494	868	75 34 24	29.4618397	1152074
819	67 07 61	28.6181760	1221001	869	75 51 61	29.4788059	1150748
820	67 24 00	28.6356421	1219512	870	75 69 00	29.4957624	1149425
821	67 40 41	28.6530976	1218027	871	75 86 41	29.5127091	1148106
822	67 56 84	28.6705424	1216545	872	76 03 84	29.5296461	1146789
823	67 73 29	28.6879766	1215067	873	76 21 29	29.5465734	1145475
824	67 89 76	28.7054002	1213592	874	76 38 76	29.5634910	1144165
825	68 06 25	28.7228132	1212121	875	76 56 25	29.5803989	1142857
826	68 22 76	28.7402157	1210654	876	76 73 76	29.5972972	1141553
827	68 39 29	28.7576077	1209190	877	76 91 29	29.6141858	1140251
828	68 55 84	28.7749891	1207729	878	77 08 84	29.6310648	1138952
829	68 72 41	28.7923601	1206273	879	77 26 41	29.6479342	1137656
830	68 89 00	28.8097206	1204819	880	77 44 00	29.6647939	1136364
831	69 05 61	28.8270706	1203369	881	77 61 61	29.6816442	1135074
832	69 22 24	28.8444102	1201923	882	77 79 24	29.6984848	1133787
833	69 38 89	28.8617394	1200480	883	77 96 89	29.7153159	1132503
834	69 55 56	28.8790582	1199041	884	78 14 56	29.7321375	1131222
835	69 72 25	28.8963666	1197605	885	78 32 25	29.7489496	1129944
836	69 88 96	28.9136646	1196172	886	78 49 96	29.7657521	1128668
837	70 05 69	28.9309523	1194743	887	78 67 69	29.7825452	1127396
838	70 22 44	28.9482297	1193317	888	78 85 44	29.7993289	1126126
839	70 39 21	28.9654967	1191895	889	79 03 21	29.8161030	1124859
840	70 56 00	28.9827535	1190476	890	79 21 00	29.8328678	1123596
841	70 72 81	29.0000000	1189061	891	79 38 81	29.8496231	1122334
842	70 89 64	29.0172363	1187648	892	79 56 64	29.8663690	1121076
843	71 06 49	29.0344623	1186240	893	79 74 49	29.8831056	1119821
844	71 23 36	29.0516781	1184834	894	79 92 36	29.8998328	1118568
845	71 40 25	29.0688837	1183432	895	80 10 25	29.9165506	1117318
846	71 57 16	29.0860791	1182033	896	80 28 16	29.9332591	1116071
847	71 74 09	29.1032644	1180638	897	80 46 09	29.9499583	1114827
848	71 91 04	29.1204396	1179245	898	80 64 04	29.9666481	1113586
849	72 08 01	29.1376046	1177856	899	80 82 01	29.9833287	1112347
850	72 25 00	29.1547595	1176471	900	81 00 00	30.0000000	1111111

No.	Square	Square Root	Reciprocal .00	No.	Square	Square Root	Reciprocal .00
901	81 18 01	30.0166620	1109878	951	90 44 01	30.8382879	1051525
902	81 36 04	30.0333148	1108647	952	90 63 04	30.8544972	1050420
903	81 54 09	30.0499584	1107420	953	90 82 09	30.8706981	1049318
904	81 72 16	30.0665928	1106195	954	91 01 16	30.8868904	1048218
905	81 90 25	30.0832179	1104972	955	91 20 25	30.9030743	1047120
906	82 08 36	30.0998339	1103753	956	91 39 36	30.9192497	1046025
907	82 26 49	30.1164407	1102536	957	91 58 49	30.9354166	1044932
908	82 44 64	30.1330383	1101322	958	91 77 64	30.9515751	1043841
909	82 62 81	30.1496269	1100110	959	91 96 81	30.9677251	1042753
910	82 81 00	30.1662063	1098901	960	92 16 00	30.9838668	1041667
911	82 99 21	30.1827765	1097695	961	92 35 21	31.0000000	1040583
912	83 17 44	30.1993377	1096491	962	92 54 44	31.0161248	1039501
913	83 35 69	30.2158899	1095290	963	92 73 69	31.0322413	1038422
914	83 53 96	30.2324329	1094092	964	92 92 96	31.0483494	1037344
915	83 72 25	30.2489669	1092896	965	93 12 25	31.0644491	1036269
916	83 90 56	30.2654919	1091703	966	93 31 56	31.0805405	1035197
917	84 08 89	30.2820079	1090513	967	93 50 89	31.0966236	1034126
918	84 27 24	30.2985148	1089325	968	93 70 24	31.1126984	1033058
919	84 45 61	30.3150128	1088139	969	93 89 61	31.1287648	1031992
920	84 64 00	30.3315018	1086957	970	94 09 00	31.1448230	1030928
921	84 82 41	30.3479818	1085776	971	94 28 41	31.1608729	1029866
922	85 00 84	30.3644529	1084599	972	94 47 84	31.1769145	1028807
923	85 19 29	30.3809151	1083424	973	94 67 29	31.1929479	1027749
924	85 37 76	30.3973683	1082251	974	94 86 76	31.2089731	1026694
925	85 56 25	30.4138127	1081081	975	95 06 25	31.2249900	1025641
926	85 74 76	30.4302481	1079914	976	95 25 76	31.2409987	1024590
927	85 93 29	30.4466747	1078749	977	95 45 29	31.2569992	1023541
928	86 11 84	30.4630924	1077586	978	95 64 84	31.2729915	1022495
929	86 30 41	30.4795013	1076426	979	95 84 41	31.2889757	1021450
930	86 49 00	30.4959014	1075269	980	96 04 00	31.3049517	1020408
931	86 67 61	30.5122926	1074114	981	96 23 61	31.3209195	1019368
932	86 86 24	30.5286750	1072961	982	96 43 24	31.3368792	1018330
933	87 04 89	30.5450487	1071811	983	96 62 89	31.3528308	1017294
934	87 23 56	30.5614136	1070664	984	96 82 56	31.3687743	1016260
935	87 42 25	30.5777697	1069519	985	97 02 25	31.3847097	1015228
936	87 60 96	30.5941171	1068376	986	97 21 96	31.4006369	1014199
937	87 79 69	30.6104557	1067236	987	97 41 69	31.4165561	1013171
938	87 98 44	30.6267857	1066098	988	97 61 44	31.4324673	1012146
939	88 17 21	30.6431069	1064963	989	97 81 21	31.4483704	1011122
940	88 36 00	30.6594194	1063830	990	98 01 00	31.4642654	1010101
941	88 54 81	30.6757233	1062699	991	98 20 81	31.4801525	1009082
942	88 73 64	30.6920185	1061571	992	98 40 64	31.4960315	1008065
943	88 92 49	30.7083051	1060445	993	98 60 49	31.5119025	1007049
944	89 11 36	30.7245830	1059322	994	98 80 36	31.5277655	1006036
945	89 30 25	30.7408523	1058201	995	99 00 25	31.5436206	1005025
946	89 49 16	30.7571130	1057082	996	99 20 16	31.5594677	1004016
947	89 68 09	30.7733651	1055966	997	99 40 09	31.5753068	1003009
948	89 87 04	30.7896086	1054852	998	99 60 04	31.5911380	1002004
949	90 06 01	30.8058436	1053741	999	99 80 01	31.6069613	1001001
950	90 25 00	30.8220700	1052632	1000	1 00 00 00	31.6227766	1000000

Appendix XIV
LOGARITHMS OF NUMBERS

The logarithm of a number (N in the table) is the power to which 10 must be raised to produce N. A logarithm is composed of two parts, the *characteristic* and the *mantissa*.

The characteristic, which is always an integer or zero, is determined by the following rule:

If $N \geq 1$, the characteristic is positive and its value is one less than the number of digits in N which are to the left of the decimal point. For example,

N	*Characteristic*
4568	3
456.8	2
45.68	1
4.568	0

If $N < 1$, the characteristic is negative and its value is one more than the number of zeros just to the right of the decimal point. For example,

N	*Characteristic*
0.4568	-1 or $9 - 10$
0.04568	-2 or $8 - 10$
0.004568	-3 or $7 - 10$
0.0004568	-4 or $6 - 10$

The mantissa, which is always a decimal or zero, is obtained from a table such as that which follows. The mantissa is the same for any given combination of digits no matter where the decimal point may be placed. Thus, for all of the eight N's just listed, the mantissa is 0.659726.

Combining the characteristic and the mantissa gives the logarithm. For the eight values of N given above,

N	*Logarithm*
4568	3.659726
456.8	2.659726
45.68	1.659726
4.568	0.659726
0.4568	$9.659726 - 10$
0.04568	$8.659726 - 10$
0.004568	$7.659726 - 10$
0.0004568	$6.659726 - 10$

Table of Logarithms

N.	0	1	2	3	4	5	6	7	8	9	D.
100	000000	000434	000868	001301	001734	002166	002598	003029	003461	003891	432
1	4321	4751	5181	5609	6038	6466	6894	7321	7748	8174	423
2	8600	9026	9451	9876	010300	010724	011147	011570	011993	012415	424
3	012837	013259	013680	014100	4521	4940	5360	5779	6197	6616	420
4	7033	7451	7868	8284	8700	9116	9532	9947	020361	020775	416
105	021189	021603	022016	022428	022841	023252	023664	024075	4486	4896	412
6	5306	5715	6125	6533	6942	7350	7757	8164	8571	8978	408
7	9384	9789	030195	030600	031004	031408	031812	032216	032619	033021	404
8	033424	033826	4227	4628	5029	5430	5830	6230	6629	7028	400
9	7426	7825	8223	8620	9017	9414	9811	040207	040602	040998	397
110	041393	041787	042182	042576	042969	043362	043755	044148	044540	044932	393
1	5323	5714	6105	6495	6885	7275	7664	8053	8442	8830	390
2	9218	9606	9993	050380	050766	051153	051538	051924	052309	052694	386
3	053078	053463	053846	4230	4613	4996	5378	5760	6142	6524	383
4	6905	7286	7666	8046	8426	8805	9185	9563	9942	060320	379
115	060698	061075	061452	061829	062206	062582	062958	063333	063709	4083	376
6	4458	4832	5206	5580	5953	6326	6699	7071	7443	7815	373
7	8186	8557	8928	9298	9668	070038	070407	070776	071145	071514	370
8	071882	072250	072617	072985	073352	3718	4085	4451	4816	5182	366
9	5547	5912	6276	6640	7004	7368	7731	8094	8457	8819	363
120	079181	079543	079904	080266	080626	080987	081347	081707	082067	082426	360
1	082785	083144	083503	3861	4219	4576	4934	5291	5647	6004	357
2	6360	6716	7071	7426	7781	8136	8490	8845	9198	9552	355
3	9905	090258	090611	090963	091315	091667	092018	092370	092721	093071	352
4	093422	3772	4122	4471	4820	5169	5518	5866	6215	6562	349
125	6910	7257	7604	7951	8298	8644	8990	9335	9681	100026	346
6	100371	100715	101059	101403	101747	102091	102434	102777	103119	3462	343
7	3804	4146	4487	4828	5169	5510	5851	6191	6531	6871	341
8	7210	7549	7888	8227	8565	8903	9241	9579	9916	110253	338
9	110590	110926	111263	111599	111934	112270	112605	112940	113275	3609	335
130	113943	114277	114611	114944	115278	115611	115943	116276	116608	116940	333
1	7271	7603	7934	8265	8595	8926	9256	9586	9915	120245	330
2	120574	120903	121231	121560	121888	122216	122544	122871	123198	3525	328
3	3852	4178	4504	4830	5156	5481	5806	6131	6456	6781	325
4	7105	7429	7753	8076	8399	8722	9045	9368	9690	130012	323
135	130334	130655	130977	131298	131619	131939	132260	132580	132900	3219	321
6	3539	3858	4177	4496	4814	5133	5451	5769	6086	6403	318
7	6721	7037	7354	7671	7987	8303	8618	8934	9249	9564	316
8	9879	140194	140508	140822	141136	141450	141763	142076	142389	142702	314
9	143015	3327	3639	3951	4263	4574	4885	5196	5507	5818	311
140	146128	146438	146748	147058	147367	147676	147985	148294	148603	148911	309
1	9219	9527	9835	150142	150449	150756	151063	151370	151676	151982	307
2	152288	152594	152900	3205	3510	3815	4120	4424	4728	5032	305
3	5336	5640	5943	6246	6549	6852	7154	7457	7759	8061	303
4	8362	8664	8965	9266	9567	9868	160168	160469	160769	161068	301
145	161368	161667	161967	162266	162564	162863	3161	3460	3758	4055	299
6	4353	4650	4947	5244	5541	5838	6134	6430	6726	7022	297
7	7317	7613	7908	8203	8497	8792	9086	9380	9674	9968	295
8	170262	170555	170848	171141	171434	171726	172019	172311	172603	172895	293
9	3186	3478	3769	4060	4351	4641	4932	5222	5512	5802	291
150	176091	176381	176670	176959	177248	177536	177825	178113	178401	178689	289
1	8977	9264	9552	9839	180126	180413	180699	180986	181272	181558	287
2	181844	182129	182415	182700	2985	3270	3555	3839	4123	4407	285
3	4691	4975	5259	5542	5825	6108	6391	6674	6956	7239	283
4	7521	7803	8084	8366	8647	8928	9209	9490	9771	190051	281
155	190332	190612	190892	191171	191451	191730	192010	192289	192567	2846	279
6	3125	3403	3681	3959	4237	4514	4792	5069	5346	5623	278
7	5900	6176	6453	6729	7005	7281	7556	7832	8107	8382	276
8	8657	8932	9206	9481	9755	200029	200303	200577	200850	201124	274
9	201397	201670	201943	202216	202488	2761	3033	3305	3577	3848	272
N.	0	1	2	3	4	5	6	7	8	9	D.

Log e = 0.434295; log π = 0.497150; log $\sqrt{\pi}$ = 0.248575.

N.	0	1	2	3	4	5	6	7	8	9	D.
160	204120	204391	204663	204934	205204	205475	205746	206016	206286	206556	271
1	6826	7096	7365	7634	7904	8173	8441	8710	8979	9247	269
2	9515	9783	210051	210319	210586	210853	211121	211388	211654	211921	267
3	212188	212454	2720	2986	3252	3518	3783	4049	4314	4579	266
4	4844	5109	5373	5638	5902	6166	6430	6694	6957	7221	264
165	7484	7747	8010	8273	8536	8798	9060	9323	9585	9846	262
6	220108	220370	220631	220892	221153	221414	221675	221936	222196	222456	261
7	2716	2976	3236	3496	3755	4015	4274	4533	4792	5051	259
8	5309	5568	5826	6084	6342	6600	6858	7115	7372	7630	258
9	7887	8144	8400	8657	8913	9170	9426	9682	9938	230193	256
170	230449	230704	230960	231215	231470	231724	231979	232234	232488	232742	255
1	2996	3250	3504	3757	4011	4264	4517	4770	5023	5276	253
2	5528	5781	6033	6285	6537	6789	7041	7292	7544	7795	252
3	8046	8297	8548	8799	9049	9299	9550	9800	240050	240300	250
4	240549	240799	241048	241297	241546	241795	242044	242293	2541	2790	249
175	3038	3286	3534	3782	4030	4277	4525	4772	5019	5266	248
6	5513	5759	6006	6252	6499	6745	6991	7237	7482	7728	246
7	7973	8219	8454	8709	8954	9198	9443	9687	9932	250176	245
8	250420	250664	250908	251151	251395	251638	251881	252125	252368	2610	243
9	2853	3096	3338	3580	3822	4064	4306	4548	4790	5031	242
180	255273	255514	255755	255996	256237	256477	256718	256958	257198	257439	241
1	7679	7918	8158	8398	8637	8877	9116	9355	9594	9833	239
2	260071	260310	260548	260787	261025	261263	261501	261739	261976	262214	238
3	2451	2688	2925	3162	3399	3636	3873	4109	4346	4582	237
4	4818	5054	5290	5525	5761	5996	6232	6467	6702	6937	235
185	7172	7406	7641	7875	8110	8344	8578	8812	9046	9279	234
6	9513	9746	9980	270213	270446	270679	270912	271144	271377	271609	233
7	271842	272074	272306	2538	2770	3001	3233	3464	3696	3927	232
8	4158	4389	4620	4850	5081	5311	5542	5772	6002	6232	230
9	6462	6692	6921	7151	7380	7609	7838	8067	8296	8525	229
190	278754	278982	279211	279439	279667	279895	280123	280351	280578	280806	228
1	281033	281261	281488	281715	281942	282169	2396	2622	2849	3075	227
2	3301	3527	3753	3979	4205	4431	4656	4882	5107	5332	226
3	5557	5782	6007	6232	6456	6681	6905	7130	7354	7578	225
4	7802	8026	8249	8473	8696	8920	9143	9366	9589	9812	223
195	290035	290257	290480	290702	290925	291147	291369	291591	291813	292034	222
6	2256	2478	2699	2920	3141	3363	3584	3804	4025	4246	221
7	4466	4687	4907	5127	5347	5567	5787	6007	6226	6446	220
8	6665	6884	7104	7323	7542	7761	7979	8198	8416	8635	219
9	8853	9071	9289	9507	9725	9943	300161	300378	300595	300813	218
200	301030	301247	301464	301681	301898	302114	302331	302547	302764	302980	217
1	3196	3412	3628	3844	4059	4275	4491	4706	4921	5136	216
2	5351	5566	5781	5996	6211	6425	6639	6854	7068	7282	215
3	7496	7710	7924	8137	8351	8564	8778	8991	9204	9417	213
4	9630	9843	310056	310268	310481	310693	310906	311118	311330	311542	212
205	311754	311966	2177	2389	2600	2812	3023	3234	3445	3656	211
6	3867	4078	4289	4499	4710	4920	5130	5340	5551	5760	210
7	5970	6180	6390	6599	6809	7018	7227	7436	7646	7854	209
8	8063	8272	8481	8689	8898	9106	9314	9522	9730	9938	208
9	320146	320354	320562	320769	320977	321184	321391	321598	321805	322012	207
210	322219	322426	322633	322839	323046	323252	323458	323665	323871	324077	206
1	4282	4488	4694	4899	5105	5310	5516	5721	5926	6131	205
2	6336	6541	6745	6950	7155	7359	7563	7767	7972	8176	204
3	8380	8583	8787	8991	9194	9398	9601	9805	330008	330211	203
4	330414	330617	330819	331022	331225	331427	331630	331832	2034	2236	202
215	2438	2640	2842	3044	3246	3447	3649	3850	4051	4253	202
6	4454	4655	4856	5057	5257	5458	5658	5859	6059	6260	201
7	6460	6660	6860	7060	7260	7459	7659	7858	8058	8257	200
8	8456	8656	8855	9054	9253	9451	9650	9849	340047	340246	199
9	340444	340642	340841	341039	341237	341435	341632	341830	2028	2225	198
N.	0	1	2	3	4	5	6	7	8	9	D.

N.	0	1	2	3	4	5	6	7	8	9	D.
220	342423	342620	342817	343014	343212	343409	343606	343802	343999	344196	197
1	4392	4589	4785	4981	5178	5374	5570	5766	5962	6157	196
2	6353	6549	6744	6939	7135	7330	7525	7720	7915	8110	195
3	8305	8500	8694	8889	9083	9278	9472	9666	9860	350054	194
4	350248	350442	350636	350829	351023	351216	351410	351603	351796	1989	193
225	2183	2375	2568	2761	2954	3147	3339	3532	3724	3916	193
6	4108	4301	4493	4685	4876	5068	5260	5452	5643	5834	192
7	6026	6217	6408	6599	6790	6981	7172	7363	7554	7744	191
8	7935	8125	8316	8506	8696	8886	9076	9266	9456	9646	190
9	9835	360025	360215	360404	360593	360783	360972	361161	361350	361539	189
230	361728	361917	362105	362294	362482	362671	362859	363048	363236	363424	188
1	3612	3800	3988	4176	4363	4551	4739	4926	5113	5301	188
2	5488	5675	5862	6049	6236	6423	6610	6796	6983	7169	187
3	7356	7542	7729	7915	8101	8287	8473	8659	8845	9030	186
4	9216	9401	9587	9772	9958	370143	370328	370513	370698	370883	185
235	371068	371253	371437	371622	371806	1991	2175	2360	2544	2728	184
6	2912	3096	3280	3464	3647	3831	4015	4198	4382	4565	184
7	4748	4932	5115	5298	5481	5664	5846	6029	6212	6394	183
8	6577	6759	6942	7124	7306	7488	7670	7852	8034	8216	182
9	8398	8580	8761	8943	9124	9306	9487	9668	9849	380030	181
240	380211	380392	380573	380754	380934	381115	381296	381476	381656	381837	181
1	2017	2197	2377	2557	2737	2917	3097	3277	3456	3636	180
2	3815	3995	4174	4353	4533	4712	4891	5070	5249	5428	179
3	5606	5785	5964	6142	6321	6499	6677	6856	7034	7212	178
4	7390	7568	7746	7923	8101	8279	8456	8634	8811	8989	178
245	9166	9343	9520	9698	9875	390051	390228	390405	390582	390759	177
6	390935	391112	391288	391464	391641	1817	1993	2169	2345	2521	176
7	2697	2873	3048	3224	3400	3575	3751	3926	4101	4277	176
8	4452	4627	4802	4977	5152	5326	5501	5676	5850	6025	175
9	6199	6374	6548	6722	6896	7071	7245	7419	7592	7766	174
250	397940	398114	398287	398461	398634	398808	398981	399154	399328	399501	173
1	9674	9847	400020	400192	400365	400538	400711	400883	401056	401228	173
2	401401	401573	1745	1917	2089	2261	2433	2605	2777	2949	172
3	3121	3292	3464	3635	3807	3978	4149	4320	4492	4663	171
4	4834	5005	5176	5346	5517	5688	5858	6029	6199	6370	171
255	6540	6710	6881	7051	7221	7391	7561	7731	7901	8070	170
6	8240	8410	8579	8749	8918	9087	9257	9426	9595	9764	169
7	9933	410102	410271	410440	410609	410777	410946	411114	411283	411451	169
8	411620	1788	1956	2124	2293	2461	2629	2796	2964	3132	168
9	3300	3467	3635	3803	3970	4137	4305	4472	4639	4806	167
260	414973	415140	415307	415474	415641	415808	415974	416141	416308	416474	167
1	6641	6807	6973	7139	7306	7472	7638	7804	7970	8135	166
2	8301	8467	8633	8798	8964	9129	9295	9460	9625	9791	165
3	9956	420121	420286	420451	420616	420781	420945	421110	421275	421439	165
4	421604	1768	1933	2097	2261	2426	2590	2754	2918	3082	164
265	3246	3410	3574	3737	3901	4065	4228	4392	4555	4718	164
6	4882	5045	5208	5371	5534	5697	5860	6023	6186	6349	163
7	6511	6674	6836	6999	7161	7324	7486	7648	7811	7973	162
8	8135	8297	8459	8621	8783	8944	9106	9268	9429	9591	162
9	9752	9914	430075	430236	430398	430559	430720	430881	431042	431203	161
270	431364	431525	431685	431846	432007	432167	432328	432488	432649	432809	161
1	2969	3130	3290	3450	3610	3770	3930	4090	4249	4409	160
2	4569	4729	4888	5048	5207	5367	5526	5685	5844	6004	159
3	6163	6322	6481	6640	6799	6957	7116	7275	7433	7592	159
4	7751	7909	8067	8226	8384	8542	8701	8859	9017	9175	158
275	9333	9491	9648	9806	9964	440122	440279	440437	440594	440752	158
6	440909	441066	441224	441381	441538	1695	1852	2009	2166	2323	157
7	2480	2637	2793	2950	3106	3263	3419	3576	3732	3889	157
8	4045	4201	4357	4513	4669	4825	4981	5137	5293	5449	156
9	5604	5760	5915	6071	6226	6382	6537	6692	6848	7003	155
N.	0	1	2	3	4	5	6	7	8	9	D.

N.	0	1	2	3	4	5	6	7	8	9	D.
280	447158	447313	447468	447623	447778	447933	448088	448242	448397	448552	155
1	8706	8861	9015	9170	9324	9478	9633	9787	9941	450095	154
2	450249	450403	450557	450711	450865	451018	451172	451326	451479	1633	154
3	1786	1940	2093	2247	2400	2553	2706	2859	3012	3165	153
4	3318	3471	3624	3777	3930	4082	4235	4387	4540	4692	153
285	4845	4997	5150	5302	5454	5606	5758	5910	6062	6214	152
6	6366	6518	6670	6821	6973	7125	7276	7428	7579	7731	152
7	7882	8033	8184	8336	8487	8638	8789	8940	9091	9242	151
8	9392	9543	9694	9845	9995	460146	460296	460447	460597	460748	151
9	460898	461048	461198	461348	461499	1649	1799	1948	2098	2248	150
290	462398	462548	462697	462847	462997	463146	463296	463445	463594	463744	150
1	3893	4042	4191	4340	4490	4639	4788	4936	5085	5234	149
2	5383	5532	5680	5829	5977	6126	6274	6423	6571	6719	149
3	6868	7016	7164	7312	7460	7608	7756	7904	8052	8200	148
4	8347	8495	8643	8790	8938	9085	9233	9380	9527	9675	148
295	9822	9969	470116	470263	470410	470557	470704	470851	470998	471145	147
6	471292	471438	1585	1732	1878	2025	2171	2318	2464	2610	146
7	2756	2903	3049	3195	3341	3487	3633	3779	3925	4071	146
8	4216	4362	4508	4653	4799	4944	5090	5235	5381	5526	146
9	5671	5816	5962	6107	6252	6397	6542	6687	6832	6976	145
300	477121	477266	477411	477555	477700	477844	477989	478133	478278	478422	145
1	8566	8711	8855	8999	9143	9287	9431	9575	9719	9863	144
2	480007	480151	480294	480438	480582	480725	480869	481012	481156	481299	144
3	1443	1586	1729	1872	2016	2159	2302	2445	2588	2731	143
4	2874	3016	3159	3302	3445	3587	3730	3872	4015	4157	143
305	4300	4442	4585	4727	4869	5011	5153	5295	5437	5579	142
6	5721	5863	6005	6147	6289	6430	6572	6714	6855	6997	142
7	7138	7280	7421	7563	7704	7845	7986	8127	8269	8410	141
8	8551	8692	8833	8974	9114	9255	9396	9537	9677	9818	141
9	9958	490099	490239	490380	490520	490661	490801	490941	491081	491222	140
310	491362	491502	491642	491782	491922	492062	492201	492341	492481	492621	140
1	2760	2900	3040	3179	3319	3458	3597	3737	3876	4015	139
2	4155	4294	4433	4572	4711	4850	4989	5128	5267	5406	139
3	5544	5683	5822	5960	6099	6238	6376	6515	6653	6791	139
4	6930	7068	7206	7344	7483	7621	7759	7897	8035	8173	138
315	8311	8448	8586	8724	8862	8999	9137	9275	9412	9550	138
6	9687	9824	9962	500099	500236	500374	500511	500648	500785	500922	137
7	501059	501196	501333	1470	1607	1744	1880	2017	2154	2291	137
8	2427	2564	2700	2837	2973	3109	3246	3382	3518	3655	136
9	3791	3927	4063	4199	4335	4471	4607	4743	4878	5014	136
320	505150	505286	505421	505557	505693	505828	505964	506099	506234	506370	136
1	6505	6640	6776	6911	7046	7181	7316	7451	7586	7721	135
2	7856	7991	8126	8260	8395	8530	8664	8799	8934	9068	135
3	9203	9337	9471	9606	9740	9874	510009	510143	510277	510411	134
4	510545	510679	510813	510947	511081	511215	1349	1482	1616	1750	134
325	1883	2017	2151	2284	2418	2551	2684	2818	2951	3084	133
6	3218	3351	3484	3617	3750	3883	4016	4149	4282	4415	133
7	4548	4681	4813	4946	5079	5211	5344	5476	5609	5741	133
8	5874	6006	6139	6271	6403	6535	6668	6800	6932	7064	132
9	7196	7328	7460	7592	7724	7855	7987	8119	8251	8382	132
330	518514	518646	518777	518909	519040	519171	519303	519434	519566	519697	131
1	9828	9959	520090	520221	520353	520484	520615	520745	520876	521007	131
2	521138	521269	1400	1530	1661	1792	1922	2053	2183	2314	131
3	2444	2575	2705	2835	2966	3096	3226	3356	3486	3616	130
4	3746	3876	4006	4136	4266	4396	4526	4656	4785	4915	130
335	5045	5174	5304	5434	5563	5693	5822	5951	6081	6210	129
6	6339	6469	6598	6727	6856	6985	7114	7243	7372	7501	129
7	7630	7759	7888	8016	8145	8274	8402	8531	8660	8788	129
8	8917	9045	9174	9302	9430	9559	9687	9815	9943	530072	128
9	530200	530328	530456	530584	530712	530840	530968	531096	531223	1351	128
N.	0	1	2	3	4	5	6	7	8	9	D.

N.	0	1	2	3	4	5	6	7	8	9	D.
340	531479	531607	531734	531862	531990	532117	532245	532372	532500	532627	128
1	2754	2882	3009	3136	3264	3391	3518	3645	3772	3899	127
2	4026	4153	4280	4407	4534	4661	4787	4914	5041	5167	127
3	5294	5421	5547	5674	5800	5927	6053	6180	6306	6432	126
4	6558	6685	6811	6937	7063	7189	7315	7441	7567	7693	126
345	7819	7945	8071	8197	8322	8448	8574	8699	8825	8951	126
6	9076	9202	9327	9452	9578	9703	9829	9954	540079	540204	125
7	540329	540455	540580	540705	540830	540955	541080	541205	1330	1454	125
8	1579	1704	1829	1953	2078	2203	2327	2452	2576	2701	125
9	2825	2950	3074	3199	3323	3447	3571	3696	3820	3944	124
350	544068	544192	544316	544440	544564	544688	544812	544936	545060	545183	124
1	5307	5431	5555	5678	5802	5925	6049	6172	6296	6419	124
2	6543	6666	6789	6913	7036	7159	7282	7405	7529	7652	123
3	7775	7898	8021	8144	8257	8389	8512	8635	8758	8881	123
4	9003	9126	9249	9371	9494	9616	9739	9861	9984	550106	123
355	550228	550351	550473	550595	550717	550840	550962	551084	551206	1328	122
6	1450	1572	1694	1816	1938	2060	2181	2303	2425	2547	122
7	2668	2790	2911	3033	3155	3276	3398	3519	3640	3762	121
8	3883	4004	4126	4247	4368	4489	4610	4731	4852	4973	12.
9	5094	5215	5336	5457	5578	5699	5820	5940	6061	6182	121
360	556303	556423	556544	556664	556785	556905	557026	557146	557267	557387	120
1	7507	7627	7748	7868	7988	8108	8228	8349	8469	8589	120
2	8709	8829	8948	9068	9188	9308	9428	9548	9667	9787	120
3	9907	560026	560146	560265	560385	560504	560624	560743	560863	560982	119
4	561101	1221	1340	1459	1578	1698	1817	1936	2055	2174	119
365	2293	2412	2531	2650	2769	2887	3006	3125	3244	3362	119
6	3481	3600	3718	3837	3955	4074	4192	4311	4429	4548	119
7	4666	4784	4903	5021	5139	5257	5376	5494	5612	5730	118
8	5848	5966	6084	6202	6320	6437	6555	6673	6791	6909	118
9	7026	7144	7262	7379	7497	7614	7732	7849	7967	8084	118
370	568202	568319	568436	568554	568671	568788	568905	569023	569140	569257	117
1	9374	9491	9608	9725	9842	9959	570076	570193	570309	570426	117
2	570543	570660	570776	570893	571010	571126	1243	1359	1476	1592	117
3	1709	1825	1942	2058	2174	2291	2407	2523	2639	2755	116
4	2872	2988	3104	3220	3336	3452	3568	3684	3800	3915	116
375	4031	4147	4263	4379	4494	4610	4726	4841	4957	5072	116
6	5188	5303	5419	5534	5650	5765	5880	5996	6111	6226	115
7	6341	6457	6572	6687	6802	6917	7032	7147	7262	7377	115
8	7492	7607	7722	7836	7951	8066	8181	8295	8410	8525	115
9	8639	8754	8868	8983	9097	9212	9326	9441	9555	9669	114
380	579784	579898	580012	580126	580241	580355	580469	580583	580697	580811	114
1	580925	581039	1153	1267	1381	1495	1608	1722	1836	1950	114
2	2063	2177	2291	2404	2518	2631	2745	2858	2972	3085	114
3	3199	3312	3426	3539	3652	3765	3879	3992	4105	4218	113
4	4331	4444	4557	4670	4783	4896	5009	5122	5235	5348	113
385	5461	5574	5686	5799	5912	6024	6137	6250	6362	6475	113
6	6587	6700	6812	6925	7037	7149	7262	7374	7486	7599	112
7	7711	7823	7935	8047	8160	8272	8384	8496	8608	8720	112
8	8832	8944	9056	9167	9279	9391	9503	9615	9726	9838	112
9	9950	590061	590173	590284	590396	590507	590619	590730	590842	590953	112
390	591065	591176	591287	591399	591510	591621	591732	591843	591955	592066	111
1	2177	2288	2399	2510	2621	2732	2843	2954	3064	3175	111
2	3286	3397	3508	3618	3729	3840	3950	4061	4171	4282	111
3	4393	4503	4614	4724	4834	4945	5055	5165	5276	5380	110
4	5496	5606	5717	5827	5937	6047	6157	6267	6377	6487	110
395	6597	6707	6817	6927	7037	7146	7256	7366	7476	7586	110
6	7695	7805	7914	8024	8134	8243	8353	8462	8572	8681	110
7	8791	8900	9009	9119	9228	9337	9446	9556	9665	9774	109
8	9883	9992	600101	600210	600319	600428	600537	600646	600755	600864	109
9	600973	601082	1191	1299	1408	1517	1625	1734	1843	1951	109
N.	0	1	2	3	4	5	6	7	8	9	D.

N.	0	1	2	3	4	5	6	7	8	9	D.
400	602060	602169	602277	602386	602494	602603	602711	602819	602928	603036	108
1	3144	3253	3361	3469	3577	3686	3794	3902	4010	4118	108
2	4226	4334	4442	4550	4658	4766	4874	4982	5089	5197	108
3	5305	5413	5521	5628	5736	5844	5951	6059	6166	6274	108
4	6381	6489	6596	6704	6811	6919	7026	7133	7241	7348	107
405	7455	7562	7669	7777	7884	7991	8098	8205	8312	8419	107
6	8526	8633	8740	8847	8954	9061	9167	9274	9381	9488	107
7	9594	9701	9808	9914	610021	610128	610234	610341	610447	610554	107
8	610660	610767	610873	610979	1086	1192	1298	1405	1511	1617	106
9	1723	1829	1936	2042	2148	2254	2360	2466	2572	2678	106
410	612784	612890	612996	613102	613207	613313	613419	613525	613630	613736	106
1	3842	3947	4053	4159	4264	4370	4475	4581	4686	4792	106
2	4897	5003	5108	5213	5319	5424	5529	5634	5740	5845	105
3	5950	6055	6160	6265	6370	6476	6581	6686	6790	6895	105
4	7000	7105	7210	7315	7420	7525	7629	7734	7839	7943	105
415	8048	8153	8257	8362	8466	8571	8676	8780	8884	8989	105
6	9093	9198	9302	9406	9511	9615	9719	9824	9928	620032	104
7	620136	620240	620344	620448	620552	620656	620760	620864	620968	1072	104
8	1176	1280	1384	1488	1592	1695	1799	1903	2007	2110	104
9	2214	2318	2421	2525	2628	2732	2835	2939	3042	3146	104
420	623249	623353	623456	623559	623663	623766	623869	623973	624076	624179	103
1	4282	4385	4488	4591	4695	4798	4901	5004	5107	5210	103
2	5312	5415	5518	5621	5724	5827	5929	6032	6135	6238	103
3	6340	6443	6546	6648	6751	6853	6956	7058	7161	7263	103
4	7366	7468	7571	7673	7775	7878	7980	8082	8185	8287	102
425	8389	8491	8593	8695	8797	8900	9002	9104	9206	9308	102
6	9410	9512	9613	9715	9817	9919	630021	630123	630224	630326	102
7	630428	630530	630631	630733	630835	630936	1038	1139	1241	1342	102
8	1444	1545	1647	1748	1849	1951	2052	2153	2255	2356	101
9	2457	2559	2660	2761	2862	2963	3064	3165	3266	3367	101
430	633468	633569	633670	633771	633872	633973	634074	634175	634276	634376	101
1	4477	4578	4679	4779	4880	4981	5081	5182	5283	5383	101
2	5484	5584	5685	5785	5886	5986	6087	6187	6287	6388	100
3	6488	6588	6688	6789	6889	6989	7089	7189	7290	7390	100
4	7490	7590	7690	7790	7890	7990	8090	8190	8290	8389	100
435	8489	8589	8689	8789	8888	8988	9088	9188	9287	9387	100
6	9486	9586	9686	9785	9885	9984	640084	640183	640283	640382	99
7	640481	640581	640680	640779	640879	640978	1077	1177	1276	1375	99
8	1474	1573	1672	1771	1871	1970	2069	2168	2267	2366	99
9	2465	2563	2662	2761	2860	2959	3058	3156	3255	3354	99
440	643453	643551	643650	643749	643847	643946	644044	644143	644242	644340	98
1	4439	4537	4636	4734	4832	4931	5029	5127	5226	5324	98
2	5422	5521	5619	5717	5815	5913	6011	6110	6208	6306	98
3	6404	6502	6600	6698	6796	6894	6992	7089	7187	7285	98
4	7383	7481	7579	7676	7774	7872	7969	8067	8165	8262	98
445	8360	8458	8555	8653	8750	8848	8945	9043	9140	9237	97
6	9335	9432	9530	9627	9724	9821	9919	650016	650113	650210	97
7	650308	650405	650502	650599	650696	650793	650890	0987	1084	1181	97
8	1278	1375	1472	1569	1666	1762	1859	1956	2053	2150	97
9	2246	2343	2440	2536	2633	2730	2826	2923	3019	3116	97
450	653213	653309	653405	653502	653598	653695	653791	653888	653984	654080	96
1	4177	4273	4369	4465	4562	4658	4754	4850	4946	5042	96
2	5138	5235	5331	5427	5523	5619	5715	5810	5906	6002	96
3	6098	6194	6290	6386	6482	6577	6673	6769	6864	6960	96
4	7056	7152	7247	7343	7438	7534	7629	7725	7820	7916	96
455	8011	8107	8202	8298	8393	8488	8584	8679	8774	8870	95
6	8965	9060	9155	9250	9346	9441	9536	9631	9726	9821	95
7	9916	660011	660106	660201	660296	660391	660486	660581	660676	660771	95
8	660865	0960	1055	1150	1245	1339	1434	1529	1623	1718	95
9	1813	1907	2002	2096	2191	2286	2380	2475	2569	2663	95
N.	0	1	2	3	4	5	6	7	8	9	D.

N.	0	1	2	3	4	5	6	7	8	9	D.
460	662758	662852	662947	663041	663135	663230	663324	663418	663512	663607	94
1	3701	3795	3889	3983	4078	4172	4266	4360	4454	4548	94
2	4642	4736	4830	4924	5018	5112	5206	5299	5393	5487	94
3	5581	5675	5769	5862	5956	6050	6143	6237	6331	6424	94
4	6518	6612	6705	6799	6892	6986	7079	7173	7266	7360	94
465	7453	7546	7640	7733	7826	7920	8013	8106	8199	8293	93
6	8386	8479	8572	8665	8759	8852	8945	9038	9131	9224	93
7	9317	9410	9503	9596	9689	9782	9875	9967	670060	670153	93
8	670246	670339	670431	670524	670617	670710	670802	670895	0988	1080	93
9	1173	1265	1358	1451	1543	1636	1728	1821	1913	2005	93
470	672098	672190	672283	672375	672467	672560	672652	672744	672836	672929	92
1	3021	3113	3205	3297	3390	3482	3574	3666	3758	3850	92
2	3942	4034	4126	4218	4310	4402	4494	4586	4677	4769	92
3	4861	4953	5045	5137	5228	5320	5412	5503	5595	5687	92
4	5778	5870	5962	6053	6145	6236	6328	6419	6511	6602	92
475	6694	6785	6876	6968	7059	7151	7242	7333	7424	7516	91
6	7607	7698	7789	7881	7972	8063	8154	8245	8336	8427	91
7	8518	8609	8700	8791	8882	8973	9064	9155	9246	9337	91
8	9428	9519	9610	9700	9791	9882	9973	680063	680154	680245	91
9	680336	680426	680517	680607	680698	680789	680879	0970	1060	1151	91
480	681241	681332	681422	681513	681603	681693	681784	681874	681964	682055	90
1	2145	2235	2326	2416	2506	2596	2686	2777	2867	2957	90
2	3047	3137	3227	3317	3407	3497	3587	3677	3767	3857	90
3	3947	4037	4127	4217	4307	4396	4486	4576	4666	4756	90
4	4845	4935	5025	5114	5204	5294	5383	5473	5563	5652	90
485	5742	5831	5921	6010	6100	6189	6279	6368	6458	6547	89
6	6636	6726	6815	6904	6994	7083	7172	7261	7351	7440	89
7	7529	7618	7707	7796	7886	7975	8064	8153	8242	8331	89
8	8420	8509	8598	8687	8776	8865	8953	9042	9131	9220	89
9	9309	9398	9486	9575	9664	9753	9841	9930	690019	690107	89
490	690196	690285	690373	690462	690550	690639	690728	690816	690905	690993	89
1	1081	1170	1258	1347	1435	1524	1612	1700	1789	1877	88
2	1965	2053	2142	2230	2318	2406	2494	2583	2671	2759	88
3	2847	2935	3023	3111	3199	3287	3375	3463	3551	3639	88
4	3727	3815	3903	3991	4078	4166	4254	4342	4430	4517	88
495	4605	4693	4781	4868	4956	5044	5131	5219	5307	5394	88
6	5482	5569	5657	5744	5832	5919	6007	6094	6182	6269	87
7	6356	6444	6531	6618	6706	6793	6880	6968	7055	7142	87
8	7229	7317	7404	7491	7578	7665	7752	7839	7926	8014	87
9	8101	8188	8275	8362	8449	8535	8622	8709	8796	8883	87
500	698970	699057	699144	699231	699317	699404	699491	699578	699664	699751	87
1	9838	9924	700011	700098	700184	700271	700358	700444	700531	700617	87
2	700704	700790	0877	0963	1050	1136	1222	1309	1395	1482	86
3	1568	1654	1741	1827	1913	1999	2086	2172	2258	2344	86
4	2431	2517	2603	2689	2775	2861	2947	3033	3119	3205	86
505	3291	3377	3463	3549	3635	3721	3807	3893	3979	4065	86
6	4151	4236	4322	4408	4494	4579	4665	4751	4837	4922	86
7	5008	5094	5179	5265	5350	5436	5522	5607	5693	5778	86
8	5864	5949	6035	6120	6206	6291	6376	6462	6547	6632	85
9	6718	6803	6888	6974	7059	7144	7229	7315	7400	7485	85
510	707570	707655	707740	707826	707911	707996	708081	708166	708251	708336	85
1	8421	8506	8591	8676	8761	8846	8931	9015	9100	9185	85
2	9270	9355	9440	9524	9609	9694	9779	9863	9948	710033	85
3	710117	710202	710287	710371	710456	710540	710625	710710	710794	0879	85
4	0963	1048	1132	1217	1301	1385	1470	1554	1639	1723	84
515	1807	1892	1976	2060	2144	2229	2313	2397	2481	2566	84
6	2650	2734	2818	2902	2986	3070	3154	3238	3323	3407	84
7	3491	3575	3659	3742	3826	3910	3994	4078	4162	4246	84
8	4330	4414	4497	4581	4665	4749	4833	4916	5000	5084	84
9	5167	5251	5335	5418	5502	5586	5669	5753	5836	5920	84
N.	0	1	2	3	4	5	6	7	8	9	D.

N.	0	1	2	3	4	5	6	7	8	9	D.
520	716003	716087	716170	716254	716337	716421	716504	716588	716671	716754	83
1	6838	6921	7004	7088	7171	7254	7338	7421	7504	7587	83
2	7671	7754	7837	7920	8003	8086	8169	8253	8336	8419	83
3	8502	8585	8668	8751	8834	8917	9000	9083	9165	9248	83
4	9331	9414	9497	9580	9663	9745	9828	9911	9994	720077	83
525	720159	720242	720325	720407	720490	720573	720655	720738	720821	0903	83
6	0986	1068	1151	1233	1316	1398	1481	1563	1646	1728	82
7	1811	1893	1975	2058	2140	2222	2305	2387	2469	2552	82
8	2634	2716	2798	2881	2963	3045	3127	3209	3291	3374	82
9	3456	3538	3620	3702	3784	3866	3948	4030	4112	4194	82
530	724276	724358	724440	724522	724604	724685	724767	724849	724931	725013	82
1	5095	5176	5258	5340	5422	5503	5585	5667	5748	5830	82
2	5912	5993	6075	6156	6238	6320	6401	6483	6564	6646	82
3	6727	6809	6890	6972	7053	7134	7216	7297	7379	7460	81
4	7541	7623	7704	7785	7866	7948	8029	8110	8191	8273	81
535	8354	8435	8516	8597	8678	8759	8841	8922	9003	9084	81
6	9165	9246	9327	9408	9489	9570	9651	9732	9813	9893	81
7	9974	730055	730136	730217	730298	730378	730459	730540	730621	730702	81
8	730782	0863	0944	1024	1105	1186	1266	1347	1428	1508	81
9	1589	1669	1750	1830	1911	1991	2072	2152	2233	2313	81
540	732394	732474	732555	732635	732715	732796	732876	732956	733037	733117	80
1	3197	3278	3358	3438	3518	3598	3679	3759	3839	3919	80
2	3999	4079	4160	4240	4320	4400	4480	4560	4640	4720	80
3	4800	4880	4960	5040	5120	5200	5279	5359	5439	5519	80
4	5599	5679	5759	5838	5918	5998	6078	6157	6237	6317	80
545	6397	6476	6556	6635	6715	6795	6874	6954	7034	7113	80
6	7193	7272	7352	7431	7511	7590	7670	7749	7829	7908	79
7	7987	8067	8146	8225	8305	8384	8463	8543	8622	8701	79
8	8781	8860	8939	9018	9097	9177	9256	9335	9414	9493	79
9	9572	9651	9731	9810	9889	9968	740047	740126	740205	740284	79
550	740363	740442	740521	740600	740678	740757	740836	740915	740994	741073	79
1	1152	1230	1309	1388	1467	1546	1624	1703	1782	1860	79
2	1939	2018	2096	2175	2254	2332	2411	2489	2568	2647	79
3	2725	2804	2882	2961	3039	3118	3196	3275	3353	3431	78
4	3510	3588	3667	3745	3823	3902	3980	4058	4136	4215	78
555	4293	4371	4449	4528	4606	4684	4762	4840	4919	4997	78
6	5075	5153	5231	5309	5387	5465	5543	5621	5699	5777	78
7	5855	5933	6011	6089	6167	6245	6323	6401	6479	6556	78
8	6634	6712	6790	6868	6945	7023	7101	7179	7256	7334	78
9	7412	7489	7567	7645	7722	7800	7878	7955	8033	8110	78
560	748188	748266	748343	748421	748498	748576	748653	748731	748808	748885	77
1	8963	9040	9118	9195	9272	9350	9427	9504	9582	9659	77
2	9736	9814	9891	9968	750045	750123	750200	750277	750354	750431	77
3	750508	750586	750663	750740	0817	0894	0971	1048	1125	1202	77
4	1279	1356	1433	1510	1587	1664	1741	1818	1895	1972	77
565	2048	2125	2202	2279	2356	2433	2509	2586	2663	2740	77
6	2816	2893	2970	3047	3123	3200	3277	3353	3430	3506	77
7	3583	3660	3736	3813	3889	3966	4042	4119	4195	4272	77
8	4348	4425	4501	4578	4654	4730	4807	4883	4960	5036	76
9	5112	5189	5265	5341	5417	5494	5570	5646	5722	5799	76
570	755875	755951	756027	756103	756180	756256	756332	756408	756484	756560	76
1	6636	6712	6788	6864	6940	7016	7092	7168	7244	7320	76
2	7396	7472	7548	7624	7700	7775	7851	7927	8003	8079	76
3	8155	8230	8306	8382	8458	8533	8609	8685	8761	8836	76
4	8912	8988	9063	9139	9214	9290	9366	9441	9517	9592	76
575	9668	9743	9819	9894	9970	760045	760121	760196	760272	760347	75
6	760422	760498	760573	760649	760724	0799	0875	0950	1025	1101	75
7	1176	1251	1326	1402	1477	1552	1627	1702	1778	1853	75
8	1928	2003	2078	2153	2228	2303	2378	2453	2529	2604	75
9	2679	2754	2829	2904	2978	3053	3128	3203	3278	3353	75
N.	0	1	2	3	4	5	6	7	8	9	D.

N.	0	1	2	3	4	5	6	7	8	9	D.
580	763428	763503	763578	763653	763727	763802	763877	763952	764027	764101	75
1	4176	4251	4326	4400	4475	4550	4624	4699	4774	4848	75
2	4923	4998	5072	5147	5221	5296	5370	5445	5520	5594	75
3	5669	5743	5818	5892	5966	6041	6115	6190	6264	6338	74
4	6413	6487	6562	6636	6710	6785	6859	6933	7007	7082	74
585	7156	7230	7304	7379	7453	7527	7601	7675	7749	7823	74
6	7898	7972	8046	8120	8194	8268	8342	8416	8490	8564	74
7	8638	8712	8786	8860	8934	9008	9082	9156	9230	9303	74
8	9377	9451	9525	9599	9673	9746	9820	9894	9968	770042	74
9	770115	770189	770263	770336	770410	770484	770557	770631	770705	0778	74
590	770852	770926	770999	771073	771146	771220	771293	771367	771440	771514	74
1	1587	1661	1734	1808	1881	1955	2028	2102	2175	2248	73
2	2322	2395	2468	2542	2615	2688	2762	2835	2908	2981	73
3	3055	3128	3201	3274	3348	3421	3494	3567	3640	3713	73
4	3786	3860	3933	4006	4079	4152	4225	4298	4371	4444	73
595	4517	4590	4663	4736	4809	4882	4955	5028	5100	5173	73
6	5246	5319	5392	5465	5538	5610	5683	5756	5829	5902	73
7	5974	6047	6120	6193	6265	6338	6411	6483	6556	6629	73
8	6701	6774	6846	6919	6992	7064	7137	7209	7282	7354	73
9	7427	7499	7572	7644	7717	7789	7862	7934	8006	8079	72
600	778151	778224	778296	778368	778441	778513	778585	778658	778730	778802	72
1	8874	8947	9019	9091	9163	9236	9308	9380	9452	9524	72
2	9596	9669	9741	9813	9885	9957	780029	780101	780173	780245	72
3	780317	780389	780461	780533	780605	780677	0749	0821	0893	0965	72
4	1037	1109	1181	1253	1324	1396	1468	1540	1612	1684	72
605	1755	1827	1899	1971	2042	2114	2186	2258	2329	2401	72
6	2473	2544	2616	2688	2759	2831	2902	2974	3046	3117	72
7	3189	3260	3332	3403	3475	3546	3618	3689	3761	3832	71
8	3904	3975	4046	4118	4189	4261	4332	4403	4475	4546	71
9	4617	4689	4760	4831	4902	4974	5045	5116	5187	5259	71
610	785330	785401	785472	785543	785615	785686	785757	785828	785899	785970	71
1	6041	6112	6183	6254	6325	6396	6467	6538	6609	6680	71
2	6751	6822	6893	6964	7035	7106	7177	7248	7319	7390	71
3	7460	7531	7602	7673	7744	7815	7885	7956	8027	8098	71
4	8168	8239	8310	8381	8451	8522	8593	8663	8734	8804	71
615	8875	8946	9016	9087	9157	9228	9299	9369	9440	9510	71
6	9581	9651	9722	9792	9863	9933	790004	790074	790144	790215	70
7	790285	790356	790426	790496	790567	790637	0707	0778	0848	0918	70
8	0988	1059	1129	1199	1269	1340	1410	1480	1550	1620	70
9	1691	1761	1831	1901	1971	2041	2111	2181	2252	2322	70
620	792392	792462	792532	792602	792672	792742	792812	792882	792952	793022	70
1	3092	3162	3231	3301	3371	3441	3511	3581	3651	3721	70
2	3790	3860	3930	4000	4070	4139	4209	4279	4349	4418	70
3	4488	4558	4627	4697	4767	4836	4906	4976	5045	5115	70
4	5185	5254	5324	5393	5463	5532	5602	5672	5741	5811	70
625	5880	5949	6019	6088	6158	6227	6297	6366	6436	6505	69
6	6574	6644	6713	6782	6852	6921	6990	7060	7129	7198	69
7	7268	7337	7406	7475	7545	7614	7683	7752	7821	7890	69
8	7960	8029	8098	8167	8236	8305	8374	8443	8513	8582	69
9	8651	8720	8789	8858	8927	8996	9065	9134	9203	9272	69
630	799341	799409	799478	799547	799616	799685	799754	799823	799892	799961	69
1	800029	800098	800167	800236	800305	800373	800442	800511	800580	800648	69
2	0717	0786	0854	0923	0992	1061	1129	1198	1266	1335	69
3	1404	1472	1541	1609	1678	1747	1815	1884	1952	2021	69
4	2089	2158	2226	2295	2363	2432	2500	2568	2637	2705	68
635	2774	2842	2910	2979	3047	3116	3184	3252	3321	3389	68
6	3457	3525	3594	3662	3730	3798	3867	3935	4003	4071	68
7	4139	4208	4276	4344	4412	4480	4548	4616	4685	4753	68
8	4821	4889	4957	5025	5093	5161	5229	5297	5365	5433	68
9	5501	5569	5637	5705	5773	5841	5908	5976	6044	6112	68
N.	0	1	2	3	4	5	6	7	8	9	D.

N.	0	1	2	3	4	5	6	7	8	9	D.
640	806180	806248	806316	806384	806451	806519	806587	806655	806723	806790	68
1	6858	6926	6994	7061	7129	7197	7264	7332	7400	7467	68
2	7535	7603	7670	7738	7806	7873	7941	8008	8076	8143	68
3	8211	8279	8346	8414	8481	8549	8616	8684	8751	8818	67
4	8886	8953	9021	9088	9156	9223	9290	9358	9425	9492	67
645	9560	9627	9694	9762	9829	9896	9964	810031	810098	810165	67
6	810233	810300	810367	810434	810501	810569	810636	0703	0770	0837	67
7	0904	0971	1039	1106	1173	1240	1307	1374	1441	1508	67
8	1575	1642	1709	1776	1843	1910	1977	2044	2111	2178	67
9	2245	2312	2379	2445	2512	2579	2646	2713	2780	2847	67
650	812913	812980	813047	813114	813181	813247	813314	813381	813448	813514	67
1	3581	3648	3714	3781	3848	3914	3981	4048	4114	4181	67
2	4248	4314	4381	4447	4514	4581	4647	4714	4780	4847	67
3	4913	4980	5046	5113	5179	5246	5312	5378	5445	5511	66
4	5578	5644	5711	5777	5843	5910	5976	6042	6109	6175	66
655	6241	6308	6374	6440	6506	6573	6639	6705	6771	6838	66
6	6904	6970	7036	7102	7169	7235	7301	7367	7433	7499	66
7	7565	7631	7698	7764	7830	7896	7962	8028	8094	8160	66
8	8226	8292	8358	8424	8490	8556	8622	8688	8754	8820	66
9	8885	8951	9017	9083	9149	9215	9281	9346	9412	9478	66
660	819544	819610	819676	819741	819807	819873	819939	820004	820070	820136	66
1	820201	820267	820333	820399	820464	820530	820595	0661	0727	0792	66
2	0858	0924	0989	1055	1120	1186	1251	1317	1382	1448	66
3	1514	1579	1645	1710	1775	1841	1906	1972	2037	2103	65
4	2168	2233	2299	2364	2430	2495	2560	2626	2691	2756	65
665	2822	2887	2952	3018	3083	3148	3213	3279	3344	3409	65
6	3474	3539	3605	3670	3735	3800	3865	3930	3996	4061	65
7	4126	4191	4256	4321	4386	4451	4516	4581	4646	4711	65
8	4776	4841	4906	4971	5036	5101	5166	5231	5296	5361	65
9	5426	5491	5556	5621	5686	5751	5815	5880	5945	6010	65
670	826075	826140	826204	826269	826334	826399	826464	826528	826593	826658	65
1	6723	6787	6852	6917	6981	7046	7111	7175	7240	7305	65
2	7369	7434	7499	7563	7628	7692	7757	7821	7886	7951	65
3	8015	8080	8144	8209	8273	8338	8402	8467	8531	8595	64
4	8660	8724	8789	8853	8918	8982	9046	9111	9175	9239	64
675	9304	9368	9432	9497	9561	9625	9690	9754	9818	9882	64
6	9947	830011	830075	830139	830204	830268	830332	830396	830460	830525	64
7	830589	0653	0717	0781	0845	0909	0973	1037	1102	1166	64
8	1230	1294	1358	1422	1486	1550	1614	1678	1742	1806	64
9	1870	1934	1998	2062	2126	2189	2253	2317	2381	2445	64
680	832509	832573	832637	832700	832764	832828	832892	832956	833020	833083	64
1	3147	3211	3275	3338	3402	3466	3530	3593	3657	3721	64
2	3784	3848	3912	3975	4039	4103	4166	4230	4294	4357	64
3	4421	4484	4548	4611	4675	4739	4802	4866	4929	4993	64
4	5056	5120	5183	5247	5310	5373	5437	5500	5564	5627	63
685	5691	5754	5817	5881	5944	6007	6071	6134	6197	6261	63
6	6324	6387	6451	6514	6577	6641	6704	6767	6830	6894	63
7	6957	7020	7083	7146	7210	7273	7336	7399	7462	7525	63
8	7588	7652	7715	7778	7841	7904	7967	8030	8093	8156	63
9	8219	8282	8345	8408	8471	8534	8597	8660	8723	8786	63
690	838849	838912	838975	839038	839101	839164	839227	839289	839352	839415	63
1	9478	9541	9604	9667	9729	9792	9855	9918	9981	840043	63
2	840106	840169	840232	840294	840357	840420	840482	840545	840608	0671	63
3	0733	0796	0859	0921	0984	1046	1109	1172	1234	1297	63
4	1359	1422	1485	1547	1610	1672	1735	1797	1860	1922	63
695	1985	2047	2110	2172	2235	2297	2360	2422	2484	2547	62
6	2609	2672	2734	2796	2859	2921	2983	3046	3108	3170	62
7	3233	3295	3357	3420	3482	3544	3606	3669	3731	3793	62
8	3855	3918	3980	4042	4104	4166	4229	4291	4353	4415	62
9	4477	4539	4601	4664	4726	4788	4850	4912	4974	5036	62
N.	0	1	2	3	4	5	6	7	8	9	D.

N.	0	1	2	3	4	5	6	7	8	9	D.
700	845098	845160	845222	845284	845346	845408	845470	845532	845594	845656	62
1	5718	5780	5842	5904	5966	6028	6090	6151	6213	6275	62
2	6337	6399	6461	6523	6585	6646	6708	6770	6832	6894	62
3	6955	7017	7079	7141	7202	7264	7326	7388	7449	7511	62
4	7573	7634	7696	7758	7819	7881	7943	8004	8066	8128	62
705	8189	8251	8312	8374	8435	8497	8559	8620	8682	8743	62
6	8805	8866	8928	8989	9051	9112	9174	9235	9297	9358	61
7	9419	9481	9542	9604	9665	9726	9788	9849	9911	9972	61
8	850033	850095	850156	850217	850279	850340	850401	850462	850524	850585	61
9	0646	0707	0769	0830	0891	0952	1014	1075	1136	1197	61
710	851258	851320	851381	851442	851503	851564	851625	851686	851747	851809	61
1	1870	1931	1992	2053	2114	2175	2236	2297	2358	2419	61
2	2480	2541	2602	2663	2724	2785	2846	2907	2968	3029	61
3	3090	3150	3211	3272	3333	3394	3455	3516	3577	3637	61
4	3698	3759	3820	3881	3941	4002	4063	4124	4185	4245	61
715	4306	4367	4428	4488	4549	4610	4670	4731	4792	4852	61
6	4913	4974	5034	5095	5156	5216	5277	5337	5398	5459	61
7	5519	5580	5640	5701	5761	5822	5882	5943	6003	6064	61
8	6124	6185	6245	6306	6366	6427	6487	6548	6608	6668	60
9	6729	6789	6850	6910	6970	7031	7091	7152	7212	7272	60
720	857332	857393	857453	857513	857574	857634	857694	857755	857815	857875	60
1	7935	7995	8056	8116	8176	8236	8297	8357	8417	8477	60
2	8537	8597	8657	8718	8778	8838	8898	8958	9018	9078	60
3	9138	9198	9258	9318	9379	9439	9499	9559	9619	9679	60
4	9739	9799	9859	9918	9978	860038	860098	860158	860218	860278	60
725	860338	860398	860458	860518	860578	0637	0697	0757	0817	0877	60
6	0937	0996	1056	1116	1176	1236	1295	1355	1415	1475	60
7	1534	1594	1654	1714	1773	1833	1893	1952	2012	2072	60
8	2131	2191	2251	2310	2370	2430	2489	2549	2608	2668	60
9	2728	2787	2847	2906	2966	3025	3085	3144	3204	3263	60
730	863323	863382	863442	863501	863561	863620	863680	863739	863799	863858	59
1	3917	3977	4036	4096	4155	4214	4274	4333	4392	4452	59
2	4511	4570	4630	4689	4748	4808	4867	4926	4985	5045	59
3	5104	5163	5222	5282	5341	5400	5459	5519	5578	5637	59
4	5696	5755	5814	5874	5933	5992	6051	6110	6169	6228	59
735	6287	6346	6405	6465	6524	6583	6642	6701	6760	6819	59
6	6878	6937	6996	7055	7114	7173	7232	7291	7350	7409	59
7	7467	7526	7585	7644	7703	7762	7821	7880	7939	7998	59
8	8056	8115	8174	8233	8292	8350	8409	8468	8527	8586	59
9	8644	8703	8762	8821	8879	8938	8997	9056	9114	9173	59
740	869232	869290	869349	869408	869466	869525	869584	869642	869701	869760	59
1	9818	9877	9935	9994	870053	870111	870170	870223	870287	870345	59
2	870404	870462	870521	870579	0538	0696	0755	0813	0872	0930	58
3	0989	1047	1106	1164	1223	1281	1339	1398	1456	1515	58
4	1573	1631	1690	1748	1806	1865	1923	1981	2040	2098	58
745	2156	2215	2273	2331	2389	2448	2506	2564	2622	2681	58
6	2739	2797	2855	2913	2972	3030	3088	3146	3204	3262	58
7	3321	3379	3437	3495	3553	3611	3669	3727	3785	3844	58
8	3902	3960	4018	4076	4134	4192	4250	4308	4366	4424	58
9	4482	4540	4598	4656	4714	4772	4830	4888	4945	5003	58
750	875061	875119	875177	875235	875293	875351	875409	875466	875524	875582	58
1	5640	5698	5756	5813	5871	5929	5987	6045	6102	6160	58
2	6218	6276	6333	6391	6449	6507	6564	6622	6680	6737	58
3	6795	6853	6910	6968	7026	7083	7141	7199	7256	7314	58
4	7371	7429	7487	7544	7602	7659	7717	7774	7832	7889	58
755	7947	8004	8062	8119	8177	8234	8292	8349	8407	8464	57
6	8522	8579	8637	8694	8752	8809	8866	8924	8981	9039	57
7	9096	9153	9211	9268	9325	9383	9440	9497	9555	9612	57
8	9669	9726	9784	9841	9898	9956	880013	880070	880127	880185	57
9	880242	880299	880356	880413	880471	880528	0585	0642	0699	0756	57
N.	0	1	2	3	4	5	6	7	8	9	D.

N.	0	1	2	3	4	5	6	7	8	9	D.
760	880814	880871	880928	880985	881042	881099	881156	881213	881271	881328	57
1	1385	1442	1499	1556	1613	1670	1727	1784	1841	1898	57
2	1955	2012	2069	2126	2183	2240	2297	2354	2411	2468	57
3	2525	2581	2638	2695	2752	2809	2866	2923	2980	3037	57
4	3093	3150	3207	3264	3321	3377	3434	3491	3548	3605	57
765	3661	3718	3775	3832	3888	3945	4002	4059	4115	4172	57
6	4229	4285	4342	4399	4455	4512	4569	4625	4682	4739	57
7	4795	4852	4909	4965	5022	5078	5135	5192	5248	5305	57
8	5361	5418	5474	5531	5587	5644	5700	5757	5813	5870	57
9	5926	5983	6039	6096	6152	6209	6265	6321	6378	6434	56
770	886491	886547	886604	886660	886716	886773	886829	886885	886942	886998	56
1	7054	7111	7167	7223	7280	7336	7392	7449	7505	7561	56
2	7617	7674	7730	7786	7842	7898	7955	8011	8067	8123	56
3	8179	8236	8292	8348	8404	8460	8516	8573	8629	8685	56
4	8741	8797	8853	8909	8965	9021	9077	9134	9190	9246	56
775	9302	9358	9414	9470	9526	9582	9638	9694	9750	9806	56
6	9862	9918	9974	890030	890086	890141	890197	890253	890309	890365	56
7	890421	890477	890533	0589	0645	0700	0756	0812	0868	0924	56
8	0980	1035	1091	1147	1203	1259	1314	1370	1426	1482	56
9	1537	1593	1649	1705	1760	1816	1872	1928	1983	2039	56
780	892095	892150	892206	892262	892317	892373	892429	892484	892540	892595	56
1	2651	2707	2762	2818	2873	2929	2985	3040	3096	3151	56
2	3207	3262	3318	3373	3429	3484	3540	3595	3651	3706	56
3	3762	3817	3873	3928	3984	4039	4094	4150	4205	4261	55
4	4316	4371	4427	4482	4538	4593	4648	4704	4759	4814	55
785	4870	4925	4980	5036	5091	5146	5201	5257	5312	5367	55
6	5423	5478	5533	5588	5644	5699	5754	5809	5864	5920	55
7	5975	6030	6085	6140	6195	6251	6306	6361	6416	6471	55
8	6526	6581	6636	6692	6747	6802	6857	6912	6967	7022	55
9	7077	7132	7187	7242	7297	7352	7407	7462	7517	7572	55
790	897627	897682	897737	897792	897847	897902	897957	898012	898067	898122	55
1	8176	8231	8286	8341	8396	8451	8506	8561	8615	8670	55
2	8725	8780	8835	8890	8944	8999	9054	9109	9164	9218	55
3	9273	9328	9383	9437	9492	9547	9602	9656	9711	9766	55
4	9821	9875	9930	9985	900039	900094	900149	900203	900258	900312	55
795	900367	900422	900476	900531	0586	0640	0695	0749	0804	0859	55
6	0913	0968	1022	1077	1131	1186	1240	1295	1349	1404	55
7	1458	1513	1567	1622	1676	1731	1785	1840	1894	1948	54
8	2003	2057	2112	2166	2221	2275	2329	2384	2438	2492	54
9	2547	2601	2655	2710	2764	2818	2873	2927	2981	3036	54
800	903090	903144	903199	903253	903307	903361	903416	903470	903524	903578	54
1	3633	3687	3741	3795	3849	3904	3958	4012	4066	4120	54
2	4174	4229	4283	4337	4391	4445	4499	4553	4607	4661	54
3	4716	4770	4824	4878	4932	4986	5040	5094	5148	5202	54
4	5256	5310	5364	5418	5472	5526	5580	5634	5688	5742	54
805	5796	5850	5904	5958	6012	6066	6119	6173	6227	6281	54
6	6335	6389	6443	6497	6551	6604	6658	6712	6766	6820	54
7	6874	6927	6981	7035	7089	7143	7196	7250	7304	7358	54
8	7411	7465	7519	7573	7626	7680	7734	7787	7841	7895	54
9	7949	8002	8056	8110	8163	8217	8270	8324	8378	8431	54
810	908485	908539	908592	908646	908699	908753	908807	908860	908914	908967	54
1	9021	9074	9128	9181	9235	9289	9342	9396	9449	9503	54
2	9556	9610	9663	9716	9770	9823	9877	9930	9984	910037	53
3	910091	910144	910197	910251	910304	910358	910411	910464	910518	0571	53
4	0624	0678	0731	0784	0838	0891	0944	0998	1051	1104	53
815	1158	1211	1264	1317	1371	1424	1477	1530	1584	1637	53
6	1690	1743	1797	1850	1903	1956	2009	2063	2116	2169	53
7	2222	2275	2328	2381	2435	2488	2541	2594	2647	2700	53
8	2753	2806	2859	2913	2966	3019	3072	3125	3178	3231	53
9	3284	3337	3390	3443	3496	3549	3602	3655	3708	3761	53
N.	0	1	2	3	4	5	6	7	8	9	D.

N.	0	1	2	3	4	5	6	7	8	9	D.
820	913814	913867	913920	913973	914026	914079	914132	914184	914237	914290	53
1	4343	4396	4449	4502	4555	4608	4660	4713	4766	4819	53
2	4872	4925	4977	5030	5083	5136	5189	5241	5294	5347	53
3	5400	5453	5505	5558	5611	5664	5716	5769	5822	5875	53
4	5927	5980	6033	6085	6138	6191	6243	6296	6349	6401	53
825	6454	6507	6559	6612	6664	6717	6770	6822	6875	6927	53
6	6980	7033	7085	7138	7190	7243	7295	7348	7400	7453	53
7	7506	7558	7611	7663	7716	7768	7820	7873	7925	7978	52
8	8030	8083	8135	8188	8240	8293	8345	8397	8450	8502	52
9	8555	8607	8659	8712	8764	8816	8869	8921	8973	9026	52
830	919078	919130	919183	919235	919287	919340	919392	919444	919496	919549	52
1	9601	9653	9706	9758	9810	9862	9914	9967	920019	920071	52
2	920123	920176	920228	920280	920332	920384	920436	920489	0541	0593	52
3	0645	0697	0749	0801	0853	0906	0958	1010	1062	1114	52
4	1166	1218	1270	1322	1374	1426	1478	1530	1582	1634	52
835	1686	1738	1790	1842	1894	1946	1998	2050	2102	2154	52
6	2206	2258	2310	2362	2414	2466	2518	2570	2622	2674	52
7	2725	2777	2829	2881	2933	2985	3037	3089	3140	3192	52
8	3244	3296	3348	3399	3451	3503	3555	3607	3658	3710	52
9	3762	3814	3865	3917	3969	4021	4072	4124	4176	4228	52
840	924279	924331	924383	924434	924486	924538	924589	924641	924693	924744	52
1	4796	4848	4899	4951	5003	5054	5106	5157	5209	5261	52
2	5312	5364	5415	5467	5518	5570	5621	5673	5725	5776	52
3	5828	5879	5931	5982	6034	6085	6137	6188	6240	6291	51
4	6342	6394	6445	6497	6548	6600	6651	6702	6754	6805	51
845	6857	6908	6959	7011	7062	7114	7165	7216	7268	7319	51
6	7370	7422	7473	7524	7576	7627	7678	7730	7781	7832	51
7	7883	7935	7986	8037	8088	8140	8191	8242	8293	8345	51
8	8396	8447	8498	8549	8601	8652	8703	8754	8805	8857	51
9	8908	8959	9010	9061	9112	9163	9215	9266	9317	9368	51
850	929419	929470	929521	929572	929623	929674	929725	929776	929827	929879	51
1	9930	9981	930032	930083	930134	930185	930236	930287	930338	930389	51
2	930440	930491	0542	0592	0643	0694	0745	0796	0847	0898	51
3	0949	1000	1051	1102	1153	1204	1254	1305	1356	1407	51
4	1458	1509	1560	1610	1661	1712	1763	1814	1865	1915	51
855	1966	2017	2068	2118	2169	2220	2271	2322	2372	2423	51
6	2474	2524	2575	2626	2677	2727	2778	2829	2879	2930	51
7	2981	3031	3082	3133	3183	3234	3285	3335	3386	3437	51
8	3487	3538	3589	3639	3690	3740	3791	3841	3892	3943	51
9	3993	4044	4094	4145	4195	4246	4296	4347	4397	4448	51
860	934498	934549	934599	934650	934700	934751	934801	934852	934902	934953	50
1	5003	5054	5104	5154	5205	5255	5306	5356	5406	5457	50
2	5507	5558	5608	5658	5709	5759	5809	5860	5910	5960	50
3	6011	6061	6111	6162	6212	6262	6313	6363	6413	6463	50
4	6514	6564	6614	6665	6715	6765	6815	6865	6916	6966	50
865	7016	7066	7117	7167	7217	7267	7317	7367	7418	7468	50
6	7518	7568	7618	7668	7718	7769	7819	7869	7919	7969	50
7	8019	8069	8119	8169	8219	8269	8320	8370	8420	8470	50
8	8520	8570	8620	8670	8720	8770	8820	8870	8920	8970	50
9	9020	9070	9120	9170	9220	9270	9320	9369	9419	9469	50
870	939519	939569	939619	939669	939719	939769	939819	939869	939918	939968	50
1	940018	940068	940118	940168	940218	940267	940317	940367	940417	940467	50
2	0516	0566	0616	0666	0716	0765	0815	0865	0915	0964	50
3	1014	1064	1114	1163	1213	1263	1313	1362	1412	1462	50
4	1511	1561	1611	1660	1710	1760	1809	1859	1909	1958	50
875	2008	2058	2107	2157	2207	2256	2306	2355	2405	2455	50
6	2504	2554	2603	2653	2702	2752	2801	2851	2901	2950	50
7	3000	3049	3099	3148	3198	3247	3297	3346	3396	3445	49
8	3495	3544	3593	3643	3692	3742	3791	3841	3890	3939	49
9	3989	4038	4088	4137	4186	4236	4285	4335	4384	4433	49
N.	0	1	2	3	4	5	6	7	8	9	D.

N.	0	1	2	3	4	5	6	7	8	9	D.
880	944483	944532	944581	944631	944680	944729	944779	944828	944877	944927	49
1	4976	5025	5074	5124	5173	5222	5272	5321	5370	5419	49
2	5469	5518	5567	5616	5665	5715	5764	5813	5862	5912	49
3	5961	6010	6059	6108	6157	6207	6256	6305	6354	6403	49
4	6452	6501	6551	6600	6649	6698	6747	6796	6845	6894	49
885	6943	6992	7041	7090	7140	7189	7238	7287	7336	7385	49
6	7434	7483	7532	7581	7630	7679	7728	7777	7826	7875	49
7	7924	7973	8022	8070	8119	8168	8217	8266	8315	8364	49
8	8413	8462	8511	8560	8609	8657	8706	8755	8804	8853	49
9	8902	8951	8999	9048	9097	9146	9195	9244	9292	9341	49
890	949390	949439	949488	949536	949585	949634	949683	949731	949780	949829	49
1	9878	9926	9975	950024	950073	950121	950170	950219	950267	950316	49
2	950365	950414	950462	0511	0560	0608	0657	0706	0754	0803	49
3	0851	0900	0949	0997	1046	1095	1143	1192	1240	1289	49
4	1338	1386	1435	1483	1532	1580	1629	1677	1726	1775	49
895	1823	1872	1920	1969	2017	2066	2114	2163	2211	2260	48
6	2308	2356	2405	2453	2502	2550	2599	2647	2696	2744	48
7	2792	2841	2889	2938	2986	3034	3083	3131	3180	3228	48
8	3276	3325	3373	3421	3470	3518	3566	3615	3663	3711	48
9	3760	3808	3856	3905	3953	4001	4049	4098	4146	4194	48
900	954243	954291	954339	954387	954435	954484	954532	954580	954628	954677	48
1	4725	4773	4821	4869	4918	4966	5014	5062	5110	5158	48
2	5207	5255	5303	5351	5399	5447	5495	5543	5592	5640	48
3	5688	5736	5784	5832	5880	5928	5976	6024	6072	6120	48
4	6168	6216	6265	6313	6361	6409	6457	6505	6553	6601	48
905	6649	6697	6745	6793	6840	6888	6936	6984	7032	7080	48
6	7128	7176	7224	7272	7320	7368	7416	7464	7512	7559	48
7	7607	7655	7703	7751	7799	7847	7894	7942	7990	8038	48
8	8086	8134	8181	8229	8277	8325	8373	8421	8468	8516	48
9	8564	8612	8659	8707	8755	8803	8850	8898	8946	8994	48
910	959041	959089	959137	959185	959232	959280	959328	959375	959423	959471	48
1	9518	9566	9614	9661	9709	9757	9804	9852	9900	9947	48
2	9995	960042	960090	960138	960185	960233	960280	960328	960376	960423	48
3	960471	0518	0566	0613	0661	0709	0756	0804	0851	0899	48
4	0946	0994	1041	1089	1136	1184	1231	1279	1326	1374	48
915	1421	1469	1516	1563	1611	1658	1706	1753	1801	1848	47
6	1895	1943	1990	2038	2085	2132	2180	2227	2275	2322	47
7	2369	2417	2464	2511	2559	2606	2653	2701	2748	2795	47
8	2843	2890	2937	2985	3032	3079	3126	3174	3221	3268	47
9	3316	3363	3410	3457	3504	3552	3599	3646	3693	3741	47
920	963788	963835	963882	963929	963977	964024	964071	964118	964165	964212	47
1	4260	4307	4354	4401	4448	4495	4542	4590	4637	4684	47
2	4731	4778	4825	4872	4919	4966	5013	5061	5108	5155	47
3	5202	5249	5296	5343	5390	5437	5484	5531	5578	5625	47
4	5672	5719	5766	5813	5860	5907	5954	6001	6048	6095	47
925	6142	6189	6236	6283	6329	6376	6423	6470	6517	6564	47
6	6611	6658	6705	6752	6799	6845	6892	6939	6986	7033	47
7	7080	7127	7173	7220	7267	7314	7361	7408	7454	7501	47
8	7548	7595	7642	7688	7735	7782	7829	7875	7922	7969	47
9	8016	8062	8109	8156	8203	8249	8296	8343	8390	8436	47
930	968483	968530	968576	968623	968670	968716	968763	968810	968856	968903	47
1	8950	8996	9043	9090	9136	9183	9229	9276	9323	9369	47
2	9416	9463	9509	9556	9602	9649	9695	9742	9789	9835	47
3	9882	9928	9975	970021	970068	970114	970161	970207	970254	970300	47
4	970347	970393	970440	0486	0533	0579	0626	0672	0719	0765	46
935	0812	0858	0904	0951	0997	1044	1090	1137	1183	1229	46
6	1276	1322	1369	1415	1461	1508	1554	1601	1647	1693	46
7	1740	1786	1832	1879	1925	1971	2018	2064	2110	2157	46
8	2203	2249	2295	2342	2388	2434	2481	2527	2573	2619	46
9	2666	2712	2758	2804	2851	2897	2943	2989	3035	3082	46
N.	0	1	2	3	4	5	6	7	8	9	D.

N.	0	1	2	3	4	5	6	7	8	9	D.
940	973128	973174	973220	973266	973313	973359	973405	973451	973497	973543	46
1	3590	3636	3682	3728	3774	3820	3866	3913	3959	4005	46
2	4051	4097	4143	4189	4235	4281	4327	4374	4420	4466	46
3	4512	4558	4604	4650	4696	4742	4788	4834	4880	4926	46
4	4972	5018	5064	5110	5156	5202	5248	5294	5340	5386	46
945	5432	5478	5524	5570	5616	5662	5707	5753	5799	5845	46
6	5891	5937	5983	6029	6075	6121	6167	6212	6258	6304	46
7	6350	6396	6442	6488	6533	6579	6625	6671	6717	6763	46
8	6808	6854	6900	6946	6992	7037	7083	7129	7175	7220	46
9	7266	7312	7358	7403	7449	7495	7541	7586	7632	7678	46
950	977724	977769	977815	977861	977906	977952	977998	978043	978089	978135	46
1	8181	8226	8272	8317	8363	8409	8454	8500	8546	8591	46
2	8637	8683	8728	8774	8819	8865	8911	8956	9002	9047	46
3	9093	9138	9184	9230	9275	9321	9366	9412	9457	9503	46
4	9548	9594	9639	9685	9730	9776	9821	9867	9912	9958	46
955	980003	980049	980094	980140	980185	980231	980276	980322	980367	980412	45
6	0458	0503	0549	0594	0640	0685	0730	0776	0821	0867	45
7	0912	0957	1003	1048	1093	1139	1184	1229	1275	1320	45
8	1366	1411	1456	1501	1547	1592	1637	1683	1728	1773	45
9	1819	1864	1909	1954	2000	2045	2090	2135	2181	2226	45
960	982271	982316	982362	982407	982452	982497	982543	982588	982633	982678	45
1	2723	2769	2814	2859	2904	2949	2994	3040	3085	3130	45
2	3175	3220	3265	3310	3356	3401	3446	3491	3536	3581	45
3	3626	3671	3716	3762	3807	3852	3897	3942	3987	4032	45
4	4077	4122	4167	4212	4257	4302	4347	4392	4437	4482	45
965	4527	4572	4617	4662	4707	4752	4797	4842	4887	4932	45
6	4977	5022	5067	5112	5157	5202	5247	5292	5337	5382	45
7	5426	5471	5516	5561	5606	5651	5696	5741	5786	5830	45
8	5875	5920	5965	6010	6055	6100	6144	6189	6234	6279	45
9	6324	6369	6413	6458	6503	6548	6593	6637	6682	6727	45
970	986772	986817	986861	986906	986951	986996	987040	987085	987130	987175	45
1	7219	7264	7309	7353	7398	7443	7488	7532	7577	7622	45
2	7666	7711	7756	7800	7845	7890	7934	7979	8024	8068	45
3	8113	8157	8202	8247	8291	8336	8381	8425	8470	8514	45
4	8559	8604	8648	8693	8737	8782	8826	8871	8916	8960	45
975	9005	9049	9094	9138	9183	9227	9272	9316	9361	9405	45
6	9450	9494	9539	9583	9628	9672	9717	9761	9806	9850	44
7	9895	9939	9983	990028	990072	990117	990161	990206	990250	990294	44
8	990339	990383	990428	0472	0516	0561	0605	0650	0694	0738	44
9	0783	0827	0871	0916	0960	1004	1049	1093	1137	1182	44
980	991226	991270	991315	991359	991403	991448	991492	991536	991580	991625	44
1	1669	1713	1758	1802	1846	1890	1935	1979	2023	2067	44
2	2111	2156	2200	2244	2288	2333	2377	2421	2465	2509	44
3	2554	2598	2642	2686	2730	2774	2819	2863	2907	2951	44
4	2995	3039	3083	3127	3172	3216	3260	3304	3348	3392	44
985	3436	3480	3524	3568	3613	3657	3701	3745	3789	3833	44
6	3877	3921	3965	4009	4053	4097	4141	4185	4229	4273	44
7	4317	4361	4405	4449	4493	4537	4581	4625	4669	4713	44
8	4757	4801	4845	4889	4933	4977	5021	5065	5108	5152	44
9	5196	5240	5284	5328	5372	5416	5460	5504	5547	5591	44
990	995635	995679	995723	995767	995811	995854	995898	995942	995986	996030	44
1	6074	6117	6161	6205	6249	6293	6337	6380	6424	6468	44
2	6512	6555	6599	6643	6687	6731	6774	6818	6862	6906	44
3	6949	6993	7037	7080	7124	7168	7212	7255	7299	7343	44
4	7386	7430	7474	7517	7561	7605	7648	7692	7736	7779	44
995	7823	7867	7910	7954	7998	8041	8085	8129	8172	8216	44
6	8259	8303	8347	8390	8434	8477	8521	8564	8608	8652	44
7	8695	8739	8782	8826	8869	8913	8956	9000	9043	9087	44
8	9131	9174	9218	9261	9305	9348	9392	9435	9479	9522	44
9	9565	9609	9652	9696	9739	9783	9826	9870	9913	9957	43
N.	0	1	2	3	4	5	6	7	8	9	D.

INDEX

Adler, Franz, 276
Ages, reporting, 47–49
Age-specific death rates, 9
American Journal of Botany, 227
American Journal of Public Health, 50
American Journal of the Medical Sciences, 115
Appendix, reference tables in, 12
Archives of Internal Medicine, 40
Areas under normal curve:
  determining, 191–195
  tables, 322–325
Arithmetic graph paper, 25
Arithmetic mean, 59–66
  averaging percentages or averages, 65–66
  compared with median and mode, 72–74
  concept of, 74
  confidence limits of $\bar{X}_\wp$, 231–235
  defined, 72
  difference between $\bar{X}$ and $\bar{X}_\wp$, 219–231
  difference between $\bar{X}_1$ and $\bar{X}_2$, 235–242
  grouped data, 61–65
  obtaining, 59–61
  reliability of, 209–219
  sample (*see* Sample means)
  of series of sample means, 211
  significance of, 219–242
  ungrouped data, 59–61
Arithmetic progression, 25–26
Arithmetic scales, line diagrams using, 18–24
Array, nature of, 40–41
Average, the, 59
Average comparisons vs. relative comparisons, 3
Average deviation, 84
Averages:
  averaging percentages or, 65–66
  use of, in correlation, 129–131

Bar charts, 18, 31–33
Barlow's Tables, 131
Base, defined, 4
Belk, William P., 115
Berkson, J., 203, 205, 206
Bi-modal frequency distribution, 72
Binomial, 180, 196–201, 247–252, 254–257, 259–263
  fitting of, 196–201
  normal curve and, 180–183
  Poisson distribution and, 201–206
Biometrica, 326–327, 330, 332, 341, 342
Birth-death ratio, 3
Bi-serial r, 143
Body of table, 11
Box head of table, 10–11
Brinton, W. C., 18
Britten, R. H., 54, 55
Burks, Barbara S., 51

Cain, James C., 115
California, University of, Medical School, 151
Camp-Meidell inequality, $90n$.
Casale, W., 231, 236, 296, 305
Causation, and correlation, 127–128
Cause-specific death rates, 9
Census of the United States, 36, 37
Central tendency, measures of, 57–79
  arithmetic mean, 59–66
  comparison of arithmetic mean, median, and mode, 72–77
    algebraic treatment, 76
    basic ideas, 72–74
    extremes of unknown value, effect of, 77
    mathematical properties, 76
    rearrangement and classification of raw data, 76–77
    skewness, 74–76
    unequal class intervals, effect of, 77

Central tendency (*Cont.*):
  geometric mean, 78–79
  median, 59, 66–70
  mode, 59, 70–72
  no best measure of, 72–73
Characteristic, 353
Charts, 18–38
  bar, 18, 31–33
  carelessly drawn, 18, 20
  column diagram, 42
  guide lines on, 21
  kinds of, 18
  lettering, 20, 21–22
  line diagrams, 18–30 (*see also* Line diagrams)
  pictographs, 18, 33–38
  pie diagrams, 18, 31, 35
  preparation of, for publication, 21
  proportions in, 22
  ratio, 25, 27
  reduction of size, 21
  reproduction of, 21
  scale-breaks in, 24
  scatter plot, 112–114
  semi-logarithmic, 25
  source notes, 18–19
  tics in, 21
  titles of, 18, 19
  two frequency curves on one chart, 53
  wall, 21
Ching, Richard E., 267
Chi-square, table of values, 328–329
Chi-square test, 1, 267–283, 288–293
  distribution, 268–269, 282
    interrelations between normal, t, χ^2, and F, 310–311
  "goodness of fit," 282–283
  1×2 table, 267–271
    identity with $p - \pi$ test, 270
    large numbers, 267–269
    small numbers, 271
  1×3 table, 279–280
  2×2 table, 271–278
    identity with $p_1 - p_2$ test, 274
    large numbers, 271–274
    small numbers, 275–278
      exact procedure, 276–278
      Yates' correction, 275–276
  2×3 and larger tables, 280–282

Cholesterol intake, *graphs*, 19, 20, 22, 23, 24
Chronological data, 14
Classes:
  for frequency distribution, 46–52
    number of, 46
    writing, 46–52
  mid-values of, 88, 90
Class intervals, 64–65
  unequal, effect of, 77
Clopper, C. J., 263
Cochran, W. G., 280, 283
Coefficient of correlation (*see* Correlation)
Coin-tossing, and normal curve, 181–182
Colorado, University of, School of Medicine, 149, 160
Column diagram, 42, 49
Comparisons, absolute vs. relative, 3
Confidence limits:
  of π, 257–263
  of σ^2, 291–293
  of $\bar{X}_{\varphi}$, 233–235
  of $\bar{X}_{\varphi_1} - \bar{X}_{\varphi_2}$, 239
  of r, 316
Correlation:
  analysis, objectives of, 114
  and causation, 127–128
  cautions concerning, 127–131
  coefficients of:
    confidence limits, 316
    multiple, 169–174
    non-linear, 156–159
    partial, 172–174
    two-variable linear, 120–126, 133–136
  estimates of, in population, 315–316
  estimating equations:
    multiple, 163–168, 174, 175–176
    non-linear, 152–155, 157, 159
    two-variable linear, 114–119, 136–137
  fortuitous, 127
  intraclass, 138–140
  multiple, 159–178
    four variables, 174–178
    three variables, 159–161, 163–174
  non-linear, 148–159, 163n
  rank, 140–143
  scatter plot, 109–114, 128–130, 149–150, 153
  significance of coefficients, 312–318

INDEX 371

Correlation (*Cont.*):
  simple, 161–163 (*see also* Correlation, two-variable linear)
  standard error of estimate:
    multiple, 168–169, 174, 177
    non-linear, 156, 158, 159
    two-variable linear, 119–120, 137–138
  two-variable linear, 109–143
    grouped data, 131–138
    ungrouped data, 112–131
Cowden, D. J., 10, 24, 38, 45, 71, 79, 91, 97, 117, 133, 163, 186, 212, 213, 228, 236, 263, 335
Croxton, F. E., 10, 24, 38, 45, 71, 79, 91, 97, 117, 133, 163, 186, 212, 213, 228, 236, 263, 323, 324, 335
Crude death rate, 8
Crumpler, T. B., 183
Cumulative frequency distributions (*see* Ogives)
Curves (*see also* Line diagrams):
  approximately symmetrical, 49
  asymmetrical, or skewed, 51, 186
  exactly symmetrical, 49, 51
  frequency distribution, 42–43, 49–52
  "goodness of fit" of, 184, 187, 196, 213, 282–283
  leptokurtic, 101, 103, 104
  normal (*see* Normal curve)
  platykurtic, 101
  skewed, 51, 186 (*see also* Skewness)
  symmetrical, 186

Dahlberg, Gunnar, 253, 279
Data:
  grouped (*see* Grouped data)
  heterogeneous, 128–129
  raw, 39–40
    rearranging or classifying, 76–77
  rigged, 280
  statistics differentiated from, 1
  ungrouped (*see* Ungrouped data)
Death rates, 8–9
Deciles, 68–70
Decimals, misplaced, 6–7
Degrees of freedom, 230, 238, 268, 272–273
Dependent variable, 114
Determination, coefficient of (*see* Correlation, coefficients of)

Deviation:
  average, 84
  explained, 120–122
  standard (*see* Standard deviation)
  total, 120–122
  unexplained, 120–122
Dispersion, measures of, 82–93
  absolute, 82–91
  average deviation, 84
  defined, 59
  measures based on quartiles and percentiles, 83–84
  range, 82–83
  relative, 91–93
  sample means, 211–212
  semi-interquartile range, 83–84
  standard deviation, 84–91
    (*see also* Standard deviation)
  two or more series, compared, 91–93
Distribution:
  binomial, 180, 196–201, 247–252, 254–257, 259–263
  normal (*see* Normal curve)
  of p:
    when $\pi = 0.50$, 247–250
    when $\pi \neq 0.50$, 250–252
  Poisson, 201–206
  sample means, 211–219
Dixon, W. J., 309
Doyle, Rodger P., 233–235, 292

Equation:
  estimating (*see* Estimating equation)
  normal (*see* Normal equations)
  normal curve, 180–183
  regression (*see* Estimating equation)
Errors:
  normal curve of, 183
  standard (*see* Standard error)
  Type I, 223–225, 244
  Type II, 223–225
Estimate, unbiased, 228
Estimated variance (*see under* Variance)
Estimating equation:
  linear correlation, two-variable, 114–120
  multiple, three variables, 163–168
  multiple, four variables, 175–176
  non-linear correlation, 152–159, 163n.

Explained variation, 122–125, 170, 171
Ezekiel, Mordecai, 175

F, tables of values, 334–340
F distribution, 293–295
  interrelationships between normal, t, χ^2, and F, 310–311
Fiducial limits (see Confidence limits)
Fisher, R. A., 199, 314, 326, 329
Footnotes:
  of charts, 20
  of tables, 11, 15
Four-variable correlation, formulas for, 174–178
Freed, S. Charles, 32
Freedom, degrees of, 230, 238, 268, 272–273
Frequency distribution, 39–56
  array, 40–41
  bi-modal, 72
  classes for, 46–49
    number of, 46
    writing, 46–49
  constructing, 43–45
  cumulative (see Ogives)
  graphic comparison of, 53–56
  graphic forms of, 49–52
  graphic portrayal of, 42–43
  ogives, 52–53
  raw data, 39–40
Friedman, Meyer, 32

Gaussian curve (see Normal curve)
Geissler, Arthur, 199
Geometric mean, 59, 78–79
Geometric progression, 26–27
Girshick, Meyer A., 172
"Goodness of fit," test of, 184, 187, 196, 213, 282–283
Goulden, C. H., 281
Grand mean, 296
Graphs, 18–38 (see also charts):
  frequency distribution, 42–43, 49–52
Grouped data:
  arithmetic mean, 59–61
  correlation of, 131–138
  median, 67–68
  mode, 71–72
  standard deviation, 87–91
Grove, R. D., 8
Guide lines on charts, 21

Harding, Paul, 109, 241
Harmonic mean, 59, 78, 79
Haskins, H. D., 40
Headings, in tables, 10–11, 15
Heath, Clark W., 85
Heterogeneity in data, 128–129
Hinton, J. W., 231, 236, 296, 305
Huffman, M., 7
Hurn, M., 203, 205, 206

Independent variable, 114
Interaction, computation of, 307
Interclass correlation, 138
Intraclass correlation, 138–140
Iowa State College Journal of Science, 280, 283

Journal of the American Statistical Association, 51, 203, 276
Judgments based on probabilities, 222

Kendall, Maurice G., 182, 238
Keys, Ancel, 19, 20, 22, 23, 24
Kurtosis, 101–106
  defined, 59, 101
  of sample means, 212–214
  testing significance of, 318–319, 341, 342

Lettering in charts, 20, 21–22
Libby, Raymond L., 110
Linder, F. E., 8
Linear correlation, two-variable (see Correlation: two-variable linear)
Line diagrams:
  using arithmetic scales, 18–24
  using logarithmic vertical scale, 24–30
Localio, S. A., 231, 236, 296, 305
Logarithmic horizontal scale, use of, 152, 153
Logarithmic vertical and horizontal scales, use of, 152, 158
Logarithmic vertical scale, use of, 24–30, 152, 157
Logarithms:
  of numbers, 353
  table of, 354–368
London Mathematical Society, Proceedings of the, 91
Lowenstein, Dyno, 35

INDEX

Magath, T. B., 203, 205, **206**
Mantissa, 353
Maps, statistical, 18, 38
Maresh, Marion M., 160
Marks, Herbert H., 50
Martin, Pete, 7
Marvin, James, 227
Massey, Frank J., Jr., 309
Mather, K., 311
Mean, 59
  arithmetic, 59–66 (*see also* Arithmetic mean)
  designated, 63
  geometric, 59, 78–79
  grand, 296
  harmonic, 59, 78, 79
  population, 210–211
  quadratic, 78, 79
  sample (*see* Sample means)
Median, 59, 66–70
  compared with arithmetic mean and mode, 72–74
  defined, 72
  grouped data, 67–68
  related measures, 68–70
  ungrouped data, 66–67
Medical Statistics Division, Office of Surgeon General, U. S. Army, 49, 50, 51, 95, 99
Medicine, statistics and, 1–3
Merrington, Maxine, 336
Metropolitan Life Insurance Company, 11, 12, 13–14, 15, 16, 17, 31, 32, 33, 35, 38
Meyers, Aldula J., 149
Mid-values of classes, 88, 90
Milbank Memorial Fund, 197
Mode, 70–72
  bi-modality, 72
  compared with arithmetic mean and median, 72–74
  defined, 70
  grouped data, 71–72
  Pearsonian method of determining, 94n.
  ungrouped data, 70–71
  when not measure of central tendency, 73
Modley, Rudolph, 35
Monthly Labor Review, 141
Multiple correlation, 159–178 (*see also* Correlation: multiple)

Multiple determination, coefficient of, 169–170, 172–173, 177

National Office of Vital Statistics, 8, 13, 28, 29, 32
New York Times, The, 267
New Zealand, Dominion of, *Population Census*, 201
Non-linear correlation, 148–159, 163n.
Normal curve, 101, 102, 103, 180–196
  applications, 183–187
  areas under, *table*, 322–325
  distribution, interrelations between, normal, t, χ^2, and F, 310–311
  equation, 180–183
  of error, 183
  fitting process, 187–195
    computing ordinates, 188–191
    determining areas, 191–195
  Gaussian curve, 183
  ordinates of, *table*, 321
  when to fit, 195–196
  Yates' correction for continuity of, 254, 255–256, 265, 275, 276
Normal equations, 116–118, 153–154, 157–159, 161, 162, 164–168, 175–176

O'Brien, Ruth, 132, 172
Ogives, 52–53
Open-end classes, in frequency distributions, 77
Ordinates, normal curve:
  computing, 188–191
  table, 321
Osgood, Edwin E., 40, 188

Page, Ernest W., 151
Partial correlation, 170–173, **177–178**
Pearl, Raymond, 243–244
Pearson, Egon S., 263, 341, 342
Pearson, Karl, 94, 204, 321
  product-moment formula, 125–126
Pearsonian skewness, 80, 94
Percentages:
  computation of, 4–5
    misplaced decimals, 6–7
    rounding, 5–6
    size of base, 7
  ratios and, 4
Percentiles, 68–70
  measures of dispersion based on, 83, 84

Pictographs, 18, 33–38
Pie diagrams, 18, 31, 35
Poisson distribution, 201–206
Population, 209, 210, 226, 246
Prefatory note of table, 11
Probability:
 and suitable criterion of significance, 222–226
 judgment based on, 222
 understatement of, 254
Product-moment formula, 125–126
Proportions:
 confidence limits of π, 257–263
 of non-occurrences, 246
 of occurrences, 246
 reliability and significance of, 246–265
 standard error of, 247
 Yates' correction, 255–256
Public Health Bulletin No. 162, 54, 55
Punch-card equipment, 132n.

Quadratic mean, 78, 79
Quartiles, 68–70
 measures of dispersion based on, 83
Quintiles, 68–70

Race-specific death rates, 9
Random samples:
 arithmetic means from, 210–219
 defined, 209
 proportions from, 247–252
  distribution of p:
   when $\pi = 0.50$, 247–250
   when $\pi \neq 0.50$, 250–252
Range, 82–83
 semi-interquartile, 83–84
Rank correlation, 140–143
Rates:
 defined, 3
 vs. ratios, 3–4
Ratio chart, 24–30
Ratios:
 computation of, 4–5
 defined, 4
 medical, 7–8
 percentages and, 4
 rates vs., 3–4
Reciprocals, squares, and square roots, table, 343–352
Reference tables, 11–12
 in appendix, 12

Reference tables (*Cont.*):
 defined, 11
 designing, 12–13
Regression equation (*see* Estimating equation)
Relative comparisons, absolute, vs., 3
Reliability and significance:
 arithmetic means, 209–244
 correlation coefficients, 312–318
 criterion, suitable, 222–225
 kurtosis, measures of, 318–319
 proportions, 246–265, 270, 274
 skewness, measures of, 318–319
 standard deviations, 288–295
 statistical vs. biological significance, 242–244
 variances, 288–310
Resident death rate, 8–9
Residual variation, 303
Revised death rate, 9
Richardson, C. H., 182
Rider, Paul R., 275
Rietz, H. L., 91
Robbins, W. J., 34
Rounding, 5–6, 91
Rugg, H. O., 321, 322
Ruling:
 in charts, 20–21
 in tables, 16–18

Sample:
 random (*see* Random sample; Sample means)
 standard deviation of, 84–90
Sample means:
 behavior of, 210–219
 dispersion of, 211–212
 expected distribution of, 217–219
 illustrative distributions of, 214–219
 significance of difference, 235–242
  independent samples, 235–239
  non-independent samples, 240–242
 skewness and kurtosis of, 212–214
 standard error of, 212
Sample variances, 288–295
Sampling, reasons for, 209
Scale-breaks, in charts, 24
Scatter, use of, in correlation, 119
Scatter plots, 109, 110, 111, 112–114
Science, 19, 20, 22, 23, 24, 110
Semi-interquartile range, 83–84

INDEX

Semi-logarithmic chart, 25, 28–30
Semi-logarithmic paper, 26, 27, 28, 30
Sex-specific death rates, 9
Sharp & Dohme, Inc., 301
Shelton, William C., 132
Sheppard, W. F., 90–91
Sheppard's correction, 80, 90–91, 100, 103, 319
Shewhart, Walter A., 184, 210, 213, 214, 219, 221, 288
Significance (*see* Reliability and significance)
Significance ratio, 220, 228–229
Simple correlation (*see* Correlation, two-variable linear)
Skewed curves, 186
Skewness, 51, 93–101
  absolute, 94
  defined, 59, 93
  relative, 93–101
  of sample means, 212–214
  testing significance of, 318–319
Snedecor, G. W., 46
Source note:
  of chart, 18–19
  of table, 11, 16
Specific death rates, 9
Spiegelman, Mortimer, 50
Squares, square roots, and reciprocals, *table*, 343–352
Standard deviation, 79, 84–91
  grouped data, 87–90
  Sheppard's correction, 90–91
  ungrouped data, 86–87
Standard error, 119
  of estimate (*see under* Correlation)
  of proportion, 247
  of the mean, 212
Statistical charts (*see* Charts)
Statistical maps, 18, 38
Statistics:
  defined, 1
  differentiated from *data*, 1
  medicine and, 1–3
Stub of table, 10
Surgery, Gynecology, and Obstetrics, 231, 296, 305
Symmetrical curve, 186

t, table of values, 326–327
t distribution, 228–230
  interrelations between normal, t, χ^2, and F, 310–311

Tables, 10–16
  in Appendix, 321–368
    areas under normal curve, 322–325
    logarithms, 354–368
    ordinates of normal curve, 321
    squares, square roots, and reciprocals, 343–352
    upper and lower 0.05 and 0.01 limits of β_2, 342
    upper 0.10 and 0.02 limits of β_1, 341
    values of χ^2, 328–329
    values of F, 334–340
    values of $\frac{\hat{\sigma}^2}{\sigma^2}$, 330–331
    values of $\frac{\sigma^2}{\hat{\sigma}^2}$, 332–333
    values of t, 326–327
  footnotes in, 11, 15
  headings, 10–11, 15
  parts of, 10–11, 14–18
  reference (*see* Reference tables)
  ruling in, 16–18
  source notes in, 11, 16
  text (*see* Text tables)
  titles of, 10, 14–15
  typewritten, 16, 17–18
  units of measurement in, 15
Tchebycheff's inequality, 89–90*n*.
Text tables, 11–12
  defined, 11–12
  designing, 13–14
Thompson, Catherine M., 330, 332, 336
Thompson, L. R., 54, 55
Three-variable correlation, 148, 159–161, 163–168 (*see also* Correlation: multiple)
Tics, in charts, 21
Title:
  of chart, 18
  of table, 10, 14–15
Total variation, 156, 297–298, 300–302, 304
Two-variable correlation, 161–163
  linear, 109–143 (*see also* Correlation: two-variable linear)
Typewritten tables, 16, 17–18

Unexplained variation, 122–125, 170–171

Ungrouped data:
  arithmetic mean, 59–61
  correlation of, 112–114
  median, 66–67
  mode, 70–71
  standard deviation, 86–87
United States Army, 49, 50, 51
United States Bureau of the Census, 36–37
United States Children's Bureau, 104
United States Department of Agriculture, 109, 132, 172, 241
United States Fruit Company, 271
Units of measurement, in tables, 15

Variables:
  continuous, 46–47
  dependent, 114
  discrete, 46–47
  independent, 114
  interdependent, 127
  one variable, as cause of other, 127
Variance, 84n., 228, 295–310
  analysis of, 295–310
    estimated variance, 298–299, 303–304, 307–310
      between column means, 298–299, 303–304, 307–310
      between row means, 303–304, 307–310
      interaction, 307–310
      residual, 303–304
      within boxes, 307–310
      within columns, 298–299
    one criterion of classification, 295–300
    two criteria of classification, 300–310
      more than one entry in each box, 304–310
      one entry in each box, 300–304
    variation (see Variation)
  estimate of population variance, 228, 299
  population variance, 288–291
  reliability and significance of, 288–295
    confidence limits of σ^2, 291–293
    difference between $\hat{\sigma}^2$ and σ^2, 288–291
    difference between $\hat{\sigma}_1^2$ and $\hat{\sigma}_2^2$, 293–295

Variation:
  between column means, 295–297, 302, 304–306
  between row means, 302, 306
  explained, 122–125, 156, 170–171
  interaction, 307
  residual, 303
  total, 156, 297–298, 300–302, 304
  unexplained, 122–125, 170–171
  within boxes, 306–307
  within columns, 297
Vital rates, 8–9
Vital Statistics, National Office of, Public Health Service, 8, 13, 28, 29, 32

Wall charts, 21
Wilks, S. S., 201
Wingfield, Alex H., 111
Woodbury, Robert Morse, 104

$\bar{X}_\mathcal{P}$, confidence limits of, 231–235
χ^2, values of, table, 328–329
χ^2 test (see Chi-square test)
$\bar{X}$ and $\bar{X}_\mathcal{P}$, significance of differences between:
  population values known 219–226
    non-significant difference, 219–221
    significant difference, 221–222
    suitable criterion of significance, 222–226
  when σ is not known, 226–231
$\bar{X}_1$ and $\bar{X}_2$, significance of differences between:
  independent samples, 235–239
  non-independent samples, 240–242

Yates, F., 326, 329
Yates correction, 254, 255–256, 265, 275, 276
Yoe, J. H., 183
Yule, G. U., 182

Zero:
  correlation, 111–112, 114
  on scatter-plot scales, 113–114
  on vertical scale of chart, 22

CATALOGUE OF DOVER BOOKS

Catalogue of Dover Books

BOOKS EXPLAINING SCIENCE AND MATHEMATICS

General

WHAT IS SCIENCE?, Norman Campbell. This excellent introduction explains scientific method, role of mathematics, types of scientific laws. Contents: 2 aspects of science, science & nature, laws of science, discovery of laws, explanation of laws, measurement & numerical laws, applications of science. 192pp. 5⅜ x 8. S43 Paperbound **$1.25**

THE COMMON SENSE OF THE EXACT SCIENCES, W. K. Clifford. Introduction by James Newman, edited by Karl Pearson. For 70 years this has been a guide to classical scientific and mathematical thought. Explains with unusual clarity basic concepts, such as extension of meaning of symbols, characteristics of surface boundaries, properties of plane figures, vectors, Cartesian method of determining position, etc. Long preface by Bertrand Russell. Bibliography of Clifford. Corrected, 130 diagrams redrawn. 249pp. 5⅜ x 8. T61 Paperbound **$1.60**

SCIENCE THEORY AND MAN, Erwin Schrödinger. This is a complete and unabridged reissue of SCIENCE AND THE HUMAN TEMPERAMENT plus an additional essay: "What is an Elementary Particle?" Nobel laureate Schrödinger discusses such topics as nature of scientific method, the nature of science, chance and determinism, science and society, conceptual models for physical entities, elementary particles and wave mechanics. Presentation is popular and may be followed by most people with little or no scientific training. "Fine practical preparation for a time when laws of nature, human institutions . . . are undergoing a critical examination without parallel," Waldemar Kaempffert, N. Y. TIMES. 192pp. 5⅜ x 8. T428 Paperbound **$1.35**

FADS AND FALLACIES IN THE NAME OF SCIENCE, Martin Gardner. Examines various cults, quack systems, frauds, delusions which at various times have masqueraded as science. Accounts of hollow-earth fanatics like Symmes; Velikovsky and wandering planets; Hoerbiger; Bellamy and the theory of multiple moons; Charles Fort; dowsing, pseudoscientific methods for finding water, ores, oil. Sections on naturopathy, iridiagnosis, zone therapy, food fads, etc. Analytical accounts of Wilhelm Reich and orgone sex energy; L. Ron Hubbard and Dianetics; A. Korzybski and General Semantics; many others. Brought up to date to include Bridey Murphy, others. Not just a collection of anecdotes, but a fair, reasoned appraisal of eccentric theory. Formerly titled IN THE NAME OF SCIENCE. Preface. Index. x + 384pp. 5⅜ x 8. T394 Paperbound **$1.50**

A DOVER SCIENCE SAMPLER, edited by George Barkin. 64-page book, sturdily bound, containing excerpts from over 20 Dover books, explaining science. Edwin Hubble, George Sarton, Ernst Mach, A. d'Abro, Galileo, Newton, others, discussing island universes, scientific truth, biological phenomena, stability in bridges, etc. Copies limited; no more than 1 to a customer, **FREE**

POPULAR SCIENTIFIC LECTURES, Hermann von Helmholtz. Helmholtz was a superb expositor as well as a scientist of genius in many areas. The seven essays in this volume are models of clarity, and even today they rank among the best general descriptions of their subjects ever written. "The Physiological Causes of Harmony in Music" was the first significant physiological explanation of musical consonance and dissonance. Two essays, "On the Interaction of Natural Forces" and "On the Conservation of Force," were of great importance in the history of science, for they firmly established the principle of the conservation of energy. Other lectures include "On the Relation of Optics to Painting," "On Recent Progress in the Theory of Vision," "On Goethe's Scientific Researches," and "On the Origin and Significance of Geometrical Axioms." Selected and edited with an introduction by Professor Morris Kline. xii + 286pp. 5⅜ x 8½. T799 Paperbound **$1.45**

BOOKS EXPLAINING SCIENCE AND MATHEMATICS

Physics

CONCERNING THE NATURE OF THINGS, Sir William Bragg. Christmas lectures delivered at the Royal Society by Nobel laureate. Why a spinning ball travels in a curved track; how uranium is transmuted to lead, etc. Partial contents: atoms, gases, liquids, crystals, metals, etc. No scientific background needed; wonderful for intelligent child. 32pp. of photos, 57 figures. xii + 232pp. 5⅜ x 8. T31 Paperbound **$1.35**

THE RESTLESS UNIVERSE, Max Born. New enlarged version of this remarkably readable account by a Nobel laureate. Moving from sub-atomic particles to universe, the author explains in very simple terms the latest theories of wave mechanics. Partial contents: air and its relatives, electrons & ions, waves & particles, electronic structure of the atom, nuclear physics. Nearly 1000 illustrations, including 7 animated sequences. 325pp. 6 x 9. T412 Paperbound **$2.00**

Catalogue of Dover Books

FROM EUCLID TO EDDINGTON: A STUDY OF THE CONCEPTIONS OF THE EXTERNAL WORLD, Sir Edmund Whittaker. A foremost British scientist traces the development of theories of natural philosophy from the western rediscovery of Euclid to Eddington, Einstein, Dirac, etc. The inadequacy of classical physics is contrasted with present day attempts to understand the physical world through relativity, non-Euclidean geometry, space curvature, wave mechanics, etc. 5 major divisions of examination: Space; Time and Movement; the Concepts of Classical Physics; the Concepts of Quantum Mechanics; the Eddington Universe. 212pp. 5⅜ x 8. T491 Paperbound **$1.35**

PHYSICS, THE PIONEER SCIENCE, L. W. Taylor. First thorough text to place all important physical phenomena in cultural-historical framework; remains best work of its kind. Exposition of physical laws, theories developed chronologically, with great historical, illustrative experiments diagrammed, described, worked out mathematically. Excellent physics text for self-study as well as class work. Vol. 1: Heat, Sound: motion, acceleration, gravitation, conservation of energy, heat engines, rotation, heat, mechanical energy, etc. 211 illus. 407pp. 5⅜ x 8. Vol. 2: Light, Electricity: images, lenses, prisms, magnetism, Ohm's law, dynamos, telegraph, quantum theory, decline of mechanical view of nature, etc. Bibliography. 13 table appendix. Index. 551 illus. 2 color plates. 508pp. 5⅜ x 8.
Vol. 1 S565 Paperbound **$2.00**
Vol. 2 S566 Paperbound **$2.00**
The set **$4.00**

A SURVEY OF PHYSICAL THEORY, Max Planck. One of the greatest scientists of all time, creator of the quantum revolution in physics, writes in non-technical terms of his own discoveries and those of other outstanding creators of modern physics. Planck wrote this book when science had just crossed the threshold of the new physics, and he communicates the excitement felt then as he discusses electromagnetic theories, statistical methods, evolution of the concept of light, a step-by-step description of how he developed his own momentous theory, and many more of the basic ideas behind modern physics. Formerly "A Survey of Physics." Bibliography. Index. 128pp. 5⅜ x 8. S650 Paperbound **$1.15**

THE ATOMIC NUCLEUS, M. Korsunsky. The only non-technical comprehensive account of the atomic nucleus in English. For college physics students, etc. Chapters cover: Radioactivity, the Nuclear Model of the Atom, the Mass of Atomic Nuclei, the Disintegration of Atomic Nuclei, the Discovery of the Positron, the Artificial Transformation of Atomic Nuclei, Artificial Radioactivity, Mesons, the Neutrino, the Structure of Atomic Nuclei and Forces Acting Between Nuclear Particles, Nuclear Fission, Chain Reaction, Peaceful Uses, Thermonuclear Reactions. Slightly abridged edition. Translated by G. Yankovsky. 65 figures. Appendix includes 45 photographic illustrations. 413 pp. 5⅜ x 8. S1052 Paperbound **$2.00**

PRINCIPLES OF MECHANICS SIMPLY EXPLAINED, Morton Mott-Smith. Excellent, highly readable introduction to the theories and discoveries of classical physics. Ideal for the layman who desires a foundation which will enable him to understand and appreciate contemporary developments in the physical sciences. Discusses: Density, The Law of Gravitation, Mass and Weight, Action and Reaction, Kinetic and Potential Energy, The Law of Inertia, Effects of Acceleration, The Independence of Motions, Galileo and the New Science of Dynamics, Newton and the New Cosmos, The Conservation of Momentum, and other topics. Revised edition of "This Mechanical World." Illustrated by E. Kosa, Jr. Bibliography and Chronology. Index. xiv + 171pp. 5⅜ x 8½. T1067 Paperbound **$1.00**

THE CONCEPT OF ENERGY SIMPLY EXPLAINED, Morton Mott-Smith. Elementary, non-technical exposition which traces the story of man's conquest of energy, with particular emphasis on the developments during the nineteenth century and the first three decades of our own century. Discusses man's earlier efforts to harness energy, more recent experiments and discoveries relating to the steam engine, the engine indicator, the motive power of heat, the principle of excluded perpetual motion, the bases of the conservation of energy, the concept of entropy, the internal combustion engine, mechanical refrigeration, and many other related topics. Also much biographical material. Index. Bibliography. 33 illustrations. ix + 215pp. 5⅜ x 8½. T1071 Paperbound **$1.25**

HEAT AND ITS WORKINGS, Morton Mott-Smith. One of the best elementary introductions to the theory and attributes of heat, covering such matters as the laws governing the effect of heat on solids, liquids and gases, the methods by which heat is measured, the conversion of a substance from one form to another through heating and cooling, evaporation, the effects of pressure on boiling and freezing points, and the three ways in which heat is transmitted (conduction, convection, radiation). Also brief notes on major experiments and discoveries. Concise, but complete, it presents all the essential facts about the subject in readable style. Will give the layman and beginning student a first-rate background in this major topic in physics. Index. Bibliography. 50 illustrations. x + 165pp. 5⅜ x 8½. T978 Paperbound **$1.00**

THE STORY OF ATOMIC THEORY AND ATOMIC ENERGY, J. G. Feinberg. Wider range of facts on physical theory, cultural implications, than any other similar source. Completely non-technical. Begins with first atomic theory, 600 B.C., goes through A-bomb, developments to 1959. Avogadro, Rutherford, Bohr, Einstein, radioactive decay, binding energy, radiation danger, future benefits of nuclear power, dozens of other topics, told in lively, related, informal manner. Particular stress on European atomic research. "Deserves special mention . . . authoritative," Saturday Review. Formerly "The Atom Story." New chapter to 1959. Index. 34 illustrations. 251pp. 5⅜ x 8. T625 Paperbound **$1.45**

Catalogue of Dover Books

THE STRANGE STORY OF THE QUANTUM, AN ACCOUNT FOR THE GENERAL READER OF THE GROWTH OF IDEAS UNDERLYING OUR PRESENT ATOMIC KNOWLEDGE, B. Hoffmann. Presents lucidly and expertly, with barest amount of mathematics, the problems and theories which led to modern quantum physics. Dr. Hoffmann begins with the closing years of the 19th century, when certain trifling discrepancies were noticed, and with illuminating analogies and examples takes you through the brilliant concepts of Planck, Einstein, Pauli, de Broglie, Bohr, Schroedinger, Heisenberg, Dirac, Sommerfeld, Feynman, etc. This edition includes a new, long postscript carrying the story through 1958. "Of the books attempting an account of the history and contents of our modern atomic physics which have come to my attention, this is the best," H. Margenau, Yale University, in "American Journal of Physics.". 32 tables and line illustrations. Index. 275pp. 5⅜ x 8. T518 Paperbound **$1.50**

THE EVOLUTION OF SCIENTIFIC THOUGHT FROM NEWTON TO EINSTEIN, A. d'Abro. Einstein's special and general theories of relativity, with their historical implications, are analyzed in non-technical terms. Excellent accounts of the contributions of Newton, Riemann, Weyl, Planck, Eddington, Maxwell, Lorentz and others are treated in terms of space and time, equations of electromagnetics, finiteness of the universe, methodology of science. 21 diagrams. 482pp. 5⅜ x 8. T2 Paperound **$2.00**

THE RISE OF THE NEW PHYSICS, A. d'Abro. A half-million word exposition, formerly titled THE DECLINE OF MECHANISM, for readers not versed in higher mathematics. The only thorough explanation, in everyday language, of the central core of modern mathematical physical theory, treating both classical and modern theoretical physics, and presenting in terms almost anyone can understand the equivalent of 5 years of study of mathematical physics. Scientifically impeccable coverage of mathematical-physical thought from the Newtonian system up through the electronic theories of Dirac and Heisenberg and Fermi's statistics. Combines both history and exposition; provides a broad yet unified and detailed view, with constant comparison of classical and modern views on phenomena and theories. "A must for anyone doing serious study in the physical sciences," JOURNAL OF THE FRANKLIN INSTITUTE. "Extraordinary faculty . . . to explain ideas and theories of theoretical physics in the language of daily life," ISIS. First part of set covers philosophy of science, drawing upon the practice of Newton, Maxwell, Poincaré, Einstein, others, discussing modes of thought, experiment, interpretations of causality, etc. In the second part, 100 pages explain grammar and vocabulary of mathematics, with discussions of functions, groups, series, Fourier series, etc. The remainder is devoted to concrete, detailed coverage of both classical and quantum physics, explaining such topics as analytic mechanics, Hamilton's principle, wave theory of light, electromagnetic waves, groups of transformations, thermodynamics, phase rule, Brownian movement, kinetics, special relativity, Planck's original quantum theory, Bohr's atom, Zeeman effect, Broglie's wave mechanics, Heisenberg's uncertainty, Eigen-values, matrices, scores of other important topics. Discoveries and theories are covered for such men as Alembert, Born, Cantor, Debye, Euler, Foucault, Galois, Gauss, Hadamard, Kelvin, Kepler, Laplace, Maxwell, Pauli, Rayleigh, Volterra, Weyl, Young, more than 180 others. Indexed. 97 illustrations. ix + 982pp. 5⅜ x 8.
T3 Volume 1, Paperbound **$2.00**
T4 Volume 2, Paperbound **$2.00**

SPINNING TOPS AND GYROSCOPIC MOTION, John Perry. Well-known classic of science still unsurpassed for lucid, accurate, delightful exposition. How quasi-rigidity is induced in flexible and fluid bodies by rapid motions; why gyrostat falls, top rises; nature and effect on climatic conditions of earth's precessional movement; effect of internal fluidity on rotating bodies, etc. Appendixes describe practical uses to which gyroscopes have been put in ships, compasses, monorail transportation. 62 figures. 128pp. 5⅜ x 8. T416 Paperbound **$1.00**

THE UNIVERSE OF LIGHT, Sir William Bragg. No scientific training needed to read Nobel Prize winner's expansion of his Royal Institute Christmas Lectures. Insight into nature of light, methods and philosophy of science. Explains lenses, reflection, color, resonance, polarization, x-rays, the spectrum, Newton's work with prisms, Huygens' with polarization, Crookes' with cathode ray, etc. Leads into clear statement of 2 major historical theories of light, corpuscule and wave. Dozens of experiments you can do. 199 illus., including 2 full-page color plates. 293pp. 5⅜ x 8. S538 Paperbound **$1.85**

THE STORY OF X-RAYS FROM RÖNTGEN TO ISOTOPES, A. R. Bleich. Non-technical history of x-rays, their scientific explanation, their applications in medicine, industry, research, and art, and their effect on the individual and his descendants. Includes amusing early reactions to Röntgen's discovery, cancer therapy, detections of art and stamp forgeries, potential risks to patient and operator, etc. Illustrations show x-rays of flower structure, the gall bladder, gears with hidden defects, etc. Original Dover publication. Glossary. Bibliography. Index. 55 photos and figures. xiv + 186pp. 5⅜ x 8. T662 Paperbound **$1.35**

ELECTRONS, ATOMS, METALS AND ALLOYS, Wm. Hume-Rothery. An introductory-level explanation of the application of the electronic theory to the structure and properties of metals and alloys, taking into account the new theoretical work done by mathematical physicists. Material presented in dialogue-form between an "Old Metallurgist" and a "Young Scientist." Their discussion falls into 4 main parts: the nature of an atom, the nature of a metal, the nature of an alloy, and the structure of the nucleus. They cover such topics as the hydrogen atom, electron waves, wave mechanics, Brillouin zones, co-valent bonds, radioactivity and natural disintegration, fundamental particles, structure and fission of the nucleus, etc. Revised, enlarged edition. 177 illustrations. Subject and name indexes. 407pp. 5⅜ x 8½. S1046 Paperbound **$2.25**

Catalogue of Dover Books

OUT OF THE SKY, H. H. Nininger. A non-technical but comprehensive introduction to "meteoritics", the young science concerned with all aspects of the arrival of matter from outer space. Written by one of the world's experts on meteorites, this work shows how, despite difficulties of observation and sparseness of data, a considerable body of knowledge has arisen. It defines meteors and meteorites; studies fireball clusters and processions, meteorite composition, size, distribution, showers, explosions, origins, craters, and much more. A true connecting link between astronomy and geology. More than 175 photos, 22 other illustrations. References. Bibliography of author's publications on meteorites. Index. viii + 336pp. 5⅜ x 8. T519 Paperbound **$1.85**

SATELLITES AND SCIENTIFIC RESEARCH, D. King-Hele. Non-technical account of the manmade satellites and the discoveries they have yielded up to the autumn of 1961. Brings together information hitherto published only in hard-to-get scientific journals. Includes the life history of a typical satellite, methods of tracking, new information on the shape of the earth, zones of radiation, etc. Over 60 diagrams and 6 photographs. Mathematical appendix. Bibliography of over 100 items. Index. xii + 180pp. 5⅜ x 8½. T703 Paperbound **$2.00**

BOOKS EXPLAINING SCIENCE AND MATHEMATICS

Mathematics

CHANCE, LUCK AND STATISTICS: THE SCIENCE OF CHANCE, Horace C. Levinson. Theory of probability and science of statistics in simple, non-technical language. Part I deals with theory of probability, covering odd superstitions in regard to "luck," the meaning of betting odds, the law of mathematical expectation, gambling, and applications in poker, roulette, lotteries, dice, bridge, and other games of chance. Part II discusses the misuse of statistics, the concept of statistical probabilities, normal and skew frequency distributions, and statistics applied to various fields—birth rates, stock speculation, insurance rates, advertising, etc. "Presented in an easy humorous style which I consider the best kind of expository writing," Prof. A. C. Cohen, Industry Quality Control. Enlarged revised edition. Formerly titled "The Science of Chance." Preface and two new appendices by the author. Index. xiv + 365pp. 5⅜ x 8. T1007 Paperbound **$1.85**

PROBABILITIES AND LIFE, Emile Borel. Translated by M. Baudin. Non-technical, highly readable introduction to the results of probability as applied to everyday situations. Partial contents: Fallacies About Probabilities Concerning Life After Death; Negligible Probabilities and the Probabilities of Everyday Life; Events of Small Probability; Application of Probabilities to Certain Problems of Heredity; Probabilities of Deaths, Diseases, and Accidents; On Poisson's Formula. Index. 3 Appendices of statistical studies and tables. vi + 87pp. 5⅜ x 8½. T121 Paperbound **$1.00**

GREAT IDEAS OF MODERN MATHEMATICS: THEIR NATURE AND USE, Jagjit Singh. Reader with only high school math will understand main mathematical ideas of modern physics, astronomy, genetics, psychology, evolution, etc., better than many who use them as tools, but comprehend little of their basic structure. Author uses his wide knowledge of non-mathematical fields in brilliant exposition of differential equations, matrices, group theory, logic, statistics, problems of mathematical foundations, imaginary numbers, vectors, etc. Original publication. 2 appendices. 2 indexes. 65 illustr. 322pp. 5⅜ x 8. S587 Paperbound **$1.75**

MATHEMATICS IN ACTION, O. G. Sutton. Everyone with a command of high school algebra will find this book one of the finest possible introductions to the application of mathematics to physical theory. Ballistics, numerical analysis, waves and wavelike phenomena, Fourier series, group concepts, fluid flow and aerodynamics, statistical measures, and meteorology are discussed with unusual clarity. Some calculus and differential equations theory is developed by the author for the reader's help in the more difficult sections. 88 figures. Index. viii + 236pp. 5⅜ x 8. T440 Clothbound **$3.50**

THE FOURTH DIMENSION SIMPLY EXPLAINED, edited by H. P. Manning. 22 essays, originally Scientific American contest entries, that use a minimum of mathematics to explain aspects of 4-dimensional geometry: analogues to 3-dimensional space, 4-dimensional absurdities and curiosities (such as removing the contents of an egg without puncturing its shell), possible measurements and forms, etc. Introduction by the editor. Only book of its sort on a truly elementary level, excellent introduction to advanced works. 82 figures. 251pp. 5⅜ x 8. T711 Paperbound **$1.35**

Catalogue of Dover Books

MATHEMATICS—INTERMEDIATE TO ADVANCED

General

INTRODUCTION TO APPLIED MATHEMATICS, Francis D. Murnaghan. A practical and thoroughly sound introduction to a number of advanced branches of higher mathematics. Among the selected topics covered in detail are: vector and matrix analysis, partial and differential equations, integral equations, calculus of variations, Laplace transform theory, the vector triple product, linear vector functions, quadratic and bilinear forms, Fourier series, spherical harmonics, Bessel functions, the Heaviside expansion formula, and many others. Extremely useful book for graduate students in physics, engineering, chemistry, and mathematics. Index. 111 study exercises with answers. 41 illustrations. ix + 389pp. 5 3/8 x 8 1/2.
S1042 Paperbound **$2.00**

OPERATIONAL METHODS IN APPLIED MATHEMATICS, H. S. Carslaw and J. C. Jaeger. Explanation of the application of the Laplace Transformation to differential equations, a simple and effective substitute for more difficult and obscure operational methods. Of great practical value to engineers and to all workers in applied mathematics. Chapters on: Ordinary Linear Differential Equations with Constant Coefficients;; Electric Circuit Theory; Dynamical Applications; The Inversion Theorem for the Laplace Transformation; Conduction of Heat; Vibrations of Continuous Mechanical Systems; Hydrodynamics; Impulsive Functions; Chains of Differential Equations; and other related matters. 3 appendices. 153 problems, many with answers. 22 figures. xvi + 359pp. 5 3/8 x 8 1/2.
S1011 Paperbound **$2.25**

APPLIED MATHEMATICS FOR RADIO AND COMMUNICATIONS ENGINEERS, C. E. Smith. No extraneous material here!—only the theories, equations, and operations essential and immediately useful for radio work. Can be used as refresher, as handbook of applications and tables, or as full home-study course. Ranges from simplest arithmetic through calculus, series, and wave forms, hyperbolic trigonometry, simultaneous equations in mesh circuits, etc. Supplies applications right along with each math topic discussed. 22 useful tables of functions, formulas, logs, etc. Index. 166 exercises, 140 examples, all with answers. 95 diagrams. Bibliography. x + 336pp. 5 3/8 x 8.
S141 Paperbound **$1.75**

Algebra, group theory, determinants, sets, matrix theory

ALGEBRAS AND THEIR ARITHMETICS, L. E. Dickson. Provides the foundation and background necessary to any advanced undergraduate or graduate student studying abstract algebra. Begins with elementary introduction to linear transformations, matrices, field of complex numbers; proceeds to order, basal units, modulus, quaternions, etc.; develops calculus of linears sets, describes various examples of algebras including invariant, difference, nilpotent, semi-simple. "Makes the reader marvel at his genius for clear and profound analysis," Amer. Mathematical Monthly. Index. xii + 241pp. 5 3/8 x 8.
S616 Paperbound **$1.50**

THE THEORY OF EQUATIONS WITH AN INTRODUCTION TO THE THEORY OF BINARY ALGEBRAIC FORMS, W. S. Burnside and A. W. Panton. Extremely thorough and concrete discussion of the theory of equations, with extensive detailed treatment of many topics curtailed in later texts. Covers theory of algebraic equations, properties of polynomials, symmetric functions, derived functions, Horner's process, complex numbers and the complex variable, determinants and methods of elimination, invariant theory (nearly 100 pages), transformations, introduction to Galois theory, Abelian equations, and much more. Invaluable supplementary work for modern students and teachers. 759 examples and exercises. Index in each volume. Two volume set. Total of xxiv + 604pp. 5 3/8 x 8.
S714 Vol I Paperbound **$1.85**
S715 Vol II Paperbound **$1.85**
The set **$3.70**

COMPUTATIONAL METHODS OF LINEAR ALGEBRA, V. N. Faddeeva, translated by **C. D. Benster.** First English translation of a unique and valuable work, the only work in English presenting a systematic exposition of the most important methods of linear algebra—classical and contemporary. Shows in detail how to derive numerical solutions of problems in mathematical physics which are frequently connected with those of linear algebra. Theory as well as individual practice. Part I surveys the mathematical background that is indispensable to what follows. Parts II and III, the conclusion, set forth the most important methods of solution, for both exact and iterative groups. One of the most outstanding and valuable features of this work is the 23 tables, double and triple checked for accuracy. These tables will not be found elsewhere. Author's preface. Translator's note. New bibliography and index. x + 252pp. 5 3/8 x 8.
S424 Paperbound **$1.95**

ALGEBRAIC EQUATIONS, E. Dehn. Careful and complete presentation of Galois' theory of algebraic equations; theories of Lagrange and Galois developed in logical rather than historical form, with a more thorough exposition than in most modern books. Many concrete applications and fully-worked-out examples. Discusses basic theory (very clear exposition of the symmetric group); isomorphic, transitive, and Abelian groups; applications of Lagrange's and Galois' theories; and much more. Newly revised by the author. Index. List of Theorems. xi + 208pp. 5 3/8 x 8.
S697 Paperbound **$1.45**

Catalogue of Dover Books

Differential equations, ordinary and partial; integral equations

INTRODUCTION TO THE DIFFERENTIAL EQUATIONS OF PHYSICS, L. Hopf. Especially valuable to the engineer with no math beyond elementary calculus. Emphasizing intuitive rather than formal aspects of concepts, the author covers an extensive territory. Partial contents: Law of causality, energy theorem, damped oscillations, coupling by friction, cylindrical and spherical coordinates, heat source, etc. Index. 48 figures. 160pp. 5⅜ x 8.
S120 Paperbound **$1.25**

INTRODUCTION TO THE THEORY OF LINEAR DIFFERENTIAL EQUATIONS, E. G. Poole. Authoritative discussions of important topics, with methods of solution more detailed than usual, for students with background of elementary course in differential equations. Studies existence theorems, linearly independent solutions; equations with constant coefficients; with uniform analytic coefficients; regular singularities; the hypergeometric equation; conformal representation; etc. Exercises. Index. 210pp. 5⅜ x 8. S629 Paperbound **$1.65**

DIFFERENTIAL EQUATIONS FOR ENGINEERS, P. Franklin. Outgrowth of a course given 10 years at M. I. T. Makes most useful branch of pure math accessible for practical work. Theoretical basis of D.E.'s; solution of ordinary D.E.'s and partial derivatives arising from heat flow, steady-state temperature of a plate, wave equations; analytic functions; convergence of Fourier Series. 400 problems on electricity, vibratory systems, other topics. Formerly "Differential Equations for Electrical Engineers." Index 41 illus. 307pp. 5⅜ x 8.
S601 Paperbound **$1.65**

DIFFERENTIAL EQUATIONS, F. R. Moulton. A detailed, rigorous exposition of all the nonelementary processes of solving ordinary differential equations. Several chapters devoted to the treatment of practical problems, especially those of a physical nature, which are far more advanced than problems usually given as illustrations. Includes analytic differential equations; variations of a parameter; integrals of differential equations; analytic implicit functions; problems of elliptic motion; sine-amplitude functions; deviation of formal bodies; Cauchy-Lipschitz process; linear differential equations with periodic coefficients; differential equations in infinitely many variations; much more. Historical notes. 10 figures. 222 problems. Index. xv + 395pp. 5⅜ x 8. S451 Paperbound **$2.00**

DIFFERENTIAL AND INTEGRAL EQUATIONS OF MECHANICS AND PHYSICS (DIE DIFFERENTIAL- UND INTEGRALGLEICHUNGEN DER MECHANIK UND PHYSIK), edited by P. Frank and R. von Mises. Most comprehensive and authoritative work on the mathematics of mathematical physics available today in the United States: the standard, definitive reference for teachers, physicists, engineers, and mathematicians—now published (in the original German) at a relatively inexpensive price for the first time! Every chapter in this 2,000-page set is by an expert in his field: Carathéodory, Courant, Frank, Mises, and a dozen others. Vol I, on mathematics, gives concise but complete coverages of advanced calculus, differential equations, integral equations, and potential, and partial differential equations. Index. xxiii + 916pp. Vol. II (physics): classical mechanics, optics, continuous mechanics, heat conduction and diffusion, the stationary and quasi-stationary electromagnetic field, electromagnetic oscillations, and wave mechanics. Index. xxiv + 1106pp. Two volume set. Each volume available separately. 5⅝ x 8⅜.
S787 Vol I Clothbound **$7.50**
S788 Vol II Clothbound **$7.50**
The set **$15.00**

LECTURES ON CAUCHY'S PROBLEM, J. Hadamard. Based on lectures given at Columbia, Rome, this discusses work of Riemann, Kirchhoff, Volterra, and the author's own research on the hyperbolic case in linear partial differential equations. It extends spherical and cylindrical waves to apply to all (normal) hyperbolic equations. Partial contents: Cauchy's problem, fundamental formula, equations with odd number, with even number of independent variables; method of descent. 32 figures. Index. iii + 316pp. 5⅜ x 8. S105 Paperbound **$1.75**

THEORY OF DIFFERENTIAL EQUATIONS, A. R. Forsyth. Out of print for over a decade, the complete 6 volumes (now bound as 3) of this monumental work represent the most comprehensive treatment of differential equations ever written. Historical presentation includes in 2500 pages every substantial development. Vol. 1, 2: EXACT EQUATIONS, PFAFF'S PROBLEM; ORDINARY EQUATIONS, NOT LINEAR: methods of Grassmann, Clebsch, Lie, Darboux; Cauchy's theorem; branch points; etc. Vol. 3, 4: ORDINARY EQUATIONS, NOT LINEAR; ORDINARY LINEAR EQUATIONS: Zeta Fuchsian functions, general theorems on algebraic integrals, Brun's theorem, equations with uniform periodic coffiecients, etc. Vol. 4, 5: PARTIAL DIFFERENTIAL EQUATIONS: 2 existence-theorems, equations of theoretical dynamics, Laplace transformations, general transformation of equations of the 2nd order, much more. Indexes. Total of 2766pp. 5⅜ x 8. S576-7-8 Clothbound: the set **$15.00**

PARTIAL DIFFERENTIAL EQUATIONS OF MATHEMATICAL PHYSICS, A. G. Webster. A keystone work in the library of every mature physicist, engineer, researcher. Valuable sections on elasticity, compression theory, potential theory, theory of sound, heat conduction, wave propagation, vibration theory. Contents include: deduction of differential equations, vibrations, normal functions, Fourier's series, Cauchy's method, boundary problems, method of Riemann-Volterra. Spherical, cylindrical, ellipsoidal harmonics, applications, etc. 97 figures. vii + 440pp. 5⅜ x 8. S263 Paperbound **$2.00**

Catalogue of Dover Books

ELEMENTARY CONCEPTS OF TOPOLOGY, P. Alexandroff. First English translation of the famous brief introduction to topology for the beginner or for the mathematician not undertaking extensive study. This unusually useful intuitive approach deals primarily with the concepts of complex, cycle, and homology, and is wholly consistent with current investigations. Ranges from basic concepts of set-theoretic topology to the concept of Betti groups. "Glowing example of harmony between intuition and thought," David Hilbert. Translated by A. E. Farley. Introduction by D. Hilbert. Index. 25 figures. 73pp. 5⅜ x 8. S747 Paperbound **$1.00**

Number theory

INTRODUCTION TO THE THEORY OF NUMBERS, L. E. Dickson. Thorough, comprehensive approach with adequate coverage of classical literature, an introductory volume beginners can follow. Chapters on divisibility, congruences, quadratic residues & reciprocity, Diophantine equations, etc. Full treatment of binary quadratic forms without usual restriction to integral coefficients. Covers infinitude of primes, least residues, Fermat's theorem, Euler's phi function, Legendre's symbol, Gauss's lemma, automorphs, reduced forms, recent theorems of Thue & Siegel, many more. Much material not readily available elsewhere. 239 problems. Index. I figure. viii + 183pp. 5⅜ x 8. S342 Paperbound **$1.65**

ELEMENTS OF NUMBER THEORY, I. M. Vinogradov. Detailed 1st course for persons without advanced mathematics; 95% of this book can be understood by readers who have gone no farther than high school algebra. Partial contents: divisibility theory, important number theoretical functions, congruences, primitive roots and indices, etc. Solutions to both problems and exercises. Tables of primes, indices, etc. Covers almost every essential formula in elementary number theory! Translated from Russian. 233 problems, 104 exercises. viii + 227pp. 5⅜ x 8. S259 Paperbound **$1.60**

THEORY OF NUMBERS and DIOPHANTINE ANALYSIS, R. D. Carmichael. These two complete works in one volume form one of the most lucid introductions to number theory, requiring only a firm foundation in high school mathematics. "Theory of Numbers," partial contents: Eratosthenes' sieve, Euclid's fundamental theorem, G.C.F. and L.C.M. of two or more integers, linear congruences, etc "Diophantine Analysis": rational triangles, Pythagorean triangles, equations of third, fourth, higher degrees, method of functional equations, much more. "Theory of Numbers": 76 problems. Index. 94pp. "Diophantine Analysis": 222 problems. Index. 118pp. 5⅜ x 8. S529 Paperbound **$1.35**

Numerical analysis, tables

MATHEMATICAL TABLES AND FORMULAS, Compiled by Robert D. Carmichael and Edwin R. Smith. Valuable collection for students, etc. Contains all tables necessary in college algebra and trigonometry, such as five-place common logarithms, logarithmic sines and tangents of small angles, logarithmic trigonometric functions, natural trigonometric functions, four-place antilogarithms, tables for changing from sexagesimal to circular and from circular to sexagesimal measure of angles, etc. Also many tables and formulas not ordinarily accessible, including powers, roots, and reciprocals, exponential and hyperbolic functions, ten-place logarithms of prime numbers, and formulas and theorems from analytical and elementary geometry and from calculus. Explanatory introduction. viii + 269pp. 5⅜ x 8½.
S111 Paperbound **$1.00**

MATHEMATICAL TABLES, H. B. Dwight. Unique for its coverage in one volume of almost every function of importance in applied mathematics, engineering, and the physical sciences. Three extremely fine tables of the three trig functions and their inverse functions to thousandths of radians; natural and common logarithms; squares, cubes; hyperbolic functions and the inverse hyperbolic functions; $(a^2 + b^2)$ exp. ½a; complete elliptic integrals of the 1st and 2nd kind; sine and cosine integrals; exponential integrals $Ei(x)$ and $Ei(-x)$; binomial coefficients; factorials to 250; surface zonal harmonics and first derivatives; Bernoulli and Euler numbers and their logs to base of 10; Gamma function; normal probability integral; over 60 pages of Bessel functions; the Riemann Zeta function. Each table with formulae generally used, sources of more extensive tables, interpolation data, etc. Over half have columns of differences, to facilitate interpolation. Introduction. viii + 231pp. 5⅜ x 8.
S445 Paperbound **$1.75**

TABLES OF FUNCTIONS WITH FORMULAE AND CURVES, E. Jahnke & F. Emde. The world's most comprehensive 1-volume English-text collection of tables, formulae, curves of transcendent functions. 4th corrected edition, new 76-page section giving tables, formulae for elementary functions—not in other English editions. Partial contents: sine, cosine, logarithmic integral; factorial function; error integral; theta functions; elliptic integrals, functions; Legendre, Bessel, Riemann, Mathieu, hypergeometric functions, etc. Supplementary books. Bibliography. Indexed. "Out of the way functions for which we know no other source," SCIENTIFIC COMPUTING SERVICE, Ltd. 212 figures. 400pp. 5⅜ x 8. S133 Paperbound **$2.00**

Catalogue of Dover Books

CHEMISTRY AND PHYSICAL CHEMISTRY

ORGANIC CHEMISTRY, F. C. Whitmore. The entire subject of organic chemistry for the practicing chemist and the advanced student. Storehouse of facts, theories, processes found elsewhere only in specialized journals. Covers aliphatic compounds (500 pages on the properties and synthetic preparation of hydrocarbons, halides, proteins, ketones, etc.), alicyclic compounds, aromatic compounds, heterocyclic compounds, organophosphorus and organometallic compounds. Methods of synthetic preparation analyzed critically throughout. Includes much of biochemical interest. "The scope of this volume is astonishing," INDUSTRIAL AND ENGINEERING CHEMISTRY. 12,000-reference index. 2387-item bibliography. Total of x + 1005pp. 5⅜ x 8. Two volume set.
S700 Vol I Paperbound **$2.00**
S701 Vol II Paperbound **$2.00**
The set **$4.00**

THE MODERN THEORY OF MOLECULAR STRUCTURE, Bernard Pullman. A reasonably popular account of recent developments in atomic and molecular theory. Contents: The Wave Function and Wave Equations (history and bases of present theories of molecular structure); The Electronic Structure of Atoms (Description and classification of atomic wave functions, etc.); Diatomic Molecules; Non-Conjugated Polyatomic Molecules; Conjugated Polyatomic Molecules; The Structure of Complexes. Minimum of mathematical background needed. New translation by David Antin of "La Structure Moléculaire." Index. Bibliography. vii + 87pp. 5⅜ x 8½.
S987 Paperbound **$1.00**

CATALYSIS AND CATALYSTS, Marcel Prettre, Director, Research Institute on Catalysis. This brief book, translated into English for the first time, is the finest summary of the principal modern concepts, methods, and results of catalysis. Ideal introduction for beginning chemistry and physics students. Chapters: Basic Definitions of Catalysis (true catalysis and generalization of the concept of catalysis); The Scientific Bases of Catalysis (Catalysis and chemical thermodynamics, catalysis and chemical kinetics); Homogeneous Catalysis (acid-base catalysis, etc.); Chain Reactions; Contact Masses; Heterogeneous Catalysis (Mechanisms of contact catalyses, etc.); and Industrial Applications (acids and fertilizers, petroleum and petroleum chemistry, rubber, plastics, synthetic resins, and fibers). Translated by David Antin. Index. vi + 88pp. 5⅜ x 8½.
S998 Paperbound **$1.00**

POLAR MOLECULES, Pieter Debye. This work by Nobel laureate Debye offers a complete guide to fundamental electrostatic field relations, polarizability, molecular structure. Partial contents: electric intensity, displacement and force, polarization by orientation, molar polarization and molar refraction, halogen-hydrides, polar liquids, ionic saturation, dielectric constant, etc. Special chapter considers quantum theory. Indexed. 172pp. 5⅜ x 8.
S64 Paperbound **$1.50**

THE ELECTRONIC THEORY OF ACIDS AND BASES, W. F. Luder and Saverio Zuffanti. The first full systematic presentation of the electronic theory of acids and bases—treating the theory and its ramifications in an uncomplicated manner. Chapters: Historical Background; Atomic Orbitals and Valence; The Electronic Theory of Acids and Bases; Electrophilic and Electrodotic Reagents; Acidic and Basic Radicals; Neutralization; Titrations with Indicators; Displacement; Catalysis; Acid Catalysis; Base Catalysis; Alkoxides and Catalysts; Conclusion. Required reading for all chemists. Second revised (1961) eidtion, with additional examples and references. 3 figures. 9 tables. Index. Bibliography xii + 165pp. 5⅜ x 8.
S201 Paperbound **$1.50**

KINETIC THEORY OF LIQUIDS, J. Frenkel. Regarding the kinetic theory of liquids as a generalization and extension of the theory of solid bodies, this volume covers all types of arrangements of solids, thermal displacements of atoms, interstitial atoms and ions, orientational and rotational motion of molecules, and transition between states of matter. Mathematical theory is developed close to the physical subject matter. 216 bibliographical footnotes. 55 figures. xi + 485pp. 5⅜ x 8.
S95 Paperbound **$2.55**

THE PRINCIPLES OF ELECTROCHEMISTRY, D. A. MacInnes. Basic equations for almost every subfield of electrochemistry from first principles, referring at all times to the soundest and most recent theories and results; unusually useful as text or as reference. Covers coulometers and Faraday's Law, electrolytic conductance, the Debye-Hueckel method for the theoretical calculation of activity coefficients, concentration cells, standard electrode potentials, thermodynamic ionization constants, pH, potentiometric titrations, irreversible phenomena, Planck's equation, and much more. "Excellent treatise," AMERICAN CHEMICAL SOCIETY JOURNAL. "Highly recommended," CHEMICAL AND METALLURGICAL ENGINEERING. 2 Indices. Appendix. 585-item bibliography. 137 figures. 94 tables. ii + 478pp. 5⅝ x 8⅜.
S52 Paperbound **$2.45**

THE PHASE RULE AND ITS APPLICATION, Alexander Findlay. Covering chemical phenomena of 1, 2, 3, 4, and multiple component systems, this "standard work on the subject" (NATURE, London), has been completely revised and brought up to date by A. N. Campbell and N. O. Smith. Brand new material has been added on such matters as binary, tertiary liquid equilibria, solid solutions in ternary systems, quinary systems of salts and water. Completely revised to triangular coordinates in ternary systems, clarified graphic representation, solid models, etc. 9th revised edition. Author, subject indexes. 236 figures. 505 footnotes, mostly bibliographic. xii + 494pp. 5⅜ x 8.
S91 Paperbound **$2.45**

Catalogue of Dover Books

PHYSICS

General physics

FOUNDATIONS OF PHYSICS, R. B. Lindsay & H. Margenau. Excellent bridge between semi-popular works & technical treatises. A discussion of methods of physical description, construction of theory; valuable for physicist with elementary calculus who is interested in ideas that give meaning to data, tools of modern physics. Contents include symbolism, mathematical equations; space & time foundations of mechanics; probability; physics & continua; electron theory; special & general relativity; quantum mechanics; causality. "Thorough and yet not overdetailed. Unreservedly recommended," NATURE (London). Unabridged, corrected edition. List of recommended readings. 35 illustrations. xi + 537pp. 5⅜ x 8.
S377 Paperbound **$2.75**

FUNDAMENTAL FORMULAS OF PHYSICS, ed. by D. H. Menzel. Highly useful, fully inexpensive reference and study text, ranging from simple to highly sophisticated operations. Mathematics integrated into text—each chapter stands as short textbook of field represented. Vol. 1: Statistics, Physical Constants, Special Theory of Relativity, Hydrodynamics, Aerodynamics, Boundary Value Problems in Math. Physics; Viscosity, Electromagnetic Theory, etc. Vol. 2: Sound, Acoustics, Geometrical Optics, Electron Optics, High-Energy Phenomena, Magnetism, Biophysics, much more. Index. Total of 800pp. 5⅜ x 8.
Vol. 1 S595 Paperbound **$2.00**
Vol. 2 S596 Paperbound **$2.00**

MATHEMATICAL PHYSICS, D. H. Menzel. Thorough one-volume treatment of the mathematical techniques vital for classic mechanics, electromagnetic theory, quantum theory, and relativity. Written by the Harvard Professor of Astrophysics for junior, senior, and graduate courses, it gives clear explanations of all those aspects of function theory, vectors, matrices, dyadics, tensors, partial differential equations, etc., necessary for the understanding of the various physical theories. Electron theory, relativity, and other topics seldom presented appear here in considerable detail. Scores of definitions, conversion factors, dimensional constants, etc. "More detailed than normal for an advanced text . . . excellent set of sections on Dyadics, Matrices, and Tensors," JOURNAL OF THE FRANKLIN INSTITUTE. Index. 193 problems, with answers. x + 412pp. 5⅜ x 8.
S56 Paperbound **$2.00**

THE SCIENTIFIC PAPERS OF J. WILLARD GIBBS. All the published papers of America's outstanding theoretical scientist (except for "Statistical Mechanics" and "Vector Analysis"). Vol I (thermodynamics) contains one of the most brilliant of all 19th-century scientific papers—the 300-page "On the Equilibrium of Heterogeneous Substances," which founded the science of physical chemistry, and clearly stated a number of highly important natural laws for the first time; 8 other papers complete the first volume. Vol II includes 2 papers on dynamics, 8 on vector analysis and multiple algebra, 5 on the electromagnetic theory of light, and 6 miscellaneous papers. Biographical sketch by H. A. Bumstead. Total of xxxvi + 718pp. 5⅝ x 8⅜.
S721 Vol I Paperbound **$2.00**
S722 Vol II Paperbound **$2.00**
The set **$4.00**

BASIC THEORIES OF PHYSICS, Peter Gabriel Bergmann. Two-volume set which presents a critical examination of important topics in the major subdivisions of classical and modern physics. The first volume is concerned with classical mechanics and electrodynamics: mechanics of mass points, analytical mechanics, matter in bulk, electrostatics and magnetostatics, electromagnetic interaction, the field waves, special relativity, and waves. The second volume (Heat and Quanta) contains discussions of the kinetic hypothesis, physics and statistics, stationary ensembles, laws of thermodynamics, early quantum theories, atomic spectra, probability waves, quantization in wave mechanics, approximation methods, and abstract quantum theory. A valuable supplement to any thorough course or text.
Heat and Quanta: Index. 8 figures. x + 300pp. 5⅜ x 8½. S968 Paperbound **$1.75**
Mechanics and Electrodynamics: Index. 14 figures. vii + 280pp. 5⅜ x 8½.
S969 Paperbound **$1.75**

THEORETICAL PHYSICS, A. S. Kompaneyets. One of the very few thorough studies of the subject in this price range. Provides advanced students with a comprehensive theoretical background. Especially strong on recent experimentation and developments in quantum theory. Contents: Mechanics (Generalized Coordinates, Lagrange's Equation, Collision of Particles, etc.), Electrodynamics (Vector Analysis, Maxwell's equations, Transmission of Signals, Theory of Relativity, etc.), Quantum Mechanics (the Inadequacy of Classical Mechanics, the Wave Equation, Motion in a Central Field, Quantum Theory of Radiation, Quantum Theories of Dispersion and Scattering, etc.), and Statistical Physics (Equilibrium Distribution of Molecules in an Ideal Gas, Boltzmann statistics, Bose and Fermi Distribution, Thermodynamic Quantities, etc.). Revised to 1961. Translated by George Yankovsky, authorized by Kompaneyets. 137 exercises. 56 figures. 529pp. 5⅜ x 8½. S972 Paperbound **$2.50**

ANALYTICAL AND CANONICAL FORMALISM IN PHYSICS, André Mercier. A survey, in one volume, of the variational principles (the key principles—in mathematical form—from which the basic laws of any one branch of physics can be derived) of the several branches of physical theory, together with an examination of the relationships among them. Contents: the Lagrangian Formalism, Lagrangian Densities, Canonical Formalism, Canonical Form of Electrodynamics, Hamiltonian Densities, Transformations, and Canonical Form with Vanishing Jacobian Determinant. Numerous examples and exercises. For advanced students, teachers, etc. 6 figures. Index. viii + 222pp. 5⅜ x 8½. S1077 Paperbound **$1.75**

Catalogue of Dover Books

MATHEMATICAL PUZZLES AND RECREATIONS

AMUSEMENTS IN MATHEMATICS, Henry Ernest Dudeney. The foremost British originator of mathematical puzzles is always intriguing, witty, and paradoxical in this classic, one of the largest collections of mathematical amusements. More than 430 puzzles, problems, and paradoxes. Mazes and games, problems on number manipulation, unicursal and other route problems, puzzles on measuring, weighing, packing, age, kinship, chessboards, joining, crossing river, plane figure dissection, and many others. Solutions. More than 450 illustrations. vii + 258pp. 5⅜ x 8. T473 Paperbound **$1.25**

SYMBOLIC LOGIC and THE GAME OF LOGIC, Lewis Carroll. "Symbolic Logic" is not concerned with modern symbolic logic, but is instead a collection of over 380 problems posed with charm and imagination, using the syllogism, and a fascinating diagrammatic method of drawing conclusions. In "The Game of Logic," Carroll's whimsical imagination devises a logical game played with 2 diagrams and counters (included) to manipulate hundreds of tricky syllogisms. The final section, "Hit or Miss" is a lagniappe of 101 additional puzzles in the delightful Carroll manner. Until this reprint edition, both of these books were rarities costing up to $15 each. Symbolic Logic: Index, xxxi + 199pp. The Game of Logic: 96pp. Two vols. bound as one. 5⅜ x 8. T492 Paperbound **$1.50**

MAZES AND LABYRINTHS: A BOOK OF PUZZLES, W. Shepherd. Mazes, formerly associated with mystery and ritual, are still among the most intriguing of intellectual puzzles. This is a novel and different collection of 50 amusements that embody the principle of the maze: mazes in the classical tradition; 3-dimensional, ribbon, and Möbius-strip mazes; hidden messages; spatial arrangements; etc.—almost all built on amusing story situations. 84 illustrations. Essay on maze psychology. Solutions. xv + 122pp. 5⅜ x 8. T731 Paperbound **$1.00**

MATHEMATICAL RECREATIONS, M. Kraitchik. Some 250 puzzles, problems, demonstrations of recreational mathematics for beginners & advanced mathematicians. Unusual historical problems from Greek, Medieval, Arabic, Hindu sources: modern problems based on "mathematics without numbers," geometry, topology, arithmetic, etc. Pastimes derived from figurative numbers, Mersenne numbers, Fermat numbers; fairy chess, latruncles, reversi, many topics. Full solutions. Excellent for insights into special fields of math. 181 illustrations. 330pp. 5⅜ x 8. T163 Paperbound **$1.75**

MATHEMATICAL PUZZLES OF SAM LOYD, Vol. I, selected and edited by M. Gardner. Puzzles by the greatest puzzle creator and innovator. Selected from his famous "Cyclopedia of Puzzles," they retain the unique style and historical flavor of the originals. There are posers based on arithmetic, algebra, probability, game theory, route tracing, topology, counter, sliding block, operations research, geometrical dissection. Includes his famous "14-15" puzzle which was a national craze, and his "Horse of a Different Color" which sold millions of copies. 117 of his most ingenious puzzles in all, 120 line drawings and diagrams. Solutions. Selected references. xx + 167pp. 5⅜ x 8. T498 Paperbound **$1.00**

MY BEST PUZZLES IN MATHEMATICS, Hubert Phillips ("Caliban"). Caliban is generally considered the best of the modern problemists. Here are 100 of his best and wittiest puzzles, selected by the author himself from such publications as the London Daily Telegraph, and each puzzle is guaranteed to put even the sharpest puzzle detective through his paces. Perfect for the development of clear thinking and a logical mind. Complete solutions are provided for every puzzle. x + 107pp. 5⅜ x 8½. T91 Paperbound **$1.00**

MY BEST PUZZLES IN LOGIC AND REASONING, H. Phillips ("Caliban"). 100 choice, hitherto unavailable puzzles by England's best-known problemist. No special knowledge needed to solve these logical or inferential problems, just an unclouded mind, nerves of steel, and fast reflexes. Data presented are both necessary and just sufficient to allow one unambiguous answer. More than 30 different types of puzzles, all ingenious and varied, many one of a kind, that will challenge the expert, please the beginner. Original publication. 100 puzzles, full solutions. x + 107pp. 5⅜ x 8½. T119 Paperbound **$1.00**

MATHEMATICAL PUZZLES FOR BEGINNERS AND ENTHUSIASTS, G. Mott-Smith. 188 mathematical puzzles to test mental agility. Inference, interpretation, algebra, dissection of plane figures, geometry, properties of numbers, decimation, permutations, probability, all enter these delightful problems. Puzzles like the Odic Force, How to Draw an Ellipse, Spider's Cousin, more than 180 others. Detailed solutions. Appendix with square roots, triangular numbers, primes, etc. 135 illustrations. 2nd revised edition. 248pp. 5⅜ x 8. T198 Paperbound **$1.00**

MATHEMATICS, MAGIC AND MYSTERY, Martin Gardner. Card tricks, feats of mental mathematics, stage mind-reading, other "magic" explained as applications of probability, sets, theory of numbers, topology, various branches of mathematics. Creative examination of laws and their applications with scores of new tricks and insights. 115 sections discuss tricks with cards, dice, coins; geometrical vanishing tricks, dozens of others. No sleight of hand needed; mathematics guarantees success. 115 illustrations. xii + 174pp. 5⅜ x 8. T335 Paperbound **$1.00**

Catalogue of Dover Books

RECREATIONS IN THE THEORY OF NUMBERS: THE QUEEN OF MATHEMATICS ENTERTAINS, Albert H. Beiler. The theory of numbers is often referred to as the "Queen of Mathematics." In this book Mr. Beiler has compiled the first English volume to deal exclusively with the recreational aspects of number theory, an inherently recreational branch of mathematics. The author's clear style makes for enjoyable reading as he deals with such topics as: perfect numbers, amicable numbers, Fermat's theorem, Wilson's theorem, interesting properties of digits, methods of factoring, primitive roots, Euler's function, polygonal and figurate numbers, Mersenne numbers, congruence, repeating decimals, etc. Countless puzzle problems, with full answers and explanations. For mathematicians and mathematically-inclined laymen, etc. New publication. 28 figures. 9 illustrations. 103 tables. Bibliography at chapter ends. vi + 247pp. 5⅜ x 8½.
T1096 Paperbound **$1.85**

PAPER FOLDING FOR BEGINNERS, W. D. Murray and F. J. Rigney. A delightful introduction to the varied and entertaining Japanese art of origami (paper folding), with a full crystal-clear text that anticipates every difficulty; over 275 clearly labeled diagrams of all important stages in creation. You get results at each stage, since complex figures are logically developed from simpler ones. 43 different pieces are explained: place mats, drinking cups, bonbon boxes, sailboats, frogs, roosters, etc. 6 photographic plates. 279 diagrams. 95pp. 5⅝ x 8⅜.
T713 Paperbound **$1.00**

1800 RIDDLES, ENIGMAS AND CONUNDRUMS, Darwin A. Hindman. Entertaining collection ranging from hilarious gags to outrageous puns to sheer nonsense—a welcome respite from sophisticated humor. Children, toastmasters, and practically anyone with a funny bone will find these zany riddles tickling and eminently repeatable. Sample: "Why does Santa Claus always go down the chimney?" "Because it soots him." Some old, some new—covering a wide variety of subjects. New publication. iii + 154pp. 5⅜ x 8½. T1059 Paperbound **$1.00**

EASY-TO-DO ENTERTAINMENTS AND DIVERSIONS WITH CARDS, STRING, COINS, PAPER AND MATCHES, R. M. Abraham. Over 300 entertaining games, tricks, puzzles, and pastimes for children and adults. Invaluable to anyone in charge of groups of youngsters, for party givers, etc. Contains sections on card tricks and games, making things by paperfolding—toys, decorations, and the like; tricks with coins, matches, and pieces of string; descriptions of games; toys that can be made from common household objects; mathematical recreations; word games; and 50 miscellaneous entertainments. Formerly "Winter Nights Entertainments." Introduction by Lord Baden Powell. 329 illustrations. v + 186pp. 5⅜ x 8.
T921 Paperbound **$1.00**

DIVERSIONS AND PASTIMES WITH CARDS, STRING, PAPER AND MATCHES, R. M. Abraham. Another collection of amusements and diversion for game and puzzle fans of all ages. Many new paperfolding ideas and tricks, an extensive section on amusements with knots and splices, two chapters of easy and not-so-easy problems, coin and match tricks, and lots of other parlor pastimes from the agile mind of the late British problemist and gamester. Corrected and revised version. Illustrations. 160pp. 5⅜ x 8½. T1127 Paperbound **$1.00**

STRING FIGURES AND HOW TO MAKE THEM: A STUDY OF CAT'S-CRADLE IN MANY LANDS, Caroline Furness Jayne. In a simple and easy-to-follow manner, this book describes how to make 107 different string figures. Not only is looping and crossing string between the fingers a common youthful diversion, but it is an ancient form of amusement practiced in all parts of the globe, especially popular among primitive tribes. These games are fun for all ages and offer an excellent means for developing manual dexterity and coordination. Much insight also for the anthropological observer on games and diversions in many different cultures. Index. Bibliography. Introduction by A. C. Haddon, Cambridge University. 17 full-page plates. 950 illustrations. xxiii + 407pp. 5⅜ x 8½.
T152 Paperbound **$2.00**

CRYPTANALYSIS, Helen F. Gaines. (Formerly ELEMENTARY CRYPTANALYSIS.) A standard elementary and intermediate text for serious students. It does not confine itself to old material, but contains much that is not generally known, except to experts. Concealment, Transposition, Substitution ciphers; Vigenere, Kasiski, Playfair, multafid, dozens of other techniques. Appendix with sequence charts, letter frequencies in English, 5 other languages, English word frequencies. Bibliography. 167 codes. New to this edition: solution to codes. vi + 230pp. 5⅜ x 8.
T97 Paperbound **$1.95**

MAGIC SQUARES AND CUBES, W. S. Andrews. Only book-length treatment in English, a thorough non-technical description and analysis. Here are nasik, overlapping, pandiagonal, serrated squares; magic circles, cubes, spheres, rhombuses. Try your hand at 4-dimensional magical figures! Much unusual folklore and tradition included. High school algebra is sufficient. 754 diagrams and illustrations. viii + 419pp. 5⅜ x 8.
T658 Paperbound **$1.85**

CALIBAN'S PROBLEM BOOK: MATHEMATICAL, INFERENTIAL, AND CRYPTOGRAPHIC PUZZLES, H. Phillips ("Caliban"), S. T. Shovelton, G. S. Marshall. 105 ingenious problems by the greatest living creator of puzzles based on logic and inference. Rigorous, modern, piquant, and reflecting their author's unusual personality, these intermediate and advanced puzzles all involve the ability to reason clearly through complex situations; some call for mathematical knowledge, ranging from algebra to number theory. Solutions. xi + 180pp. 5⅜ x 8.
T736 Paperbound **$1.25**

FICTION

THE LAND THAT TIME FORGOT and THE MOON MAID, Edgar Rice Burroughs. In the opinion of many, Burroughs' best work. The first concerns a strange island where evolution is individual rather than phylogenetic. Speechless anthropoids develop into intelligent human beings within a single generation. The second projects the reader far into the future and describes the first voyage to the Moon (in the year 2025), the conquest of the Earth by the Moon, and years of violence and adventure as the enslaved Earthmen try to regain possession of their planet. "An imaginative tour de force that keeps the reader keyed up and expectant," NEW YORK TIMES. Complete, unabridged text of the original two novels (three parts in each). 5 illustrations by J. Allen St. John. vi + 552pp. 5⅜ x 8½.
T1020 Clothbound **$3.75**
T358 Paperbound **$2.00**

AT THE EARTH'S CORE, PELLUCIDAR, TANAR OF PELLUCIDAR: THREE SCIENCE FICTION NOVELS BY EDGAR RICE BURROUGHS. Complete, unabridged texts of the first three Pellucidar novels. Tales of derring-do by the famous master of science fiction. The locale for these three related stories is the inner surface of the hollow Earth where we discover the world of Pellucidar, complete with all types of bizarre, menacing creatures, strange peoples, and alluring maidens—guaranteed to delight all Burroughs fans and a wide cirole of adventure lovers. Illustrated by J. Allen St. John and P. F. Berdanier. vi + 433pp. 5⅜ x 8½.
T1051 Paperbound **$2.00**

THE PIRATES OF VENUS and LOST ON VENUS: TWO VENUS NOVELS BY EDGAR RICE BURROUGHS. Two related novels, complete and unabridged. Exciting adventure on the planet Venus with Earthman Carson Napier broken-field running through one dangerous episode after another. All lovers of swashbuckling science fiction will enjoy these two stories set in a world of fascinating societies, fierce beasts, 5000-ft. trees, lush vegetation, and wide seas. Illustrations by Fortunino Matania. Total of vi + 340pp. 5⅜ x 8½.
T1053 Paperbound **$1.75**

A PRINCESS OF MARS and A FIGHTING MAN OF MARS: TWO MARTIAN NOVELS BY EDGAR RICE BURROUGHS. "Princess of Mars" is the very first of the great Martian novels written by Burroughs, and it is probably the best of them all; it set the pattern for all of his later fantasy novels and contains a thrilling cast of strange peoples and creatures and the formula of Olympian heroism amidst ever-fluctuating fortunes which Burroughs carries off so successfully. "Fighting Man" returns to the same scenes and cities—many years later. A mad scientist, a degenerate dictator, and an indomitable defender of the right clash—with the fate of the Red Planet at stake! Complete, unabridged reprinting of original editions. Illustrations by F. E. Schoonover and Hugh Hutton. v + 356pp. 5⅜ x 8½.
T1140 Paperbound **$1.75**

THREE MARTIAN NOVELS, Edgar Rice Burroughs. Contains: Thuvia, Maid of Mars; The Chessmen of Mars; and The Master Mind of Mars. High adventure set in an imaginative and intricate conception of the Red Planet. Mars is peopled with an intelligent, heroic human race which lives in densely populated cities and with fierce barbarians who inhabit dead sea bottoms. Other exciting creatures abound amidst an inventive framework of Martian history and geography. Complete unabridged reprintings of the first edition. 16 illustrations by J. Allen St. John. vi + 499pp. 5⅜ x 8½.
T39 Paperbound **$1.85**

THREE PROPHETIC NOVELS BY H. G. WELLS, edited by E. F. Bleiler. Complete texts of "When the Sleeper Wakes" (1st book printing in 50 years), "A Story of the Days to Come," "The Time Machine" (1st complete printing in book form). Exciting adventures in the future are as enjoyable today as 50 years ago when first printed. Predict TV, movies, intercontinental airplanes, prefabricated houses, air-conditioned cities, etc. First important author to foresee problems of mind control, technological dictatorships. "Absolute best of imaginative fiction," N. Y. Times. Introduction. 335pp. 5⅜ x 8.
T605 Paperbound **$1.50**

28 SCIENCE FICTION STORIES OF H. G. WELLS. Two full unabridged novels, MEN LIKE GODS and STAR BEGOTTEN, plus 26 short stories by the master science-fiction writer of all time. Stories of space, time, invention, exploration, future adventure—an indispensable part of the library of everyone interested in science and adventure. PARTIAL CONTENTS: Men Like Gods, The Country of the Blind, In the Abyss, The Crystal Egg, The Man Who Could Work Miracles, A Story of the Days to Come, The Valley of Spiders, and 21 more! 928pp. 5⅜ x 8.
T265 Clothbound **$4.50**

THE WAR IN THE AIR, IN THE DAYS OF THE COMET, THE FOOD OF THE GODS: THREE SCIENCE FICTION NOVELS BY H. G. WELLS. Three exciting Wells offerings bearing on vital social and philosophical issues of his and our own day. Here are tales of air power, strategic bombing, East vs. West, the potential miracles of science, the potential disasters from outer space, the relationship between scientific advancement and moral progress, etc. First reprinting of "War in the Air" in almost 50 years. An excellent sampling of Wells at his storytelling best. Complete, unabridged reprintings. 16 illustrations. 645pp. 5⅜ x 8½.
T1135 Paperbound **$2.00**

Catalogue of Dover Books

SEVEN SCIENCE FICTION NOVELS, H. G. Wells. Full unabridged texts of 7 science-fiction novels of the master. Ranging from biology, physics, chemistry, astronomy to sociology and other studies, Mr. Wells extrapolates whole worlds of strange and intriguing character. "One will have to go far to match this for entertainment, excitement, and sheer pleasure . . . ," NEW YORK TIMES. Contents: The Time Machine, The Island of Dr. Moreau, First Men in the Moon, The Invisible Man, The War of the Worlds, The Food of the Gods, In the Days of the Comet. 1015pp. 5⅜ x 8. T264 Clothbound **$4.50**

BEST GHOST STORIES OF J. S. LE FANU, Selected and introduced by E. F. Bleiler. LeFanu is deemed the greatest name in Victorian supernatural fiction. Here are 16 of his best horror stories, including 2 nouvelles: "Carmilla," a classic vampire tale couched in a perverse eroticism, and "The Haunted Baronet." Also: "Sir Toby's Will," "Green Tea," "Schalken the Painter," "Ultor de Lacy," "The Familiar," etc. The first American publication of about half of this material: a long-overdue opportunity to get a choice sampling of LeFanu's work. New selection (1964). 8 illustrations. 5⅜ x 8⅜. T415 Paperbound **$1.85**

THE WONDERFUL WIZARD OF OZ, L. F. Baum. Only edition in print with all the original W. W. Denslow illustrations in full color—as much a part of "The Wizard" as Tenniel's drawings are for "Alice in Wonderland." "The Wizard" is still America's best-loved fairy tale, in which, as the author expresses it, "The wonderment and joy are retained and the heartaches and nightmares left out." Now today's young readers can enjoy every word and wonderful picture of the original book. New introduction by Martin Gardner. A Baum bibliography. 23 full-page color plates. viii + 268pp. 5⅜ x 8. T691 Paperbound **$1.45**

GHOST AND HORROR STORIES OF AMBROSE BIERCE, Selected and introduced by E. F. Bleiler. 24 morbid, eerie tales—the cream of Bierce's fiction output. Contains such memorable pieces as "The Moonlit Road," "The Damned Thing," "An Inhabitant of Carcosa," "The Eyes of the Panther," "The Famous Gilson Bequest," "The Middle Toe of the Right Foot," and other chilling stories, plus the essay, "Visions of the Night" in which Bierce gives us a kind of rationale for his aesthetic of horror. New collection (1964). xxii + 199pp. 5⅜ x 8⅜. T767 Paperbound **$1.00**

HUMOR

MR. DOOLEY ON IVRYTHING AND IVRYBODY, Finley Peter Dunne. Since the time of his appearance in 1893, "Mr. Dooley," the fictitious Chicago bartender, has been recognized as America's most humorous social and political commentator. Collected in this volume are 102 of the best Dooley pieces—all written around the turn of the century, the height of his popularity. Mr. Dooley's Irish brogue is employed wittily and penetratingly on subjects which are just as fresh and relevant today as they were then: corruption and hypocrisy of politicans, war preparations and chauvinism, automation, Latin American affairs, superbombs, etc. Other articles range from Rudyard Kipling to football. Selected with an introduction by Robert Hutchinson. xii + 244pp. 5⅜ x 8½. T626 Paperbound **$1.00**

RUTHLESS RHYMES FOR HEARTLESS HOMES and MORE RUTHLESS RHYMES FOR HEARTLESS HOMES, Harry Graham ("Col. D. Streamer"). A collection of Little Willy and 48 other poetic "disasters." Graham's funniest and most disrespectful verse, accompanied by original illustrations. Nonsensical, wry humor which employs stern parents, careless nurses, uninhibited children, practical jokers, single-minded golfers, Scottish lairds, etc. in the leading roles. A precursor of the "sick joke" school of today. This volume contains, bound together for the first time, two of the most perennially popular books of humor in England and America. Index. vi + 69pp. 5⅜ x 8. T930 Paperbound **75¢**

A WHIMSEY ANTHOLOGY, Collected by Carolyn Wells. 250 of the most amusing rhymes ever written. Acrostics, anagrams, palindromes, alphabetical jingles, tongue twisters, echo verses, alliterative verses, riddles, mnemonic rhymes, interior rhymes, over 40 limericks, etc. by Lewis Carroll, Edward Lear, Joseph Addison, W. S. Gilbert, Christina Rossetti, Chas. Lamb, James Boswell, Hood, Dickens, Swinburne, Leigh Hunt, Harry Graham, Poe, Eugene Field, and many others. xiv + 221pp. 5⅜ x 8½. T195 Paperbound **$1.25**

MY PIOUS FRIENDS AND DRUNKEN COMPANIONS and MORE PIOUS FRIENDS AND DRUNKEN COMPANIONS, Songs and ballads of Conviviality Collected by Frank Shay. Magnificently illuminated by John Held, Jr. 132 ballads, blues, vaudeville numbers, drinking songs, cowboy songs, sea chanties, comedy songs, etc. of the Naughty Nineties and early 20th century. Over a third are reprinted with music. Many perennial favorites such as: The Band Played On, Frankie and Johnnie, The Old Grey Mare, The Face on the Bar-room Floor, etc. Many others unlocatable elsewhere: The Dog-Catcher's Child, The Cannibal Maiden, Don't Go in the Lion's Cage Tonight, Mother, etc. Complete verses and introductions to songs. Unabridged republication of first editions, 2 Indexes (song titles and first lines and choruses). Introduction by Frank Shay. 2 volumes bounds as 1. Total of xvi + 235pp. 5⅜ x 8½. T946 Paperbound **$1.00**

Catalogue of Dover Books

MAX AND MORITZ, Wilhelm Busch. Edited and annotated by H. Arthur Klein. Translated by H. Arthur Klein, M. C. Klein, and others. The mischievous high jinks of Max and Moritz, Peter and Paul, Ker and Plunk, etc. are delightfully captured in sketch and rhyme. (Companion volume to "Hypocritical Helena.") In addition to the title piece, it contians: Ker and Plunk; Two Dogs and Two Boys; The Egghead and the Two Cut-ups of Corinth; Deceitful Henry; The Boys and the Pipe; Cat and Mouse; and others. (Original German text with accompanying English translations.) Afterword by H. A. Klein. vi + 216pp. 5⅜ x 8½.
T181 Paperbound **$1.00**

THROUGH THE ALIMENTARY CANAL WITH GUN AND CAMERA: A FASCINATING TRIP TO THE INTERIOR, Personally Conducted by George S. Chappell. In mock-travelogue style, the amusing account of an imaginative journey down the alimentary canal. The "explorers" enter the esophagus, round the Adam's Apple, narrowly escape from a fierce Amoeba, struggle through the impenetrable Nerve Forests of the Lumbar Region, etc. Illustrated by the famous cartoonist, Otto Soglow, the book is as much a brilliant satire of academic pomposity and professional travel literature as it is a clever use of the facts of physiology for supremely comic purposes. Preface by Robert Benchley. Author's Foreword. 1 Photograph. 17 illustrations by O. Soglow. xii + 114pp. 5⅜ x 8½.
T376 Paperbound **$1.00**

THE BAD CHILD'S BOOK OF BEASTS, MORE BEASTS FOR WORSE CHILDREN, and A MORAL ALPHABET, H. Belloc. Hardly an anthology of humorous verse has appeared in the last 50 years without at least a couple of these famous nonsense verses. But one must see the entire volumes—with all the delightful original illustrations by Sir Basil Blackwood—to appreciate fully Belloc's charming and witty verses that play so subacidly on the platitudes of life and morals that beset his day—and ours. A great humor classic. Three books in one. Total of 157pp. 5⅜ x 8.
T749 Paperbound **$1.00**

THE DEVIL'S DICTIONARY, Ambrose Bierce. Sardonic and irreverent barbs puncturing the pomposities and absurdities of American politics, business, religion, literature, and arts, by the country's greatest satirist in the classic tradition. Epigrammatic as Shaw, piercing as Swift, American as Mark Twain, Will Rogers, and Fred Allen. Bierce will always remain the favorite of a small coterie of enthusiasts, and of writers and speakers whom he supplies with "some of the most gorgeous witticisms of the English language." (H. L. Mencken). Over 1000 entries in alphabetical order. 144pp. 5⅜ x 8.
T487 Paperbound **$1.00**

THE COMPLETE NONSENSE OF EDWARD LEAR. This is the only complete edition of this master of gentle madness available at a popular price. A BOOK OF NONSENSE, NONSENSE SONGS, MORE NONSENSE SONGS AND STORIES in their entirety with all the old favorites that have delighted children and adults for years. The Dong With A Luminous Nose, The Jumblies, The Owl and the Pussycat, and hundreds of other bits of wonderful nonsense. 214 limericks, 3 sets of Nonsense Botany, 5 Nonsense Alphabets. 546 drawings by Lear himself, and much more. 320pp. 5⅜ x 8.
T167 Paperbound **$1.00**

SINGULAR TRAVELS, CAMPAIGNS, AND ADVENTURES OF BARON MUNCHAUSEN, R. E. Raspe, with 90 illustrations by Gustave Doré. The first edition in over 150 years to reestablish the deeds of the Prince of Liars exactly as Raspe first recorded them in 1785—the genuine Baron Munchausen, one of the most personable personalities in English literature. Included also are the best of the many sequels, written by other hands. Introduction on Raspe by J. Carswell. Bibliography of early editions. xliv + 192pp. 5⅜ x 8. T698 Paperbound **$1.00**

HOW TO TELL THE BIRDS FROM THE FLOWERS, R. W. Wood. How not to confuse a carrot with a parrot, a grape with an ape, a puffin with nuffin. Delightful drawings, clever puns, absurd little poems point out farfetched resemblances in nature. The author was a leading physicist. Introduction by Margaret Wood White. 106 illus. 60pp. 5⅜ x 8.
T523 Paperbound **75¢**

JOE MILLER'S JESTS OR, THE WITS VADE-MECUM. The original Joe Miller jest book. Gives a keen and pungent impression of life in 18th-century England. Many are somewhat on the bawdy side and they are still capable of provoking amusement and good fun. This volume is a facsimile of the original "Joe Miller" first published in 1739. It remains the most popular and influential humor book of all time. New introduction by Robert Hutchinson. xxi + 70pp. 5⅜ x 8½.
T423 Paperbound **$1.00**

Prices subject to change without notice.

Dover publishes books on art, music, philosophy, literature, languages, history, social sciences, psychology, handcrafts, orientalia, puzzles and entertainments, chess, pets and gardens, books explaining science, intermediate and higher mathematics, mathematical physics, engineering, biological sciences, earth sciences, classics of science, etc. Write to:

                        Dept. catrr.
                        Dover Publications, Inc.
                        180 Varick Street, N.Y. 14, N.Y.